Using Nursing Research
to Shape
Health Policy

Patricia A. Grady, PhD, RN, FAAN, has been affiliated with the National Institutes of Health (NIH) since 1988, first as an extramural research program administrator in the National Institute of Neurological Disorders and Stroke (NINDS), then as a member of the NIH Task Force for Medical Rehabilitation Research and assistant director of NINDS, until 1995, when she was appointed director of the National Institute of Nursing Research. Under her leadership, the institute has more than doubled its budget and significantly increased the number of research and training grants awarded. Dr. Grady is an internationally recognized researcher on the topic of stroke. She also served as a faculty member at the University of Maryland School of Nursing and School of Medicine.

She has co-authored numerous articles and serves on many journal editorial boards, including *Stroke, Stroke and Cerebral Vascular Diseases*, and *NeuroTherapeutics*, the journal of the American Society for Experimental NeuroTherapeutics. Dr. Grady is a member of the National Academy of Medicine and has been the recipient of several prestigious awards, including the Policy Luminary Award from the American Academy of Colleges of Nursing, the Second Century Award for Excellence in Health Care from Columbia University School of Nursing, and the honorary doctor of science degree from Thomas Jefferson University and the Medical University of South Carolina.

Ada Sue Hinshaw, PhD, RN, FAAN, is dean emeritus and professor emeritus, Graduate School of Nursing, Uniformed Services, University of the Health Sciences, Bethesda, Maryland, and dean emeritus and professor, University of Michigan School of Nursing, where she served as dean from 1994 to 2006. Dr. Hinshaw was selected as an American Academy of Nursing (AAN)/American Foundation of Nursing/Institute of Medicine Senior Nurse Scholar from 2006 to 2007. She was also the first permanent director of the National Center of Nursing Research and the first director of the National Institute of Nursing Research at the National Institutes of Health (NIH). During her tenure at NIH, Dr. Hinshaw was responsible for promoting research in the areas of disease prevention, health promotion, and acute and chronic illness, as well as investigating environments that enhance nursing care and patient outcomes. She has conducted research in quality of care, patient outcomes, measurement of outcomes, and building positive work environments to enhance patient safety. Dr. Hinshaw is the recipient of many awards for her work, including the Midwest Nursing Research Society Lifetime Achievement Award, the Health Leader of the Year Award from the U.S. Public Health Service, the Award for Excellence in Nursing Research (Sigma Theta Tau), the Nurse Scientist of the Year Award (ANA Council of Nurse Researchers), the Living Legend Award from the AAN, and the Walsh McDermott Award from the National Academy of Medicine. She has received 14 honorary doctorates.

Using Nursing Research to Shape Health Policy

Patricia A. Grady, PhD, RN, FAAN

Ada Sue Hinshaw, PhD, RN, FAAN

Editors

SPRINGER PUBLISHING COMPANY

NEW YORK

Springer Publishing Company, LLC
11 West 42nd Street
New York, NY 10036
www.springerpub.com

Acquisitions Editor: Margaret Zuccarini
Senior Production Editor: Kris Parrish
Compositor: Exeter Premedia Services Private Ltd.

ISBN: 978-0-8261-7010-1
e-book ISBN: 978-0-8261-7011-8
Instructor's PowerPoints ISBN: 978-0-8261-7018-7

Instructors Materials: Qualified instructors may request supplements by e-mailing textbook@springerpub.com

16 17 18 19 20 / 5 4 3 2 1

The author and the publisher of this Work have made every effort to use sources believed to be reliable to provide information that is accurate and compatible with the standards generally accepted at the time of publication. Because medical science is continually advancing, our knowledge base continues to expand. Therefore, as new information becomes available, changes in procedures become necessary. We recommend that the reader always consult current research and specific institutional policies before performing any clinical procedure. The author and publisher shall not be liable for any special, consequential, or exemplary damages resulting, in whole or in part, from the readers' use of, or reliance on, the information contained in this book. The publisher has no responsibility for the persistence or accuracy of URLs for external or third-party Internet websites referred to in this publication and does not guarantee that any content on such websites is, or will remain, accurate or appropriate.

Library of Congress Cataloging-in-Publication Data
Names: Grady, Patricia A., editor. | Hinshaw, Ada Sue, editor.
Title: Using nursing research to shape health policy/Patricia A. Grady, Ada
  Sue Hinshaw, editors.
Description: New York, NY: Springer Publishing Company, LLC, [2017] |
  Includes bibliographical references and index.
Identifiers: LCCN 2016052494 | ISBN 9780826170101 | ISBN 9780826170118
  (e-book) | ISBN 9780826170187 (instructors PowerPoints)
Subjects: | MESH: Nursing Research | Health Policy | Policy Making | United
  States
Classification: LCC RT81.5 | NLM WY 20.5 | DDC 610.73072—dc23
LC record available at https://lccn.loc.gov/2016052494

Contact us to receive discount rates on bulk purchases.
We can also customize our books to meet your needs.
For more information please contact: sales@springerpub.com

Printed in the United States of America by McNaughton & Gunn.

To nurse scientists worldwide for their valued and productive contributions to patient care and health policy! Such efforts are providing the building blocks for a healthier nation and globe. Your successes in these endeavors enrich the quality of the lives you touch, and we are glad to be a part of that journey with you.

Contents

SECTION I: EMERGING AREAS SHAPING HEALTH POLICY

SECTION II: EXAMPLES OF NURSING SCIENCE SHAPING HEALTH POLICY

**SECTION III: CONCLUSIONS: NURSING RESEARCH—FRAMING
          THE FUTURE**

Contributors

Greg Alexander, PhD, RN, FAAN, Professor, University of Missouri Sinclair School of Nursing, Columbia, Missouri

Joan K. Austin, PhD, RN, FAAN, Distinguished Professor Emerita, Indiana University School of Nursing, Indianapolis, Indiana

Suzanne Bakken, PhD, RN, FAAN, Professor, Columbia University, New York, New York

Rhonda Cady, PhD, RN, Nursing Research Specialist, Gillette Children's Specialty Healthcare, St. Paul, Minnesota

Ann K. Cashion, PhD, RN, FAAN, Professor, University of Tennessee Health Sciences Center, Memphis, Tennessee

Yvonne Commodore-Mensah, PhD, RN, Assistant Professor, Johns Hopkins University School of Nursing, Baltimore, Maryland

Cheryl Dennison Himmelfarb, PhD, ANP, RN, FAAN, Professor, Johns Hopkins University School of Nursing, Baltimore, Maryland

Laurel Despins, PhD, RD, ACNS-BC, Assistant Professor, University of Missouri Sinclair School of Nursing, Columbia, Missouri

Victoria Vaughan Dickson, PhD, RN, FAHA, FAAN, Associate Professor, New York University Rory Meyers College of Nursing, New York, New York

Susan G. Dorsey, PhD, RN, FAAN, Professor and Chair, Department of Pain and Translational Symptom Science, University of Maryland School of Nursing, Baltimore, Maryland

Stanley Finkelstein, PhD, Professor, Department of Laboratory Medicine and Pathology/Health Informatics, University of Minnesota School of Medicine, Minneapolis, Minnesota

Colleen Galambos, PhD, ACSW, LCSW-C, FGSA, Professor, Department of Social Work, University of Missouri, Columbia, Missouri

Laura N. Gitlin, PhD, FAAN, Professor and Director, Center for Innovative Care in Aging, Johns Hopkins University School of Nursing, Baltimore, Maryland

Patricia A. Grady, PhD, RN, FAAN, Bethesda, Maryland

Margaret Grey, DrPH, RN, FAAN, Annie Goodrich Professor, Yale University School of Nursing, Orange, Connecticut

Margaret M. Heitkemper, PhD, RN, FAAN, Elizabeth Sterling Soule Chair in Nursing, Professor and Chair, Biobehavioral Health Systems, University of Washington School of Nursing, Seattle, Washington

Wendy A. Henderson, PhD, CRNP, FAAN, Bethesda, Maryland

Susan E. Hickman, PhD, Professor, Indiana University School of Nursing, and Co-Director of the IUPUI Research in Palliative and End-of-Life Communication and Training (RESPECT) Signature Center, Indianapolis, Indiana

Lanis Hicks, PhD, Professor Emerita, Health Management and Informatics, School of Medicine, University of Missouri, Columbia, Missouri

Martha Hill, PhD, RN, FAAN, Professor and Dean Emeritus, Johns Hopkins University School of Nursing, Baltimore, Maryland

Pamela S. Hinds, PhD, RN, FAAN, William and Joanne Conway Chair in Nursing Research, Director, Department of Nursing Research and Quality Outcomes; Children's Hospital, Professor of Pediatrics, George Washington University, Washington, DC

Ada Sue Hinshaw, PhD, RN, FAAN, Dean Emeritus, School of Nursing, University of Michigan, Ann Arbor, Michigan; Dean Emeritus, Daniel K. Inouye Graduate School of Nursing, Uniformed Services University of the Health Sciences, Bethesda, Maryland

James Keller, PhD, Curators' Professor, Electrical and Computer Engineering, University of Missouri College of Engineering, Columbia, Missouri

Richelle Koopman, MD, Associate Professor, Family and Community Medicine, University of Missouri School of Medicine, Columbia, Missouri

Kari R. Lane, PhD, RN, Associate Professor, University of Missouri Sinclair School of Nursing, Columbia, Missouri

Christopher S. Lee, PhD, RN, FAHA, FAAN, Carol A. Lindeman Distinguished Professor, Oregon Health & Sciences University School of Nursing, Portland, Oregon

Lisa C. Lindley, PhD, RN, Associate Professor, University of Tennessee College of Nursing, Knoxville, Tennessee

Jeri L. Miller, PhD, Bethesda, Maryland

Kim Mooney-Doyle, PhD, RN, Adjunct Assistant Professor, University of Pennsylvania School of Nursing, Philadelphia, Pennsylvania

Debra K. Moser, PhD, RN, FAAN, Professor and Linda C. Gill Chair of Cardiovascular Nursing, University of Kentucky, Lexington, Kentucky

Mary D. Naylor, PhD, RN, FAAN, Marian S. Ware Professor in Gerontology; Director, NewCourtland Center for Transitions and Health, University of Pennsylvania School of Nursing, Philadelphia, Pennsylvania

Lorraine J. Phillips, PhD, RN, FAAN, Associate Professor, University of Missouri Sinclair School of Nursing, Columbia, Missouri

Lori L. Popejoy, PhD, RN, FAAN, Professor, University of Missouri Sinclair School of Nursing, Columbia, Missouri

Mihail Popescu, PhD, Associate Professor of Health Management and Informatics, University of Missouri School of Medicine, Columbia, Missouri

Marilyn J. Rantz, PhD, RN, FAAN, Curators' Professor Emerita, University of Missouri Sinclair School of Nursing, Columbia, Missouri

Kaitlyn Rechenberg, MA, MPH, MSN, PhD Student, Yale University School of Nursing, Orange, Connecticut

Barbara Riegel, PhD, RN, FAAN, Edith Clemmer Steinbright Professor of Gerontology, University of Pennsylvania School of Nursing, Philadelphia, Pennsylvania

Clayton Shuman, PhD, RN, University of Michigan School of Nursing, Ann Arbor, Michigan

Marjorie Skubic, PhD, Professor, Electrical and Computer Engineering, University of Missouri College of Engineering, Columbia, Missouri

Sarah L. Szanton, PhD, RN, FAAN, Professor, Johns Hopkins University School of Nursing, Baltimore, Maryland

Marita Titler, PhD, RN, FAAN, Professor and Chair, Department of Systems, Population and Leadership, University of Michigan School of Nursing, Ann Arbor, Michigan

Alma Vega, PhD, MSPH, Postdoctoral Fellow, University of Pennsylvania School of Nursing, Philadelphia, Pennsylvania

Karen E. Wickersham, PhD, RN, Assistant Professor, University of Maryland School of Nursing, Baltimore, Maryland

Janet K. Williams, PhD, RN, FAAN, Professor, University of Iowa School of Nursing, Iowa City, Iowa

Foreword

The public policy/political process may seem but a far-off dream for the next generation of nursing leaders—yet those who have gone before have established an impressive foundation on which to build. Nursing continues to mature into our nation's premier health care profession, and nurses into international visionaries. Public policy possesses its own history, culture, and language, yet the majority of those involved have only a rudimentary appreciation for the intricacies of health care delivery or practice. Accordingly, it is incumbent upon nursing's best and brightest to become personally involved in shaping our nation's priorities. Who else has long championed patient-centered care, the importance of prevention and wellness, as well as a population-based focus—which are the hallmarks of President Obama's landmark Patient Protection and Affordable Care Act? Today's call for interprofessional collaboration has always been nursing's forte. Study after study consistently affirms that advanced practice registered nurses (APRNs) provide the highest quality of care, second to none. Yet, historical barriers enacted by legislative bodies and professional licensing boards still prevent those citizens most in need from having ready access to nursing care. The leaders of nursing's next generation must become intimately involved in the public policy process and thereby bring about meaningful change.

Passion alone is not sufficient. History has shown that to truly make a difference in the lives of those most in need, practitioners must have access to, and be actively engaged in, cutting-edge science. With advancing knowledge and unprecedented technological breakthroughs, many of today's "clinical truths" will soon become "tomorrow's myths." Clinicians and researchers must continuously inform each other for the greater good. There is a similar reality within the public policy arena. Only by nursing science actively engaging in the critical public policy deliberations will society ultimately benefit.

Patrick H. DeLeon, PhD, MPH, JD
Former President, American Psychological Association
Distinguished Professor, Daniel K. Inouye Graduate School of Nursing
Uniformed Services University of the Health Sciences
Bethesda, Maryland

Preface

This book, *Using Nursing Research to Shape Health Policy*, examines the crucial interrelationship between nursing research and health policy. It presents examples of specific health care policies that have been influenced, implemented, or changed as a result of nursing research, as well as a number of examples that have the potential to change policy as they move forward in their translation. This text builds on the discussion that began in an earlier book, *Shaping Health Policy Through Nursing Research* (Springer Publishing, 2011). The current book updates earlier information with new examples of nursing research by esteemed scholars. In addition, it encompasses research related to major policy statements of the decade, including the Institute of Medicine's (IOM) *Future of Nursing* report, the Affordable Care Act, and the genomic nursing science blueprint, and highlights how they have influenced, and will continue to influence, health policy.

Written for multiple audiences, including undergraduate and graduate students, faculty, and nursing professionals, the book presents information on how science shapes health policy in general, models and strategies for linking research and health policy, and multiple examples of how major nursing research has influenced health policy. The text provides both a conceptual orientation and an operational approach to strategies linking research to policy and influencing policy makers at the organizational, community, state, national, and international levels.

This text is particularly timely, as advances are being made in the efforts to translate research into health policy. The editors found a higher level of engagement and activity in this area when setting out to write this book. There are many more researchers and clinicians focusing on the importance of shaping policy than there were 5 years ago.

In addition, the complexity of the health care system continues to increase incrementally, and spawns new questions and issues over which policy has not yet been formulated. The redesign of the health care system necessitates implementation of a thoughtful approach to policy, and it is best shaped by using an evidence base related to patient satisfaction and safety. Put another way, the redesign of the health care system provides opportunity for change, and that change is best informed by the research that nurses are doing. This book provides guidance and examples.

The three major health policy directives addressed in this book—the IOM *Future of Nursing* report, the Affordable Care Act, and the genomic nursing science blueprint—are landmark documents and will continue to shape health policy for decades to come. Each of these is considered for its implications and impact.

ORGANIZATION

Using Nursing Research to Shape Health Policy is organized into three sections. The first is an introductory section composed of six chapters that deal with major concepts related to research shaping policy. In the second section, a series of research programs and models, successful strategies for implementation, and lessons learned are described. The third section consists of an analysis and summary of trends and patterns used by the contributors, which helped to guide efforts in shaping health policy.

Chapter 1, "Policy Directives, Scientific Challenges, and Patterns," sets the stage by addressing major scientific challenges, innovative clinical patterns related to those challenges, and three major policy directives that help to shape policy change. Recommendations from each of those directives are explored.

Chapter 2, "Expanding Areas of Clinical and Basic Sciences," and Chapter 4, "Integration of Genomics in Nursing Research," address how the relatively new areas of genomics are beginning to shape science and policy as we move further into the 21st century. Cashion and Austin discuss some of the new advances in Chapter 2 and describe how those advances are beginning to shape our nursing agendas, while Williams in Chapter 4 provides a historical context for and identifies ways in which genomics has become integrated into our nursing research. In Chapter 3, "Implementation Science," Titler and Shuman provide a detailed description of translational science, including definitions, and deftly identify some of the roadblocks and strategies to overcome those roadblocks.

In Chapter 5, "Team Science: Challenges and Opportunities in the 21st Century," Naylor, with co-author Vega, describes the aspects of team science that are so necessary in building a research base, identifies how to build teams, and describes ways in which her team has operationalized the concept of "interdisciplinary" in the process of carrying out their studies.

Data collection, data analysis using new and emerging strategies, and data sharing emerge as increasingly important tasks as we move further into the 21st century. Understanding both new data technologies and when and how to use them has become increasingly important for discovery. Section I concludes with Chapter 6, "Data Science." In it, Bakken describes this emerging field and, using several examples, explores how this technology promises to be instrumental in helping nursing science. The chapter describes how this particular set of approaches can facilitate the manner in which data may be obtained more quickly and more robustly, which, in turn, will facilitate its use in shaping policy.

Section II offers examples of programs and strategies that have been successful in shaping health policy. Several of these examples contain elements for future use in shaping policy. All of these are described by the senior investigators and their teams involved in carrying out the research.

As our population ages and remains relatively healthy compared to previous generations, continues to be active, and is better informed, people are increasingly prepared to take a more active role in their health and wellness. This demographic change underscores the role of self-management, a hallmark of nursing science. Chapters 7 and 8 deal with this increasingly important area. Chapter 7, "Self-Management of Illness in Teens," describes a successful program in helping teens manage their diabetes, and explicates successful strategies for translation, while Chapter 8, "Self-Management of Illness in Adults," addresses some of the pioneering work with an adult population experiencing heart failure.

Chapter 9, "Integration of Genomics in Nursing Research: An Example," provides an example of planning ahead in a rapidly developing area. A specific plan is described, starting with targeting a clinical problem (neuropathic pain), studying it from a basic science perspective, and setting the stage for a successful intervention to be translated into policy. This is a good example of going from bedside to bench to bedside, a strategy that is often discussed but difficult to achieve.

Chapter 10, "Gastrointestinal Symptom Science and Assessment," provides an example of a program of research in symptom science, a cornerstone of nursing research. This chapter begins at the inception of a program to address symptoms of gastrointestinal distress, continues through paths of discovery, and ends with testing in clinical trials.

With the aging of our population, changing requirements for care and caregiving challenge us as a society to develop new approaches. Chapter 11, "Caring for Caregivers in an Aging Society: Contributions of Nursing Research to Practice and Policy," and Chapters 12 and 13, "Aging in Place: Adapting the Environment" and "Aging in Place: Innovative Teams," describe creative ways to address these changing demographics by redefining caregiving teams and altering environmental barriers. All three researchers and their teams have used equally creative strategies to solve demographic challenges and to help shape policy.

As people live longer—with one or more chronic health problems, on average—strategies to address these issues assume a greater importance. The next three chapters deal specifically with issues related to chronic illness. Chapter 14, "Chronic Illness: Addressing Hypertension and Health Disparities in Communities," describes an early community-based program of hypertension control in an adult inner-city population of African American males. Chapter 15, "Chronic Illness: Promoting Cardiovascular Health in Socioeconomically Austere Rural Areas," describes a program designed to address cardiovascular health problems in a rural community and the challenges encountered in rural settings. Both chapters address an aspect of the health disparities that remain a challenge. Chapter 16, "Chronic Illness: Telehealth Approaches to Wellness," provides several examples of the power and potential of telehealth to revolutionize our health care system. Roadblocks and strategies are identified.

Additionally, as our population ages, end-of-life issues are becoming more urgent. Three chapters deal with palliative care and the end of life from the perspective of adult and pediatric populations, and describe the intricacies of policy implications.

These chapters describe the efforts and successes in dealing with numerous policy issues that have been influenced so far. Chapter 17, "Palliative and End-of-Life Care Issues in Adults: The Physician Orders for Life-Sustaining Treatment (POLST) Program," describes the experience of a team of investigators to develop a tool to facilitate wishes of adult patients and families at the end of life. Chapter 18, "Nursing Research and Health Policy Through the Lens of Pediatric Palliative, Hospice, and End-of-Life Care," describes innovative approaches with pediatric populations and their families. Finally, Chapter 19, "Palliative and End-of-Life Care Issues: Policy Perspective," elucidates many of the policy considerations that are currently being dealt with or that will emerge as our health care system begins to address this important phase of the life span.

Section III consists of a single chapter that summarizes and analyzes the strategies and models used throughout the text, noting the unique characteristics and similarities in the approaches and strategies used by the researchers in both setting the stage for and actually shaping policy. Various levels of change have been effected, and several researchers have broken new ground that anticipates potential policy change as they and the next generation of researchers and policy experts move forward.

Qualified instructors may obtain access to ancillary PowerPoints by contacting textbook@springerpub.com.

FEATURES

As evidenced by the titles and descriptions of the chapters, a number of distinguishing features characterize this book.

- It offers examples of cutting-edge nursing research that provide a foundation for practice and policy.
- It incorporates major policy directives of this decade and highlights how nursing research has influenced health policy.
- It demonstrates to undergraduate and graduate students, faculty, and nursing professionals how nursing research can shape health policy decisions.
- It includes perspectives, models, and strategies for using nursing research to influence health policy.
- Last but not least, it addresses how nursing research shapes policy at organizational, community, state, national, and international levels.

Patricia A. Grady
Ada Sue Hinshaw

Acknowledgments

The authors are enormously grateful to the many senior colleagues and their mentees who have been committed to producing a volume to update the accomplishments in tying nursing research to health policy. This forward-thinking cadre is pioneering innovative approaches to shaping health policy. Their span of expertise is broad, and provides a state-of-the art summary of major accomplishments and their implications. We express a special, heartfelt appreciation for their outstanding contributions to this book!

Leaders in the nursing profession are actively engaged in this important process and are instilling the inspiration for continuing it in the next generation of nurses. This important mentoring will help to ensure that the profession will be an integral part of future changes as our health care system evolves to meet the changing demands of our society.

In the 5 years that intervened between our earlier book, *Shaping Health Policy Through Nursing Research*, and this book, *Using Nursing Research to Shape Health Policy*, the authors were pleased to observe the extent to which the nursing profession has moved forward incrementally in its awareness of the importance of tying research to health policy by the actions to accomplish it.

The authors are grateful to Pat DeLeon for writing the inspiring Foreword to this text, and also for his unflagging support to the nursing community—support that has continued for more than 30 years. His strong advocacy has been an integral part of the success of the National Institute of Nursing Research from the time of its inception. We value his continued contributions.

The authors want to thank Margaret Zuccarini, Publisher, Nursing, at Springer Publishing, and her staff, particularly Amanda Devine, for their help. We are especially grateful to Margaret for her expertise, sage advice, support, and encouragement during the writing of this book. We would also like to thank Amanda for keeping us on schedule with timely, helpful reminders.

1

Policy Directives, Scientific Challenges, and Patterns

Patricia A. Grady and Ada Sue Hinshaw

This text, *Using Nursing Research to Shape Health Policy*, expands the concept of nursing research's role in informing health policy. It builds on the foundation provided by a previous text, *Shaping Health Policy Through Nursing Research* (Hinshaw & Grady, 2011), which was intended to help stimulate the reader to incorporate the idea of using nursing research to influence health policy. Successful research programs were provided as exemplars. A great deal has been accomplished in this area since that time. Increasingly, the results of nursing research are being woven into practice and are influencing health policy. We have entered an important era when seminal health policy directives that have emerged on our national landscape are influenced by and have the potential to markedly impact nursing and health care in the future. This text addresses those areas and provides a perspective on impact and potential impact for the future.

The text also outlines new clinical nursing research areas and innovative scientific patterns that are changing research in the discipline. It presents new research programs of senior scientists with funding longevity, and discusses how their research has shaped policy. Moreover, it addresses the potential for influence within other programs of research. The chapters are grouped into two sections: the first section comprises introductory chapters on policy directives; the second, scientific challenges and patterns. The text also incorporates senior scientists' presentations of their research and the ways in which that research has shaped health policy.

NATIONAL HEALTH POLICY DIRECTIVES

A number of major health policy directives of the past several years have been important in shaping health care decisions and professional programs. These include the Affordable Care Act (ACA), the Institute of Medicine/National Academy of

Medicine (IOM/NAM) *Future of Nursing* report, and the genomic nursing science blueprint. These three were selected for discussion because of their major impact on health care and the profession of nursing. In addition, these national directives have influenced or have been influenced by the discipline's research programs, and this influence will continue.

Major national health policy directives are shaped by research, as one of many factors, and research is sometimes influenced by the evidence needed for policy decisions. For these reasons, several chapters in this text address aspects of these three health policy directives.

The Affordable Care Act Policy Directive

The ACA consists of two different public laws signed by President Barack Obama in 2010: the Patient Protection and Affordable Care Act and the Health Care and Education Reconciliation Act (National Council of State Boards of Nursing, 2014). Obviously, the purpose of the ACA is to enhance the accessibility and affordability of health care to all Americans. An additional purpose evident in the provisions of the program is the improvement of health care and health systems. Because the goal is to provide access to health care for 32 million additional low-income working individuals in this country, the ACA has considerable implications for the health professional workforce and those workers' ability to function at the full scope of their education, given the increased number of people to be included in health care (National Council of State Boards of Nursing, 2014).

The provisions in the ACA are numerous and complex, as they are designed to guide national programs with multiple goals. The provisions include (a) change in payment regulations by the government, such as restricting payments to hospitals for unnecessary readmissions, value-based purchasing programs for hospitals and providers, and bundled payment plans; (b) changes in the organization of health care delivery models (e.g., accountable care organizations and shared health savings plans); and (c) primary care transformations, with, for example, increased emphasis on preventive services, community-based care, and health homes for low-income individuals with different ethnic backgrounds. The ACA also recognizes the need for evaluation and research focused on public health issues and outcomes for individuals in order to assess progress on improving health care (supplement to Blumenthal, Abrams, & Nuzium, 2015a).

According to Jost (2016), the ACA has led to or contributed to a series of successes. Economically, there are between 7.0 and 14.6 million fewer uninsured low-income working individuals. This number is larger when students who are now covered on their parents' insurance policies through age 25 and individuals who are no longer excluded from insurance due to existing preconditions of disease are considered. The early research data suggest that both access to and affordability of health care have been improved (Shartzer, Long, & Anderson, 2016). In addition, the annual rate of increase in health costs has slowed. Changes in the health care delivery system and quality indicators cannot be clearly evaluated, because most of these initiatives did not begin until later, around 2013 (Blumenthal, Abrams, & Nuzium, 2015b). However, there is a trend toward a decrease in hospital readmissions and reported high satisfaction of individuals with their insurance coverage and health care (Jost, 2016).

There is strong potential that nursing research can shape the many delivery-system and quality initiatives of the ACA. The research of Naylor and others and repeated testimonies to Congress and the National Academy of Medicine are already evident in the provisions on hospital readmissions (Naylor et al., 2013). Grey's study of self-management of teens with diabetes (Grey, Knafl, Schulman-Green, & Reynolds, 2015) and Hill's investigation (Allen et al., 2011) of adult management of chronic illness have strong policy implications for the quality initiatives of the ACA. These are just a few examples of the potential of nursing research to influence and shape the quality initiatives relating to the primary care, preventive services provisions of the ACA.

The Future of Nursing Policy Directive

The Future of Nursing: Leading Change, Advancing Health (IOM, 2011) study and policy report, a collaborative endeavor of the Institute of Medicine (IOM, now NAM or National Academy of Medicine) and the Robert Wood Johnson Foundation (RWJF), is the second major health policy directive to be discussed. The RWJF and IOM initiative is directly linked to the ACA legislation passed in 2010, as it opens health care access to an additional 32 million individuals and families. Such an influx will require extensive renovation of the health care system through interprofessional cooperation and leadership in order to provide patient-centered, quality, evidence-based, and safe care. Nursing, as the largest major health profession, needs to prepare for providing health care and leadership in enhancing the health care system in the United States. *The Future of Nursing* report (IOM, 2011) provided a blueprint and a set of recommendations for the nursing profession's movement into its roles participating in and leading the redesigned health care system. According to the ACA, the U.S. health care system needs to advance a strong community and public health system in addition to acute care and palliative care systems that cross the life span of individuals and families.

The formal charge (IOM, 2011, p. 3) of *The Future of Nursing* initiative was broad and encompassing. The committee was asked to consider the "capacity of the nursing workforce" to respond to the reformed health care system and public health system, including the delivery of nursing services; the structure and changes needed in nursing education; policy changes required in national, state, and local public institutions; and how to handle current and future nursing workforce shortages.

The Future of Nursing report (IOM, 2011) advanced four key messages that spawned a number of recommendations:

- First, nurses should practice at the full extent of their education and training (IOM, 2011, p. 4).

- Second, nurses should complete higher levels of education and training through an improved educational system that encourages and enhances progression through different levels (IOM, 2011, p. 6).
- Third, nurses should be fully involved as partners with physicians and other health professionals in redesigning the health care systems in the United States (IOM, 2011, p. 7).
- Fourth, effective workforce planning and policy making require better data collection and improved information infrastructure (IOM, 2011, p. 8).

These four key messages were based on a number of professional issues and led to several recommendations for policy makers and public institutions.

The first key message pertains to nurses with various types of degrees and preparation being able to practice at the full scope of their education and training. The most obvious example with this message is the practice of advanced practice registered nurses (APRNs). There are multiple barriers to their practice; for example, the state regulations for the practice of APRNs that are more restrictive in some states than others. Another example of not reaching full scope of practice is the nurse with his or her first professional degree who, because of transition problems from school or work, drops out of nursing within a short time. Several of the report's recommendations focused on this message.

- *Recommendation 1: Remove scope of practice barriers* (IOM, 2011, p. 9). This recommendation was specifically focused on the practice of APRNs. As such, there were subrecommendations for Congress, state legislatures, the Centers for Medicare and Medicaid Services (CMS), the Office of Personnel Management (OPM), and the Federal Trade Commission.
- *Recommendation 2: Expand opportunities for nurses to lead and diffuse interprofessional efforts in redesigning health systems* (IOM, 2011, p. 11). This concept is targeted at APRNs as partners and leaders with physicians and other health professionals as the health care systems are redesigned to accommodate an additional 32 million individuals and families.
- *Recommendation 3: Implement nurse residency programs as standard practice in health systems* (IOM, 2011, p. 11). Nurse residency programs have been shown to enhance new graduates' transition from school to work and have evidenced a decrease in turnover rates for these new professionals.

The second key message focuses on nurses being educated at higher levels within an educational system that advances academic progression for students. Reviewing the increasing complexity of health care, and the knowledge and skills required for practice, the report suggested that higher levels of education are needed. Hence, three recommendations were provided:

- *Recommendation 4: The basic education of nurses needs to be enhanced with 80% prepared at the baccalaureate level by 2020* (IOM, 2011, p. 12). This is in response to the increasing complexity involved with health care knowledge, skills, and technology.

- *Recommendation 5: Double the number of nurses with a doctorate by 2020* (IOM, 2011, p. 13). This recommendation reflects a major professional challenge; that is, the consistent faculty shortage reported by schools of nursing in this country. Nursing needs additional professionals with earned doctoral degrees for education, practice, research, and leadership purposes.
- *Recommendation 6: Ensure that nurses engage in lifelong learning* (IOM, 2011, p. 13). To advance the recommendation of *The Future of Nursing* report, lifelong learning will be a requirement; for example, leading and partnering in redesigning the country's health care systems and improving the quality, safety, and evidence base under patient-centered health care, specifically nursing care.

The third key message flows from the two prior messages and the call for greater scope of practice and higher education to meet changing dynamics and the increasing complexity of health care. Such conditions also recognize the need for nurses to be leaders and partners in changing and designing the reformed health care system. Thus, the third key message: Nurses should be fully involved as partners with physicians and other health professionals in designing the health care system for the United States.

- *Recommendation 7 simply reinforces this key message; that is, prepare and enable nurses to lead change to advance health* (IOM, 2011, p. 14).

The fourth key message addresses effective workforce planning and policy making related to current and future nursing shortages. Workforce shortages occur in all the health professions; thus, the workforce planning and policy-making initiative should be broader and more inclusive. However, the implementation of this recommendation is hampered by the lack of standardized data collection processes at the national and state levels and an adequate information infrastructure to handle such data and the reports needed. The eighth recommendation focuses on this need.

- *Recommendation 8: Build an infrastructure for the collection and analysis of interprofessional health care workforce data* (IOM, 2011, p. 14).

Following the publication of *The Future of Nursing* report in 2011, a Campaign for Action Initiative was formed through collaboration between the AARP and the RWJF to facilitate the implementation of the recommendations. The initiative is housed in the Center to Champion Nursing in America at the AARP. Fifty-one coalitions were formed, by state, under the campaign initiative.

In 2015, a follow-up report was published by the IOM, titled *Assessing Progress on the Institute of Medicine Report: The Future of Nursing* (IOM, Altman, Butler, & Shern, 2015). Ten recommendations were suggested by the assessment report, all intended to advance the campaign's endeavors in implementing the original eight recommendations of the 2011 report.

The goals of the assessment report reflect the recommendations of the initial report, *The Future of Nursing: Leading Change, Advancing Health*. They include:

- Addressing educational transformation
- Leveraging nursing leadership
- Removing barriers to practice and care
- Fostering interprofessional collaboration
- Promoting diversity
- Bolstering workforce data

The 10 recommendations of the assessment report provide data when available and address general issues as to how to further the implementation of the original report. For example, under the Scope of Practice recommendation the report suggests that progress is evident, as eight additional states now allow full scope of practice for APRNs (for a total of 21 states). However, additional effort is needed, as 29 states still have reduced or restricted practice. On the interprofessional collaboration recommendation, general issues are cited. However, the assessment report strengthens the initial recommendation by addressing the need for wider, more inclusive collaboration through leadership and a focus on communication. The assessment report also strengthens the initial report by adding a recommendation on diversity. The statistics cited for nursing education programs and workforce groups show that nursing does not meet the diverse population percentage data for the country.

Given the extensive thought and study addressing the report, *The Future of Nursing: Leading Change and Advancing Health*, it is evident how nursing research provides a base for the issues and could be influenced by the need for data in some areas. Several chapters in this text speak to redesigned ways of providing health care, such as Chapters 12 and 13, addressing aging in place.

Genomic Nursing Science Blueprint Policy Directive

The third health policy directive is more specific to the discipline and has the potential to shape nursing research just as a review of current research informed the blueprint. The genomic nursing science blueprint (Calzone et al., 2013) was developed by the Genomic Nursing State of the Science Advisory Panel, which was organized by two coordinators, Dr. Kathleen Calzone and Dr. Jean Jenkins, under the sponsorship of the National Institute of Nursing Research (NINR) at the National Institutes of Health (NIH). The blueprint is a policy statement from the experts on the advisory panel and not a formal federal document.

The aim of the genomic nursing science initiative was "to establish the Genomic Nursing Science Blueprint through analysis of the evidence and expert evaluations of the current state of the science and public comments" (Calzone et al., 2013, p. 98). Using this process, the blueprint was developed to merge with four of the NINR strategic plan areas, identifying a number of potential genomic nursing research opportunities within the areas of health promotion/disease prevention, quality of life, innovations, and investigator training. In addition, the blueprint outlined two foci for genomic nursing research: the client defined as individual, family, community, or population and the context of the genomic nursing situation that was to be studied. Several cross-cutting themes were also suggested that would have to be considered in any genomic nursing investigation.

Genomic nursing research opportunities flow from the practice of genomic nursing. Calzone, Jenkins, and colleagues define *genomic nursing* as "broad, encompassing risk assessment, risk management, treatment options and treatment decisions" (2013, p. 99). Due to the complexity of genomic nursing practice and research, both are usually interdisciplinary in nature.

Aligning the genomic nursing science blueprint with the NINR strategic plan helped nurse scientists and others understand how genomic nursing research would strengthen nursing science, as well as the reverse. Genomic nursing research opportunities suggested by the advisory panel will be cited for each of the NINR strategic areas and subareas.

A major strategic area for NINR is health promotion and disease prevention. The first subarea focuses on risk assessment. Examples of genomic nursing research topics include biological plausibility issues and comprehensive screening problems. A second subarea is communication. Several examples of genomic nursing research opportunities involve risk communication with clients and broader consumer marketing. The third subarea involves decision support with genomic nursing researcher possibilities, including studies on informed consent and the effect of decision support on decision quality.

The second NINR strategic area under which many genomic nursing research opportunities were suggested was advancing the quality of life. The first subarea focuses on the family, a key target of nursing research. Several possibilities for genomic nursing research include family functioning, structure, communication patterns, genetic makeup, and context questions, such as health providers' genetic screening and communication with clients. The second subarea is symptom management, with research opportunities involving biological plausibility, clinical and person utility, and decision making with genetic symptom treatment. The next subarea deals with disease states, and the blueprint suggests studies on genetic-based information needed for treatments and pharmacogenetics. The fourth subarea involves client self-management, with possible research studies focusing on collecting and conveying information for self-management and the decision processes needed for self-management (Calzone et al., 2013).

The third NINR strategic plan area with genomic nursing research opportunities suggested by the blueprint relates to innovation. The initial subarea, technology development, offers several nursing research possibilities such as genetic information systems and the study in applying new technologies. The second subarea focuses explicitly on facilitating cross-cutting data systems for family genetic information and point-of-care decision support for health providers and clients. The third subarea targets environmental influences, with genomic nursing research suggestions such as evidence-based guidelines for different environmental situations and policies for health care reform implications for genomic nursing science.

The fourth NINR strategic plan area linked with genomic science outlines the need for education and training of future genomic nurse researchers. The issue is complex because it involves educating current faculty for genomic nursing practice as well as research, while at the same time educating the next generation of genomic nursing scientists in both basic and applied methods.

The genomic nursing science blueprint articulates several cross-cutting themes that should be considered in genomic nursing studies. These include health disparities, cost, policy, and public education. The genomic nursing research opportunities vary from health genetic equity to quality/cost ratio of genetic-based care to the interplay of public health policy and science to health/genetic literacy (Calzone et al., 2013).

Three major health policy directives of the past 5 years have been considered in relation to nursing research and its role in shaping health policy as well as being informed by such policies. Several of the authors and chapters in this text address this interrelationship.

SCIENTIFIC CHALLENGES AND PATTERNS

A number of significant challenges and patterns can be identified as nursing science moves forward into the 21st century. Many of these challenges reflect the great success achieved in the past, as a number of public health issues have been addressed, and highly effective ways have been found to prevent and manage many of the acute illnesses that presented major health problems for prior generations. It is important to note that many of the forward-looking concepts in health care are those that nursing has embodied for many years. Chief among these are wellness and prevention of disease, self-management, caregiving issues, team science, integration of genomics into nursing research, technology, and data science. Everywhere you look, the nursing community is leading the way to culturally appropriate, readily accessible, high-quality, interdisciplinary, evidence-based health care; and everywhere nurse leaders are acting as dynamic agents for positive change. This text provides examples that illustrate the importance of the work, and the positive changes that it can bring to the lives of individuals, families, and communities through shaping health policy.

Wellness and Prevention of Disease

Over the course of the past century, much progress has been made in determining what constitutes a healthy lifestyle. Research has shown that alterations in lifestyle and behavior can have positive health consequences. This has implications for both practice and policy. Wellness and disease prevention are important over the course of the life span, in primary, secondary, and even tertiary prevention. For example, because of nursing research, young men and women are able to reduce their risk of HIV/AIDS (Jemmott, Jemmott, & O'Leary, 2007; Villarruel, Jemmott, Jemmott, & Ronis, 2007), teens can better manage their diabetes and live healthier lifestyles (Grey et al., 2013), and women are more aware of cardiovascular risk (McSweeney et al., 2003). For example, the American Heart Association recently released a State of the Science statement in which McSweeney is the lead author, and the statement includes this work (McSweeney et al., 2016).

Largely as a result of improvements informed by research, our populations are living longer. Because people are living longer, they have begun to manifest signs of chronic illnesses not seen with shorter life spans. In fact, the majority of individuals older than the age of 45 are living with one or more chronic illnesses (Fried, Bernstein, & Bush, 2012; Ford, Croft, Posner, Goodman, & Giles, 2013). Consequently, a large percentage of the population is managing symptoms related to such illnesses or disorders. These demographics underscore the importance of symptom science, the determination of specific causation of symptoms, and self-management to improve quality of life. With the aging populations, self-management is visible with the emergence of new types of living arrangements, such as aging in place (Rantz et al., 2011; Szanton et al., 2015). This text addresses examples of such strategies. In addition, we are keenly aware that we have not successfully eliminated health disparities in our nation and that there are many who cannot readily access health care; others face financial difficulty because of the burden of health care costs. Underlying these issues are health care systems and services that must be better linked to improvements in health outcomes and quality of care, which is a key component of the ACA.

An example of research linked to better outcomes and quality of care that became incorporated into the ACA is that of a nurse-led clinical research team focused on transitional care for seniors with multiple comorbidities—a highly vulnerable population cohort. Working together with colleagues from other disciplines and health care professions, this team conducted a series of clinical trials which proved that transitional care improves individual outcomes, enhances quality of life, and reduces hospital readmissions and health care costs (Naylor et al., 2013).

Self-Management

The science of self-management examines strategies to help individuals across the life span with acute and chronic conditions and their caregivers better understand and manage their illness and improve their health behaviors (Lorig & Holman, 2003). Self-management is patient-centered in that it empowers individuals to identify and manage their illnesses in order to take charge of their own health. Increasingly, we are learning that patients want to be involved in managing their own health. Self-management research also explores the patient–caregiver dyad and seeks to develop interventions that manage caregiver burden while maintaining or improving the patient's and caregiver's health.

With rates of multiple chronic conditions and comorbidities on the rise and a growing older population as an increasingly health literate population, the need for self-management strategies is critically important. This research addresses the adaption of treatments to individual circumstances, accounting for social, cultural, economic, and emotional factors that can influence patients' health and quality of life. There are good examples including patient populations with cancer, HIV/AIDS, and diabetes.

In patients with cancer, it has been shown that ongoing survivorship means patients and their families are assuming a greater role in managing their follow-up care and that self-management may act as a model of cancer care where providers, patients, and families enter partnerships to manage care across all aspects of cancer treatment (McCorkle et al., 2011). New measures of self-management specific to HIV/AIDS are being developed and validated so that targeted behavioral interventions can be advanced, permitting future researchers and clinicians to assess and integrate HIV/AIDS self-management in a variety of populations and settings (Webel & Okonsky, 2012). Self-management of diabetes requires patients' integration of numerous actions into their daily life, and we know that the identification of obstacles to diabetes self-management, such as literacy and access to care, are vital, especially in diverse and vulnerable populations (Wallace, Carlson, Malone, Joyner, & Dewalt, 2010).

In addition, researchers are contributing substantially to the science of self-management for patients with asthma (Rhee, Belyea, Hunt, & Brasch, 2011), arthritis (Parker et al., 2012), irritable bowel syndrome (IBS; Deechakawan, Cain, Jarrett, Burr, & Heitkemper, 2013), and chronic obstructive pulmonary disease (COPD; Nguyen et al., 2013).

A good example of self-management for teens is the Creating Opportunities for Personal Empowerment (COPE) Healthy Lifestyles Thinking, Emotions, Exercise, and Nutrition (TEEN) program (Melnyk et al., 2013). COPE TEEN has been tested recently as an intervention for adolescents, targeting obesity, social skills, and mental health. The program, conducted by high school health teachers, included education and cognitive behavioral skill development, as well as a variety of physical activities, and had positive outcomes. The COPE TEEN program may be an effective way to prevent and treat excess weight gain and obesity in teens and could lead to improved physical health, psychosocial skills, and academic outcomes. This intervention can be used widely and may be particularly useful in rural areas with fewer health care resources, as well as increasingly cash-strapped health care systems across the country. The National Cancer Institute (NCI) featured COPE TEEN on its Research to Reality (R2R) webpage recently and included COPE TEEN in its updated list of Research-Tested Intervention Programs (RTIPs) in an effort to help speed the translation of research into practice (Melnyk et al., 2015).

Caregiver Issues

Long-term care for those with disabilities is often provided by informal caregivers. The act of caregiving is known to negatively affect caregiver health, which, in turn, can affect adherence to recommendations for the care recipients' medical care. The impact of this has negative health implications for both patient and caregiver. In one study of informal caregiving, the relationship of informal caregivers to receipt of preventive health services (flu vaccination, routine physicals, and cholesterol screening) was studied. Among the large study population of caregiver/care recipient pairs, it was found that care recipients whose caregivers reported their own functional limitations received fewer preventive health services. The researchers noted that several potential caregiver factors, such as psychological distress, depression, and mobility issues, could influence care recipients' use of preventive health services, as well as their overall quality of care (Thorpe, Thorpe, Schulz, Van Houtven, & Schleiden, 2015).

Team Science

Team science is growing in stature, primarily because it is a necessity. The researcher or policy maker working in isolation has become obsolete. The questions and problems challenging us have become too complex for any one individual or small group of like-minded individuals to master. Increasingly, multi- and interdisciplinary teams are required. The optimal size and composition of teams are still evolving and heavily influenced by discipline and the type of issue being tackled (Guimerà, Uzzi, Spiro, & Nunes Amaral, 2005). However, with the exception of arts and humanities, the proportion of papers written in teams and the mean size of teams have been steadily increasing over time (Wuchty, Jones, & Uzzi, 2007). With regard to performance, teams with less diversity typically have lower levels of performance (Guimerà et al., 2005).

Nurse scientists are in pivotal positions in the transformation of health care science. They have become essential leaders and participants in cross-disciplinary team science, working in partnership with physicians, engineers, environmental scientists, information technology specialists, and others in designing and testing solutions for a broad range of health care issues. To maintain and expand their roles as leaders in the research community, nurse scientists must keep pace with the latest techniques, initiatives, and innovations in science. For example, the nurse scientist of the future must be well versed in data science, emerging health technologies, and the latest methodologies in clinical trials such as pragmatic trials. With these tools and their clinical expertise, nurse scientists are poised to build the scientific foundation for improving clinical practice and influencing policy.

It is important that all members of the team function up to their potential. This reinforces the recommendation of the IOM/NAM *Future of Nursing* report, and it also applies to all nursing and interdisciplinary members of the team. Clinicians assimilate scientific research into their professional toolkits—embracing opportunities to participate in research projects and building working relationships with colleagues in research. Research scientists must develop and enhance their relationships with practicing nurses and other health care professionals and integrate their clinical observations and data into research projects.

Nurse scientists also have a special relationship with a broad array of stakeholders to address their interests and needs with effective implementation of basic, translational, and clinical research. Involvement of community and industry representatives in the early stages of research projects can provide valuable information on financial and logistical feasibility, gaps and needs in the community and health care practice, and end users' openness to innovations.

One example of teams developing a path to the future includes the Clinical and Translational Science Awards (CTSA) Program, which was launched in 2006 as part of the NIH Roadmap for Medical Research. It has created a nationwide consortium of institutions that use multidisciplinary approaches to improve the way clinical and translational research is conducted to enhance its efficiency and quality. The CTSA Program's goals are to accelerate the process of translating laboratory discoveries into treatments for patients, to engage communities in clinical research efforts, and to train a new generation of clinical and translational researchers.

Although there are geographical and local logistical differences among individual CTSAs, nurse scientists have been integral to them from their inception (Sampselle, Knafl, Jacob, & McCloskey, 2013). The majority of the CTSAs are affiliated with nursing schools. In a 2011 survey, three key areas emerged in which nurse scientists have made significant contributions to CTSA efforts: development of community partnerships to enhance community-based models of care, expertise in implementation science to facilitate the translation of basic and clinical research into clinical care research training that includes mentoring and co-mentoring nonnurse trainees, and the identification of best practices from CTSAs in developing multidisciplinary translational and clinical science research collaborations.

Another large-scale example of team science is the Precision Medicine Initiative (PMI), launched by President Obama in January 2015 (www.nih.gov/precision-medicine-initiative-cohort-program). This initiative is a research effort to develop a new model of patient-centered and patient-driven research that will accelerate biomedical discoveries and provide clinicians with new tools, knowledge, and therapies to select which treatments will work best for individual patients. The program will seek to extend precision medicine's success to many diseases, including common diseases as well as rare diseases. Importantly for nursing, the cohort will focus not just on disease, but also on ways to increase an individual's chances of remaining healthy throughout life.

The goal of the PMI Cohort Program is to set the foundation for a new way of doing research that fosters open, responsible data sharing with the highest regard for participant privacy, and that puts engaged participants at the center of research efforts. Because Americans are improving their health and participating in health research more than ever before, electronic health records (EHRs) have been widely adopted, genomic analysis costs have dropped significantly, data science has become increasingly sophisticated, and health technologies have become mobile; it is now feasible to carry out an initiative of this kind. Nursing has an opportunity to stimulate research using the cohort data, such as: identifying new targets for prevention and intervention; testing whether mobile devices can encourage healthy behaviors; monitoring and managing symptoms and side effects; and laying the scientific foundation for precision or personalized health.

The area of team science does provide challenges, and these will continue to be addressed as efforts move forward. These include the following: the current system of academic advancement favors the independent investigator; most institutions house scientists in discrete departments; interdisciplinary science requires interdisciplinary peer review; project management and oversight are currently performed by discrete departments; and interdisciplinary research teams take time to assemble and require unique resources.

Integration of Genomics Into Nursing Research

Symptom Science

New advances in genomics and other fields have allowed nurse scientists to better understand both the basic and clinical components of genetics, including the symptoms of chronic illness, such as pain, fatigue, gastrointestinal symptoms, and disordered sleep. Recently, the intramural program of NINR developed the NIH Symptom Science Model to guide research. The model begins by identifying a complex symptom, which is then characterized into a phenotype with biological and clinical data, followed by the application of genomics and other discovery methodologies to illuminate targets for therapeutic and clinical interventions (Cashion & Grady, 2015).

Although there is an understanding that genomics plays a hugely important role in our future, it is sometimes overlooked that genetic screening may be viewed as yet another tool in the process of history taking and risk assessment that nurses have done for generations (Sigmon, Grady, & Amende, 1997). Historically, nurses began working in genetics through their involvement in genetic clinics, particularly with children who had single-gene chromosomal disorders, such as cystic fibrosis, Down syndrome, and enzymatic disorders. Some of these nurses became genetic counselors. However, that role was eclipsed with the emergence of academic programs for dedicated genetic counselors. Nurses then began addressing genetic risks, predominately in oncology clinics.

In the early 2000s, some nurse scientists turned their focus to the legal, ethical, and social issues associated with genetics. As genetic technologies became readily available, nurse scientists have embarked on studies using the more advanced approaches and technologies to address topics in symptom science that emerged in clinical care.

One goal of nurse scientists in genetics research is to identify and isolate markers and risk factors for individuals and families with inherited conditions. Progress in this area of research would enable clinicians to tailor and personalize preventive strategies and interventions. Genomics is an area in which nurse scientists play pivotal roles in bridging basic and applied research, and translating the findings to clinical care (Calzone, 2013). They are in key positions for organizing cross-disciplinary teams to link genetics research with biological, environmental, and behavioral influences. Moreover, they are leading change in health care environments through evidence-based practice.

Incorporation of genomic research into health care is still in the early stages, and nurse scientists are part of it. As noted earlier, nurse scientists were at the forefront of ethical issues of genomic research in clinical care. They continue to investigate and evaluate delivery of information about genetic testing, test results, and genetic factors in disease risk and symptom management, to help guide patients and their families in health-related decisions. As we move forward, it is important that a blueprint for genomic nursing science be developed to stimulate and guide future progress (Calzone et al., 2013).

Technology

Technology is also an important part of future endeavors. Technology can provide improvements in care, as seen in both acute and long-term care settings, and improved access to care as seen in the increase of programs delivered by Internet and other telehealth approaches. A good example of improving access to care includes programs to increase health of rural populations. Examples include improving cardiovascular health (Chapter 14) and weight loss and maintenance for older rural women (Hageman, Pullen, Hertzog, Boeckner, & Walker, 2011). Increasingly, research is defining programs that can be scaled up and successfully delivered using technology (Grey et al., 2013). Telehealth nursing programs for children and families have been tested successfully and are finding their way into practice (Cady, Kelly, Finkelstein, Looman, & Garwick, 2014; Looman et al., 2013, 2015).

In-person self-management and education programs have demonstrated efficacy; however, there are numerous issues, such as time, resources, and consistent quality, that can interfere with access to clinically delivered programs. Internet programs have been shown to be effective with youth for managing various health problems. In addition, Internet-based interventions pose fewer barriers to accessibility, particularly in light of financial, time, and geographical constraints, and there are opportunities for better standardization of delivered materials (Grey et al., 2013).

In a Small Business Innovation Research (SBIR) success story, Dr. Kathryn Bowles of the University of Pennsylvania and colleagues developed the Discharge Decision Support System (D2S2), a tool that is embedded in EHR systems to identify patients in need of follow-up after hospital discharge, with the goal of improving health outcomes and reducing hospital readmission costs (Holland, Rhudy, Vanderboom, & Bowles, 2012). Large-scale testing (three hospitals, thousands of patients) yielded significant reduction in hospital readmissions, which garnered venture capital funding (Holland, Knafl, & Bowles, 2013).

Health care technology is advancing at a breathtaking pace. The future will place a greater emphasis on research that aims to use new tools, such as telehealth and Internet-based communication for patients and health care professionals, including tablet and smartphone applications and wearable activity monitors, as innovative ways to provide better health care. This includes designing technologies for self-management with multiple data categories, including longitudinal assessment of interventions. Nursing science has developed, and continues to develop novel applications for these mobile health (mHealth) technologies.

Data Science

As mentioned previously, in keeping with the trends in health care and the development of the scientific body of knowledge with continually emerging scientific areas, it is critical that researchers stay up to date on the latest scientific trends and methodologies as they develop and maintain their programs of research. Examples include the emerging field of data science, new approaches to clinical trials, including pragmatic trials, dealing with large cohorts, and using common data elements (CDEs). This next section concerns data science and CDEs.

CDEs are variables that are operationalized and measured in identical ways across studies (Redecker et al., 2015). The use of CDEs enables comparison of data across studies and results in larger sample sizes. It also provides for secondary data analysis that might not otherwise be possible. This approach allows for aggregation across disciplines and centers of activity and affords efficiency and cost-effectiveness not offered by other approaches (Nahm et al., 2010). Using CDEs offers potential benefits for nursing science, in that many of the early studies used small samples, and it can be difficult to find large populations that fit the criteria for many studies in any one location or circumscribed geographical area.

Large cohorts and collaborative centers are beginning to become more common. It is not always possible or practical to assemble large patient cohorts for single-question studies. Ideally, if large cohorts are available, it would be helpful to be able to ask questions of such groups. Examples of this include the health maintenance organization (HMO) collaboratory efforts pioneered by NIH and the PCORNet effort recently launched by the Patient-Centered Outcomes Research Institute (PCORI). Certain types of health issues or questions for study are more easily adapted to these cohorts than others.

Increasingly, collaborative groups are emerging, using a variety of actual and virtual strategies. One example of a collaborative is the Palliative Care Research Cooperative (PCRC). The NINR-supported PCRC is a comprehensive, multicenter resource developing structures and processes to enable and support end-of-life and palliative care research more rapidly and with access to large populations at multiple sites across the United States. Its mission is to develop scientifically based methods that will lead to meaningful evidence for decreasing the suffering of patients with advanced and/or potentially life-limiting illnesses, and their caregivers, including family members and providers of care (Abernathy et al., 2010).

Concomitant with all of these efforts is the emerging field of data science, which will be increasingly important to nursing (Brennan & Bakken, 2015). Large amounts of data are being generated by health care systems and research enterprises, especially with the advent of the EHR and new measurement approaches. Although mastery may not be required, having some working knowledge of the building blocks—such as new data management methodologies, collection, analysis, secondary analyses, data warehouses, and so on—will be helpful moving forward. This is another benefit of teams; everyone does not need to be an expert in all aspects of an endeavor.

CONCLUSION

In summary, translating research results into practice or policy remains a challenge. This text contains many good examples of approaches that have been successful and hold promise for future impact. For example, as important as developing the scientific evidence that transitional care was a viable solution to care coordination issues were the actions to incorporate it into health care systems. This team took their clinical observations and research findings directly to health care providers, insurers, and leaders in health policy in order to facilitate the translation of their findings into evidence-based practice and policy in real-world settings.

There are many examples in this text that serve as exemplars of translating research into practice and policy. These examples not only demonstrate ways in which it can be done, but also serve to underscore the importance of doing it, as seen by the strong impact of translating such information in ways that can shape the future of health care.

REFERENCES

Abernathy, A., Aziz, N. M., Basch, E., Bull, J., Cleeland, C. S., Currow, D. C., . . . Kutner, J. S. (2010). A strategy to advance the evidence base in palliative medicine: Formation of a palliative care research cooperative group. *Journal of Palliative Medicine, 13,* 1407–1413.

Allen, J. K., Dennison Himmelfarb, C. R., Szanton, S. L., Bone, L., Hill, M. N., Levine, D. M., . . . Anderson, K. (2011). Community Outreach and Cardiovascular Health (COACH) trial: A randomized, controlled trial of nurse practitioner/community health worker cardiovascular disease risk reduction in urban community health centers. *Circulation: Cardiovascular Quality and Outcomes, 4,* 595–602. doi:10.1161/CIRCOUTCOMES.111.961573

Blumenthal, D., Abrams, M., & Nuzium, R. (2015a). Supplementary appendix to the Affordable Care Act at 5 years. *New England Journal of Medicine, 372*(25), 1–14.

Blumenthal, D., Abrams, M., & Nuzium, R. (2015b). The Affordable Care Act at 5 years. *New England Journal of Medicine, 372,* 2451–2458.

Brennan, P. F., & Bakken, S. (2015). Nursing needs big data and big data needs nursing. *Journal of Nursing Scholarship, 47*(5), 477–484.

Cady, R. G., Kelly, A. M., Finkelstein, S. M., Looman, W. S., & Garwick, A. W. (2014). Attributes of advanced practice registered nurse care coordination for children with medical complexity. *Journal of Pediatric Health Care, 28*(4), 305–312.

Calzone, K. (2013). *Integration of genomics into nursing practice.* Suburban Hospital. Retrieved from https://www.youtube.com/watch?v=Su1kZVXgNFw

Calzone, K. A., Jenkins, J., Bakos, A. D., Cashion, A. K., Donaldson, D., Feero, W. G., . . . Webb J. A. (2013). A blueprint for genomic nursing science. *Journal of Nursing Scholarship, 45,* 96–104.

Cashion, A. K., & Grady, P. A. (2015). The NIH/NINR intramural research program and the development of the NIH Symptom Science Model. *Nursing Outlook, 63,* 484–487.

Deechakawan, W., Cain, K. C., Jarrett, M. E., Burr, R. L., & Heitkemper, M. M. (2013). Effect of self-management intervention on cortisol and daily stress levels in irritable bowel syndrome. *Biologic Research in Nursing, 15*(1), 26–36.

Ford, E. S., Croft, J. B., Posner, S. F., Goodman, R. A., & Giles, W. H. (2013). Co-occurrence of leading lifestyle-related chronic conditions among adults in the United States, 2002–2009. *Prevention of Chronic Diseases, 10,* 120316.

Fried, V. M., Bernstein, A. B., & Bush, M. A. (2012). *Multiple chronic conditions among adults 45 and over: Trends over the past 10 years.* Hyattsville, MD: National Center for Health Statistics.

Grey, M., Knafl, K., Schulman-Green, D., & Reynolds, N. (2015). A revised self and family management framework. *Nursing Outlook, 63*(2), 162–170.

Grey, M., Whittemore, R., Jeon, S., Murphy, K., Faulkner, M. S., & TeenCope study group. (2013). Internet psycho-education programs improve outcomes in youth with type 1 diabetes. *Diabetes Care, 36*(9), 2475–2482.

Guimerà, R., Uzzi, B., Spiro, J., & Nunes Amaral, L. A. (2005). Team assembly mechanisms determine collaboration network structure and team performance. *Science, 308,* 697–702.

Hageman, P. A., Pullen, C. H., Hertzog, M., Boeckner, L. S., & Walker, S. N. (2011). Web based interventions for weight loss and weight maintenance among rural midlife and older women: Protocol for a randomized controlled clinical trial. *BMC Public Health, 11,* 521.

Hinshaw, A. S., & Grady, P. A. (Eds.). (2011). *Shaping health policy through research.* New York, NY: Springer Publishing.

Holland, D. E., Knafl, G. J., & Bowles, K. H. (2013). Targeting hospitalized patients for early discharge planning intervention. *Journal of Clinical Nursing, 22*(19–20), 2696–2703.

Holland, D. E., Rhudy, L. M., Vanderboom, C. E., & Bowles, K. H. (2012). Feasibility of discharge planning in intensive care units: A pilot study. *American Journal of Critical Care, 21*(4), e94–e101.

Institute of Medicine. (2011). *The future of nursing: Leading change, advancing health.* Washington, DC: National Academies Press.

Institute of Medicine, Altman, H. A., Butler, A. S., & Shern, L. (Eds.). (2015). *Assessing progress on the Institute of Medicine report: The future of nursing.* Washington, DC: National Academies Press.

Jemmott, L. S., Jemmott III, J. B., & O'Leary, A. (2007). Effects on sexual risk behavior and STD rate of brief HIV/STD prevention interventions for African American women in primary care settings. *American Journal of Public Health, 97,* 1034–1040.

Jost, T. S. (2016). A critical year for the Affordable Care Act. *Health Affairs, 35*(1), 8–11.

Looman, W. S., Antolick, M., Cady, R. G., Lunos, S. A., Garwick, A. E., & Finkelstein, S. M. (2015). Effects of a telehealth care coordination intervention on perceptions of health care by caregivers of children with medical complexity: A randomized controlled trial. *Journal of Pediatric Health Care, 29*(4), 352–363.

Looman, W. S., Presler, E., Erickson, M. M., Garwick, A. W., Cady, R. G., Kelly, A. M., & Finkelstein, S. M. (2013). Care coordination for children with complex special health care needs: The value of the advanced practice nurse's enhanced scope of knowledge and practice. *Journal of Pediatric Health Care, 27*(4), 293–303.

Lorig, K. R., & Holman, H. (2003). Self-management and education: History, definition, outcomes, and mechanisms. *Annals of Behavioral Medicine, 26*(1), 1–7.

McCorkle, R., Ercolano, E., Lazenby, M., Schulman-Green, D., Schilling, L. S., Lorig, K., & Wagner, E. H. (2011). Self-management: Enabling and empowering patients living with cancer as a chronic illness. *Cancer Journal Clinics, 61,* 50–62.

McSweeney, J. C., Cody, M., O'Sullivan, P., Elberson, K., Moser, D. K., & Garvin, B. J. (2003). Women's early warning symptoms of acute myocardial infarction. *Circulation, 108*(21), 2619–2623.

McSweeney, J. C., Rosenfeld, A. G., Abel, W. M., Braun, L. T., Burke, L. E., Daugherty, S. L., . . . Reckelhoff, J. F. (2016). Preventing and experiencing heart disease as a woman: State of the science: A scientific statement from the American Heart Association. *Circulation, 133,* 1302–1331.

Melnyk, B. M., Jacobson, D., Kelly, S., Belyea, M., Shaibi, G., Small, L., . . . Marsiglia, F. F. (2013). Promoting healthy lifestyles in high school adolescents: A randomized controlled trial. *American Journal of Preventive Medicine, 45*(4), 407–415.

Melnyk, B. M., Jacobson, D., Kelly, S., Belyea, M., Shaibi, G., Small, L., . . . Marsiglia, F. F. (2015). Twelve-month effects of the COPE healthy lifestyles TEEN program on overweight and depressive symptoms in high school adolescents. *Journal of School Health, 85*(12), 861–870.

Nahm, M., Walden, A., McCourt, B., Pieper, K., HoneyCutt, E., Hamilton, C. D., & Hammond, E. (2010). Standardizing clinical data elements. *International Journal of Functional Informatics and Personalized Medicine, 3*, 314–341.

National Council of State Boards of Nursing. (2014). Implications of the Affordable Care Act on nursing regulation and practice. *Journal of Nursing Regulation, 5*(1), 26–32.

Naylor, M. D., Bowles, K. H., McCauley, K. M., Maccoy, M. C., Maislin, G., Pauly, M. V., & Krakauer, R. (2013). High-value transitional care: Translation of research into practice. *Journal of Evaluation of Clinical Practice, 19*(5), 727–733.

Nguyen, H. Q., Donetsy, D., Reinke, L. F., Wolpin, S., Chyall, L., Benditt, J. O., . . . Carrieri-Kohlman, V. (2013). Internet-based dyspnea self-management support for patients with chronic obstructive pulmonary disease. *Journal of Pain and Symptom Management, 46*(1), 43–55.

Parker, S. J., Chen, E. K., Pillemer, K., Filiberto, D., Laureano, E., Piper, J., . . . Reid, M. C. (2012). Participatory adaptation of an evidence-based, arthritis self-management program: Making changes to improve program fit. *Family and Community Health, 35*(3), 236–245.

Rantz, M. J., Phillips, L., Aud, M., Marek, K. D., Hicks, L. L., Zaniletti, I., & Miller, S. J. (2011). Evaluation of an aging in place model with home care services and registered nurse care coordination in senior housing. *Nursing Outlook, 59*(1), 27–46.

Redecker, N. S., Anderson, R., Bakken, S., Corwin, E., Docherty, S., Dorsey, S. G., . . . Grady, P. (2015). Advancing symptom science through use of common data elements. *Journal of Nursing Scholarship, 47*(5), 379–388.

Rhee, H., Belyea, M. J., Hunt, J. F., & Brasch, J. (2011). Effects of a peer-led asthma self-management program for adolescents. *Archives of Pediatric Adolescent Medicine, 165*(6), 513–519.

Sampselle, C. M., Knafl, K. A., Jacob, J. D., & McCloskey, D. J. (2013). Nurse engagement and contributions to the clinical and translational science awards initiative. *Clinical and Translational Science, 6*(3), 191–195.

Shartzer, A., Long, S. K., & Anderson, N. (2016). Access to care and affordability have improved following Affordable Care Act implementation: Problems remain. *Health Affairs, 35*(1), 161–168.

Sigmon, H. D., Grady, P. A., & Amende, L. M. (1997). The National Institute of Nursing Research explores opportunities in genetics research. *Nursing Outlook, 45*(5), 215–219.

Szanton, S. L., Wolff, J. W., Roberts, L., Leff, B. L., Thorpe, R. J., Tanner, E. K., . . . Gitlin, L. N. (2015). Preliminary data from CAPABLE, a patient directed team-based intervention to improve physical function and decrease nursing home utilization: The first 100 completers of a CMS innovations project. *Journal of the American Geriatrics Society, 63*(2), 371–374.

Thorpe, J. M., Thorpe, C. T., Schulz, R., Van Houtven, C. H., & Schleiden, L. (2015). Informal caregiver disability and access to preventive care in care recipients. *American Journal of Preventive Medicine, 49*(3), 370–379.

Villarruel, A. M., Jemmott III, J. B., Jemmott, L. S., & Ronis, D. L. (2007). Predicting condom use among sexually experienced Latino adolescents. *Western Journal of Nursing Research, 29*(6), 724–738.

Wallace, A. S., Carlson, J. R., Malone, R. M., Joyner, J., & Dewalt, D. A. (2010). The influence of literacy on patient-reported experiences of diabetes self-management support. *Nursing Research, 59*(5), 356–363.

Webel, A. R., & Okonsky, J. (2012). Measuring HIV self-management in women living with HIV/AIDS: A psychometric evaluation study of the HIV Self-Management Scale. *Journal of Acquired Immune Deficiency Syndrome, 60*(3), e72–e81.

Wuchty, F., Jones, B. F., & Uzzi, B. (2007). The increasing dominance of teams in the production of knowledge. *Science, 316*, 1036–1039.

2

Expanding Areas of Clinical and Basic Sciences

Ann K. Cashion and Joan K. Austin

Translating the rapidly emerging scientific and technological advances from the basic science and clinical research arenas into improved patient care practices requires significant policy changes, and has been a major challenge. It has been suggested that it takes 17 years to translate science into practice (Morris, Wooding, & Grant, 2011); reasons for this extended lag time are multifactorial and include time for research-related processes as well as time for translating the research to the clinical setting. Science led and conducted by nurse scientists is key to building the body of basic science and clinical knowledge that can lead to more rapid integration into patient care practices. The purpose of this chapter is to present ways in which inclusion of basic science and clinical studies into nursing science agendas can shape and guide health policy, and to provide examples of how nurse scientists active in basic and clinical research are actively participating in the formation of health policy.

WHY ARE NURSE SCIENTISTS UNIQUELY QUALIFIED TO CONDUCT CLINICAL AND BASIC SCIENCE RESEARCH THAT TRANSLATES TO POLICY?

Nursing science has changed over the years, especially in regard to developing science that is relevant for changing nursing practice. Early research in nursing primarily focused on nurses, including the nursing role, nursing process, and quality of care (Gortner, 1983, 2000). About 40 years ago, the focus of nursing research shifted to nursing practice issues especially in adults, with about two thirds of the studies being assessment of patient populations and one third being interventions. Approximately half of early nursing studies tested a theory or framework from another discipline, with most coming from the discipline of psychology (Moody et al., 1988). In the 1970s and 1980s, progress in building nursing science was evident. Increases in multiauthored publications demonstrated that nurses were engaging in more team science, the larger number of references to funding sources on publications reflected that nursing studies were being funded by outside sources, and the larger number of studies in one area by the same author indicated that nurses were developing programs of research rather than doing isolated studies (Gortner, 2000; Moody et al., 1988).

A review of nursing research between 1985 and 2010 (Yarcheski, Mahon, & Yarcheski, 2012) showed growth in the building of nursing science related to patient care. There was a decline in use of theories from other disciplines and an increase in use of empirical findings from prior research to provide a foundation for nursing studies. Although psychological variables continued to be prominent, there was more diversity in the type of variables investigated, with more biological, physiological, and biopsychosocial variables being included in studies. In addition, there was continued growth in team science and external research funding. For example, 91% of publications had multiple authors and 72% of published articles cited funding sources in 2010. Finally, the review showed greater numbers of methodological studies, qualitative studies, and use of multivariate statistics by nurse scientists, which indicated advances in the research methods being used (Yarcheski et al., 2012).

The National Institute of Nursing Research (NINR) and its predecessor, the National Center for Nursing Research, which was created in 1986, have played a key role in stimulating nursing research that addresses important health and illness challenges such as promoting health and healthy lifestyles, reducing risk factors, enhancing quality of life in persons with chronic conditions, and improving care at the end of life (Gortner, 2000). In 2016, the NINR, which is a part of the National Institutes of Health (NIH), celebrated its 30th anniversary. NINR continues to set the national agenda for nursing research through regularly developing a strategic plan that addresses current and future health care challenges. NINR is the primary funder of basic and clinical research in nursing. Research at NINR is focused on four broad areas: symptom science, which is providing a foundation for personalized health strategies; wellness, which is identifying strategies to promote health and prevent illness; self-management, which is enhancing quality of life in persons with chronic illness; and end-of-life and palliative care, which is enhancing the quality of life at the end of life for patients and their families. There are also two cross-cutting areas of innovation promotion and technology that improve health (Grady & Gough, 2015).

Nurse scientists are especially qualified to lead and conduct clinical and basic research studies that are translated to policy for a number of reasons, and we explore four of those reasons here. First, nurses are trained in a caring profession that puts at the center the patient/client who is embedded within a network of a larger family and community. Therefore, nurse scientists use a clinical lens when developing all parts of the research process, from the research question to the interpretation of findings. For nurse scientists, research questions typically originate in practice emanating from clinical problems that they have encountered, regardless of where they practice (e.g., community, hospital settings). Although research questions vary depending on the individual nurse scientist's interest, they usually have the common goal of improving clinical outcomes for patients and their families.

Second, today's science is best conducted within teams where each team member brings a unique skill set to the table. Nurses are especially well suited to work in a team; they understand team dynamics and are known to be successful at building, leading, and functioning effectively within teams. We have found this to be particularly true today because many research teams are interdisciplinary, and in addition to nurses often include a wide range of people from other disciplines, such as bioinformaticians, biomedical engineers, neuropsychologists, dietitians, and physicians. Nurses have vast experience with working in multidisciplinary teams, and have been successful team leaders. Over time, nurse scientists have continued to gain confidence in their ability to serve as leaders of large interdisciplinary research teams engaged in multisite studies.

Third, a PhD in nursing is thought of by some as a PhD in clinical research because of the type of courses offered and the amount of time and focus on clinical research. In doctoral nursing programs, the focus is most commonly on clinical research. All nurse scientists should have a PhD as well as a nursing degree. With the PhD comes a significant knowledge of research design and methods that those with only a clinical degree would not have. Prior to the availability of doctoral nursing programs, nurse scientists typically had a master's degree in nursing and PhD preparation in another field such as physiology, psychology, anthropology, or education. As a result, nurse scientists gained knowledge of theory, research design, and methods from other fields and used these methods in early nursing research. Since the establishment of PhD programs in nursing, however, research preparation in nursing has had a strong clinical focus.

Last, not only do nurse scientists use a clinical lens for identifying important research questions, they also use that clinical lens, which is patient-centered and takes into consideration the context of the family and larger community, for interpretation of data and in the implementation of findings into clinical practice. Whether or not the nurse scientist is conducting a clinical study within a hospital setting or using an animal model in a laboratory, for many nurse scientists there is a clear and distinct link to improved patient outcomes. Understanding and discussing the findings of a study within the framework of the patient's condition can help move the study findings more quickly to changes in clinical recommendations and ultimately policy changes. Many doctoral-prepared individuals have the skill to design a study and collect data, but it is the understanding of what the data mean and the relevance of the data to people and their health that is the challenge for all health care researchers. For example, a psychologist might have in-depth knowledge about how perceptions affect behaviors, but not particularly interpret findings to be relevant for the influence of illness perceptions on behaviors related to self-management of a chronic illness.

GROWTH OF NURSE SCIENTISTS CONDUCTING CLINICAL AND BASIC SCIENCE RESEARCH

We have had a shift in the types of research conducted by nurse scientists, with one trend being for nurse scientists to incorporate more biological measures and themes into their research. Recently, the Council for the Advancement of Nursing Science Idea Festival identified seven science emerging areas, one of which was omics and the microbiome (Wyman & Henly, 2015). Increasing the number of doctoral programs that include content on omics was identified as a priority (Conley et al., 2015) because currently few doctoral programs include content in this area (Wyman & Henly, 2015). Nursing research on omics is considered critical to increasing our understanding of biological mechanisms that help explain how and why nursing interventions lead to desired outcomes (Henly et al., 2015).

The commitment of NINR to basic and clinical research as well as the increased emphasis on investigating biological mechanisms are also reflected in recommendations for future research as a result of the Innovative Question Initiative that NINR initiated in 2013. The goal of the initiative was for leading scientists in the field to identify important scientific research questions in symptom science, wellness, self-management, end-of-life and palliative care, and the cross-cutting area of technology (Grady, 2014). More than half of the final innovative questions in the areas of symptom science, wellness, and self-management will have to be addressed by nurse scientists who conduct basic and clinical research. In addition, an indication of the importance of biological variables in furthering important work in nursing science was the frequency with which biological variables were identified in two emphasis areas. Specifically, references to biological variables were mentioned in six of the 11 final innovative questions in symptom science and in three of the eight in wellness.

Nurse scientists from several institutes at the NIH, including NINR, have been actively involved in discussions, which led to recommendations for tailored research topics that would use basic and clinical research to build the evidence base to inform integration of genomics into nursing practice and regulation. This led to the publication of "A Blueprint for Genomic Nursing Science" (Calzone et al., 2013), which has been widely used to drive basic and clinical research questions posed by nurse scientists. Because these research topics were developed by nurse scientists, findings from these studies and others have the potential to be moved into clinical practice in a timelier manner than what is currently experienced.

While nurse scientists are conducting clinical and basic science research in various ways, from genomic to animal models to protein measures, the example used in this section comes from genomic research initiatives by nurse scientists. Figure 2.1 presents data from a recent bibliometric review conducted by Williams et al. (Williams, Tripp-Reimer, Daack-Hirsch, & DeBerg, 2016). The authors reviewed data-based genomic nursing research articles to profile the focus, dissemination, and impact of genomic nursing science articles from 2010 to 2014. Of the almost 200 articles that they found, more than 60% addressed biological results, illustrating that nurses are

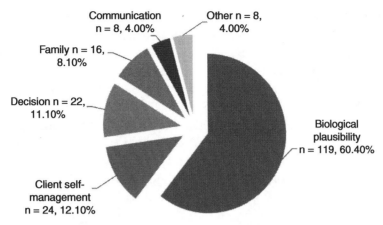

FIGURE 2.1   Blueprint topics of nursing science data-based publications, 2010 to 2014. Of the almost 200 articles found, more than 60% addressed biological results. This illustrates that nurses are interested in and publishing on biological mechanisms, among a range of topics such as family and communication that have more traditionally been topics in nursing publications.

Source: Williams et al. (2016).

interested in and publishing on biological mechanisms, among a range of topics such as family and communication, which have more traditionally been topics in nursing publications. Of note, more than 70% of the studies were conducted by interdisciplinary teams. Clearly there is evidence that the field has shifted and that nurse scientists in the area of genomics are publishing on biological data in such a way that it can be understood and used by policy makers to translate to health policy and clinical recommendations.

STRATEGIES FOR DEVELOPING A SUCCESSFUL PROGRAM OF CLINICAL OR BASIC RESEARCH THAT CAN INFORM POLICY

A Compelling Patient Story That Is Generalizable

Starting a research program by answering a patient-centered problem makes it more likely that the findings will be useful to the patient population, and hopefully generalizable to other groups. This would result in an increased chance of translation into health policy or clinical recommendations.

Obtaining Funding

Funding for a program of research is important in order to more quickly conduct the study (so that the results are relevant to policy makers) and to hire interdisciplinary team members to conduct the study and interpret the findings. Funding is important when the nurse scientist is interested in addressing questions that are most relevant to policy. Funding is also generally needed to conduct randomized clinical trials with large samples in order to generate the best levels of evidence, which are the strongest foundations on which to base clinical practice (Melnyk & Fineout-Overholt, 2015). In addition, disseminating study findings in venues where they can be found by policy makers is necessary. For example, findings from nursing studies that are published in refereed journals that are included in commonly searched databases are most likely to be included in a systematic review of the evidence in an area and therefore used to influence policy guidelines. In addition, a substantial body of studies with high levels of evidence are generally needed for research to affect policy.

Obtaining Skill Set to Influence Policy

In addition to obtaining research skills during doctoral study, it is important that nurse scientists develop the skills needed to influence policy. Nurses typically learn how to systematically review the literature; however, they also need experience in developing information that can be relevant for influencing policy. Policy makers need information in a format that helps them make decisions based on the best available evidence. Most systematic reviews focus on clinical problems and do not provide evidence on the benefits and limitations of different options that is generally needed by policy makers (Nannini & Houde, 2010). To influence policy, nurses need to develop skills in writing policy briefs where information is presented in a brief format. Lavis et al. (Lavis, Permanand, Oxman, Lewin, & Fretheim, 2009) identify that policy briefs have key messages of identifying the problem, describing options to address the problems that include the benefits and harms of each option, and considerations related to implementation of each option.

There are a number of opportunities for nurses to learn more about influencing health policy. The National Academy of Medicine services four national health policy fellowships: Food and Drug Administration Tobacco Regulatory Science Fellowship, the Distinguished Nurse Scholar-in-Residence program, the Institute of Medicine Anniversary Fellows Program, and the Robert Wood Johnson Health Policy Fellows program. Each of these fellowships provides opportunities for health care professionals to participate actively in the development of health policy at the national level (http://nationalacademies.org/hmd/about-hmd/leadership-staff/hmd-staff-leadership-boards/health-policy-educational-programs-and-fellowships.aspx).

SYMPTOM SCIENCE MODEL

With training and expertise in both clinical and research enterprises, nurse scientists occupy a unique and fundamental position in health research. However, we have not been conducting basic science research for very long. Therefore, models on how to integrate basic science, clinical research, and biobehavioral knowledge into the development of interventions are emerging. One such model was developed at the NIH where a research program within the NINR conducts basic and biobehavioral symptom science research, in an environment that provides training for the next generation of nurse scientists in symptom science. The program undertakes leading-edge research to determine the underlying behavioral and molecular mechanisms of symptoms associated with a variety of disorders. The overall goal of the program is the development of novel clinical interventions to alleviate these symptoms. Recently, intramural scientists developed a novel model, the National Institutes of Health Symptom Science Model (NIH-SSM; Cashion & Grady, 2015), to provide direction and focus to the research conducted within the intramural program, with potential to inform scientific communities and policy makers.

The NIH-SSM identifies the research process of identifying symptoms (subjective experience by the individual), characterizing symptom phenotypes (characteristics determined by behavioral, biological, and clinical data), employing "omics" methodologies to identify and test biomarkers (measures of normal biological processes, pathogenic processes, or pharmacologic responses; Biomarkers Definitions Working Group, 2001), and, ultimately developing clinical interventions for individuals with, for example, cancer-related fatigue (CRF), gastrointestinal disorders, and traumatic brain injuries (Figure 2.2; Cashion & Grady, 2015).

For example, Dr. Leorey Saligan and his research team at the NIH use the NIH-SSM to specify the clinically relevant phenotypic characterization of CRF. They then

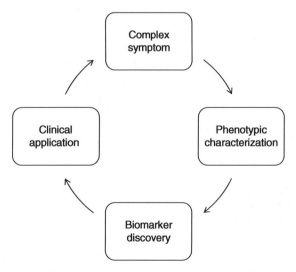

FIGURE 2.2 The National Institutes of Health Symptom Science Model. This model was developed to guide research. It begins with the presentation of a symptom; the symptom undergoes phenotypic characterization, then biomarkers are identified, and this ultimately leads to clinical applications resulting in symptom reduction and improvement.

Source: Reprinted from Cashion and Grady (2015). With permission from Elsevier.

use this knowledge to guide the identification of CRF-related biomarkers and provide a foundation for testing clinical applications. Ultimately, this will be translated into clinical interventions that alleviate the complex and debilitating symptoms of CRF experienced by many current and former patients with cancer. Recently they have identified that increases in concentrations of two proteins (apolipoprotein E and A1) and a decrease in one (transthyretin) were significantly correlated with worsening of fatigue during radiation treatment of cancer (Lukkahatai, Patel, Gucek, Hsiao, & Saligan, 2014) and that a decline in brain-derived neurotrophic factor levels during treatment is common among participants who experience high fatigue levels (Saligan, Lukkahatai, Holder, Walitt, & Machado-Vieira, 2015).

Another example comes from the work of Dr. Henderson, who is designing interventions to address complex gastrointestinal symptoms in conditions such as irritable bowel syndrome (IBS). Recent research findings suggest the presence of small noncoding ribonucleic acid (RNA) molecules that act as signatures to identify patients with IBS. The results support an underlying pathophysiology of IBS, and suggest that microRNAs may be used as either diagnostic biomarkers or targets for clinician-led, symptom-based interventions.

The final example is from Dr. Gill's lab, which is focused on complex symptoms of neurological trauma. Recent findings from Dr. Gill and her colleagues include previously unknown associations between lower health-related quality of life and inflammation with traumatic brain injury, posttraumatic stress disorder, and depression (Gill et al., 2014). Further, in another study, Dr. Gill's team found that for patients being treated for insomnia whose sleep improved, inflammatory genes were expressed differently compared to their own baseline expression, and that the differential expression was also related to reductions in depression symptoms (Livingston et al., 2015). These studies show that gene expression relates to insomnia and chronic symptoms, and that standard care (i.e., treatment for sleep disorder) can improve the condition of the patient.

Together, these three programs of research indicate that nurse scientists are making significant contributions to basic and clinical research in areas such as fatigue, gastric dysfunction, and sleep disorders that affect millions of individuals on a daily basis. Results from these research programs, and others, that have findings relevant to clinical practice should be transitioned into clinical practice and policy.

HOW TO INFLUENCE POLICY AS A NURSE SCIENTIST USING CLINICAL AND BASIC SCIENCE RESEARCH

Involvement of nurse scientists in federal and professional organizations that have as their mission to convene thought leaders, to provide clinical and regulatory recommendations, and to contribute to the policy discussion, is needed. Some organizations that have been important for nurse scientists wishing to enter the health policy arena are discussed in the following.

American Academy of Nursing Expert Panels

Nurses have the opportunity to become involved in the process of policy development through the American Academy of Nursing (AAN). AAN has an annual conference that highlights work that nurses are undertaking to influence health policy that transforms health care and improves the health of people. In addition to the conference, the AAN provides opportunities for nurses to learn about health policy through serving on expert panels that prepare position papers on compelling problems in a number of areas (e.g., quality health care, health behavior, children and families; www.aannet.org/health-policy). Expert panels were formed as working groups of the AAN. Expert panels review the current research and needs within their field to make recommendations on projects or initiatives the academy should undertake to transform health care policy and practice (www.aannet.org/expert-panels). Recently the Genomic Expert Panel published an article recognizing the importance of nurses contributing to the basic and clinical sciences in order to change practice and policy (Williams, Katapodi, et al., 2016). In this paper, Williams et al. state that nurse scientists are conducting basic science and clinical research that is providing findings that can be translated into improved health via precision health and tailored interventions. More importantly, the authors identified opportunities for action, including deriving new knowledge about disease biology, risk assessment, and treatment efficacy that can be addressed by educators, practitioners, scientists, and policy makers.

The National Academies of Sciences, Engineering, and Medicine

Recently the division of the National Academies of Sciences, Engineering, and Medicine (the Academies) that focuses on health and medicine, and was formerly known as the Institute of Medicine (IOM), was renamed the National Academy of Medicine (NAM). The NAM advises the government and the private sector in making informed decisions related to policies that are relevant to health and medicine. A number of nurses are members of the Academies, and many nurse members and nonmembers provide important service to the Academies through their membership on a committee or through providing expert testimony to a committee that is studying a particular health issue. For example, the IOM addressed the capacity of the nursing workforce to address the changes in health care that were planned with the enactment of the Affordable Care Act (ACA) in 2010. In the 2011 report *The Future of Nursing: Leading Change, Advancing Health* (IOM, 2011), there was a recommendation to double the number of nurses with doctoral degrees by 2020 because nurse scientists are needed to conduct the basic and clinical research to expand the knowledge base for the improvement of patient care.

The Academies also studies specific health conditions and makes recommendations regarding policies that would lead to better health care. For example, one of the authors, Joan K. Austin, was a member on the Institute of Medicine Committee that was asked to make recommendations for epilepsy related to public health surveillance; population and public health research; health policy, health care, and health services; and patient, provider, and public education. To accomplish these goals, the committee conducted a series of public workshops around the country in which people with epilepsy testified and experts provided information around specific areas under study. The report, *Epilepsy Across the Spectrum: Promoting Health and Understanding*, released in 2012, had 11 recommendations that would improve the power of epilepsy data, improve health care of people with epilepsy, improve community resources for epilepsy, and raise awareness and improve education about epilepsy (IOM, 2012).

Roundtable on Genomics and Precision Health (formerly the Roundtable on Translating Genomic-Based Research for Health) of the National Academies of Sciences, Engineering, and Medicine

The tremendous growth in clinical and basic science knowledge in the area of genomics and its potential impact on clinical practice led to the formation of the Roundtable on Genomics and Precision Health in 2007 (the Roundtable). In 2008, Dr. Martha Turner, a representative of the American Nurses Association, became the first nurse to obtain a seat and a voice on the Roundtable. The Roundtable is part of the Academies and brings together leaders from government, academia, industry, foundations, associations, patient communities, and other stakeholder groups. The primary purpose of the Roundtable is to convene and foster dialogue to illuminate and scrutinize critical scientific and policy issues where Roundtable engagement and input might help further the field (www.nationalacademies.org/hmd/Activities/Research/GenomicBasedResearch.aspx). To achieve its objectives, the Roundtable conducts structured discussions, public workshops, and symposia and enters into information-gathering activities, develops authored perspectives, organizes collaboratives, and publishes workshop summaries.

Previously, nurses on the Roundtable have been sponsored by the American Nurses Association, the AAN, and the NINR. Roundtable members determine the topics and speakers for their workshops, symposia, and meetings, and the influence of nurses on the Roundtable can be documented. The primary intent of nursing members of the Roundtable is to provide opportunities for nursing science and practice to inform the products of the Roundtable. Nursing engagement has resulted in more than six publications and five perspectives authored or co-authored by the nursing members. These papers speak to important issues in research, education, and practice. For example, "Genomics, Clinical Research, and Learning Health Care Systems: Strategies to Improve Patient Care" and "Using Clinical Genomics in Health Care: Strategies to Create a Prepared Workforce" present barriers and strategies to prepare APRNs and other providers to implement genomic discoveries that can benefit diverse populations in their practices (Williams & Cashion, 2015). In addition, 21% of the attendees were either nurses or worked in the nursing field for the workshop titled "Improving Genetics Education in Graduate and Continuing Health Professional Education" and more than 7% for the workshop titled "Applying an Implementation Science Approach to Genomic Medicine." Since 2010, six workshop speakers have been nurse scientists and nurse providers who have provided expertise in topics ranging from innovation in service delivery in the age of genomics to using genomic sequencing for health care decision making.

Current areas of emphasis for the Roundtable, and future opportunities for nurses, include the development of targeted therapeutics and diagnostics, clinical implementation of genomic medicine, health information technology, the use of genomic information for health care decision making, next-generation sequencing, using genomic information to generate knowledge for clinical practice and research, and education and ethical, legal, and social issues.

CONCLUSION

Our current need to quickly move research findings from basic and clinical research into policy and practice is driving scientists and policy makers to consider new models of research. Nurse scientists are emerging as a catalyst for this process because of their focus on the central role of the individual as well as their clinical lens in both identifying important clinical problems and in interpreting research findings back to the clinical setting. Interestingly, many of the skills that are found in good clinicians are often keys to being good scientists. Finally, nurses have the ability to effectively lead interdisciplinary teams. Interdisciplinary teams are necessary in order to conduct the large, multilayered, and complex studies that are needed to provide a strong foundation for influencing health policy in today's world of emerging technologies and methodologies.

ACKNOWLEDGMENTS

The authors would like to acknowledge the exciting research studies conducted by Drs. Wendy Henderson, Jessica Gill, and Leo Saligan, which were used as exemplars to illustrate key points in this chapter.

REFERENCES

Biomarkers Definitions Working Group. (2001). Biomarkers and surrogate endpoints: Preferred definitions and conceptual framework. *Clinical Pharmacology & Therapeutics, 69*(3), 89–95.

Calzone, K. A., Jenkins, J., Bakos, A. D., Cashion, A. K., Donaldson, N., Feero, W. G., . . . Webb, J. A. (2013). A blueprint for genomic nursing science. *Journal of Nursing Scholarship, 45*(1), 96–104. doi:10.1111/jnu.12007

Cashion, A. K., & Grady, P. A. (2015). The National Institutes of Health/National Institutes of Nursing Research intramural research program and the development of the National Institutes of Health Symptom Science Model. *Nursing Outlook, 63*(4), 484–487.

Conley, Y. P., Heitkemper, M., McCarthy, D., Anderson, C. M., Corwin, E. J., Daack-Hirsch, S., . . . Voss, J. (2015). Educating future nursing scientists: Recommendations for integrating omics content in PhD programs. *Nursing Outlook, 63*(4), 417–427.

Gill, J., Lee, H., Barr, T., Baxter, T., Heinzelmann, M., Rak, H., & Mysliwiec, V. (2014). Lower health related quality of life in U.S. military personnel is associated with service-related disorders and inflammation. *Psychiatry Research, 216*(1), 116–122.

Gortner, S. R. (1983). The history and philosophy of nursing science and research. *Journal of Advanced Nursing, 5*(2), 1–8.

Gortner, S. R. (2000). Knowledge development in nursing: Our historical roots and future opportunities. *Nursing Outlook, 48*(2), 60–67.

Grady, P. A. (2014). Charting future directions in nursing research: NINR's innovative questions initiative. *Journal of Nursing Scholarship, 46*(3), 143.

Grady, P. A., & Gough, L. L. (2015). Nursing science: Claiming the future. *Journal of Nursing Scholarship, 47*(6), 512–521.

Henly, S. J., McCarthy, D. O., Wyman, J. F., Stone, P. W., Redeker, N. S., McCarthy, A. M., . . . Conley, Y. P. (2015). Integrating emerging areas of nursing science into PhD programs. *Nursing Outlook, 63*(4), 408–416.

Institute of Medicine. (2011). *The future of nursing: Leading change, advancing health*. Washington, DC: National Academies Press.

Institute of Medicine. (2012). *Epilepsy across the spectrum: Promoting health and understanding*. Washington, DC: National Academies Press.

Lavis, J. N., Permanand, G., Oxman, A. D., Lewin, S., & Fretheim, A. (2009). SUPPORT Tools for evidence-informed health Policymaking (STP) 13: Preparing and using policy briefs to support evidence-informed policymaking. *Health Research Policy and Systems, 7*(1), S13.

Livingston, W. S., Rusch, H. L., Nersesian, P. V., Baxter, T., Mysliwiec, V., & Gill, J. M. (2015). Improved sleep in military personnel is associated with changes in the expression of inflammatory genes and improvement in depression symptoms. *Frontiers in Psychiatry, 6*, 59.

Lukkahatai, N., Patel, S., Gucek, M., Hsiao, C. P., & Saligan, L. N. (2014). Proteomic serum profile of fatigued men receiving localized external beam radiation therapy for non-metastatic prostate cancer. *Journal of Pain and Symptom Management, 47*(4), 748–756, e744.

Melnyk, B. M., & Fineout-Overholt, E. (2015). *Evidence-based practice in nursing and healthcare: A guide to best practice*. Philadelphia, PA: Wolters Kluwer.

Moody, L. E., Wilson, M. E., Smyth, K., Schwartz, R., Tittle, M., & Van Cott, M. L. (1988). Analysis of a decade of nursing practice research: 1977–1986. *Nursing Research, 37*(6), 374–379.

Morris, Z. S., Wooding, S., & Grant, J. (2011). The answer is 17 years, what is the question: Understanding time lags in translational research. *Journal of the Royal Society of Medicine, 104*(12), 510–520.

Nannini, A., & Houde, S. C. (2010). Translating evidence from systematic reviews for policy makers. *Journal of Gerontological Nursing, 36*(6), 22–26.

Saligan, L. N., Lukkahatai, N., Holder, G., Walitt, B., & Machado-Vieira, R. (2015). Lower brain-derived neurotrophic factor levels associated with worsening fatigue in prostate cancer patients during repeated stress from radiation therapy. *World Journal of Biological Psychiatry, 17*, 608–614.

Williams, J. K., & Cashion, A. K. (2015). Using clinical genomics in health care: Strategies to create a prepared workforce. *Nursing Outlook, 63*(5), 607–609.

Williams, J. K., Katapodi, M. C., Starkweather, A., Badzek, L., Cashion, A. K., Coleman, B., . . . Hickey, K. T. (2016). Advanced nursing practice and research contributions to precision medicine. *Nursing Outlook, 64*(2), 117–123.

Williams, J. K., Tripp-Reimer, T., Daack-Hirsch, S., & DeBerg, J. (2016). Five-year bibliometric review of genomic nursing science research. *Journal of Nursing Scholarship, 48*(2), 179–186.

Wyman, J. F., & Henly, S. J. (2015). PhD programs in nursing in the United States: Visibility of American Association of Colleges of Nursing core curricular elements and emerging areas of science. *Nursing Outlook, 63*(4), 390–397.

Yarcheski, A., Mahon, N. E., & Yarcheski, T. J. (2012). A descriptive study of research published in scientific nursing journals from 1985 to 2010. *International Journal of Nursing Studies, 49*(9), 1112–1121. doi:10.1016/j.ijnurstu.2012.03.004

3

Implementation Science

Marita Titler and Clayton Shuman

OVERVIEW

Since the late 1990s, implementation science has gained widespread acceptance as a field of research. Over time, increased attention has been directed toward developing an evidence base that informs health care delivery and population health. The Clinical and Translational Science Awards (CTSA) Program of the National Institutes of Health (NIH), by definition, focuses on clinical and translational research, including translation of clinical trial results and other research findings into practices and communities (Institute of Medicine [IOM], 2013a). The CTSAs are expected to partner with communities, practices, and clinicians not only in setting strategic directions for research but also in translating findings from research into health and health care.

Findings from clinical trials and effectiveness studies provide evidence that can be summarized and packaged for use in policy and clinical decision making. Examples of resources developed over the past two decades and made available to policy makers, health care organizations, and clinicians include numerous evidence-based clinical practice guidelines and practice recommendations, systematic reviews, and evidence-summary reports.

Despite the availability of evidence-based recommendations for health policy and practice, the *2014 National Healthcare Quality and Disparities Report* demonstrated that evidence-based care is delivered only 70% of the time, an improvement of just 4% since 2005 (Agency for Healthcare Research and Quality [AHRQ], 2015). This problem demonstrates the gap between the availability of evidence-based recommendations and application to improve population health. This gap can lead to poor health outcomes such as obesity, poor nutrition, health care–acquired infections, injurious falls, and pressure ulcers (Centers for Disease Control and Prevention, 2016; Conway, Pogorzelska, Larson, & Stone, 2012; Shever, Titler, Mackin, & Kueny, 2010; Sving, Gunningberg, Högman, & Mamhidir, 2012; Titler, 2011).

The terms *evidence-based practice* (EBP) and *implementation science* are sometimes used interchangeably, but they are different. EBP is the conscientious and judicious use of current best evidence in conjunction with clinical expertise and patient values to guide health care decisions (Titler, 2014a). Best evidence includes findings from randomized controlled trials, and evidence from other types of science such as descriptive and qualitative research, as well as information from case reports and scientific principles. In contrast, implementation science is a field of research that focuses on testing implementation interventions to improve uptake and use of evidence to improve patient outcomes and population health, and to explicate what implementation strategies work for whom, in what settings, and why (Eccles & Mittman, 2006; Titler, 2010, 2014b). An emerging body of knowledge in implementation science provides an empirical base for guiding the selection of implementation strategies to promote adoption of evidence in real-world settings (Mark, Titler, & Latimer, 2014). Thus, EBP and implementation science, though related, are not interchangeable terms; EBP is the actual application of evidence in practice and policy (the "doing of" EBP), whereas implementation science is the study of implementation interventions, factors, and contextual variables that affect knowledge uptake and use in practices, communities, and policy decision making (Titler, 2014b).

As noted in the National Institute of Nursing Research's (NINR's) 2016 strategic plan, the knowledge advanced from implementation science coupled with health care environments that promote the use of evidence-based practices and policies will help close the evidence–practice gap (NINR, 2016). Advancements in implementation science can expedite and sustain the successful integration of evidence in practice and policy to improve care delivery, population health, and health outcomes (Henly et al., 2015).

The purpose of this chapter is to provide a discussion about implementation science and health policy. First, examples are briefly described that illustrate how scientific findings have informed health policy. An overview of barriers to evidence-informed health policy is provided, and strategies to promote uptake and use of evidence by policy makers are described. Challenges in evidence-informed policy development and implementation are identified. Reflections about the future of implementation science and health policy are discussed.

EXAMPLES OF EVIDENCE-INFORMED HEALTH POLICIES

Addressing many health problems in the United States requires research-based knowledge in concert with policies from government and regulatory agencies (Nilsen, Stahl, Roback, & Cairney, 2013). Many of the public health achievements such as seat-belt laws, car seats for infants and children, and workplace regulations to decrease environmental exposures were influenced by public policies (Nilsen et al., 2013). Health policies can be conceptualized as "Big P" policies in the form of laws, rules, and regulations, or "small p" health policies such as management decisions that affect use of research by clinicians or people served within a local setting (Nilsen et al., 2013). The rules and regulations of the Joint Commission for Accreditation of Healthcare Organizations (JCAHO) and the Centers for Medicare and Medicaid Services (CMS) are examples of "Big P" health policies. Examples of "small p" health policies are those adopted by local communities and school systems to reduce childhood obesity.

Centers for Medicare and Medicaid Services

The CMS's value-based programs (VBPs) reward health care systems with incentive payments for the quality of care they give to people with Medicare coverage. These programs are part of the larger CMS quality strategy to reform how health care is delivered and paid for. VBPs also support the three-part aim of better care for individuals, better health for populations, and lower cost. The VBPs include items such as using incentives to improve care, tying payment to value through new payment models, changing how care is delivered through better coordination across health care settings, and more attention to population health. There are four original VBPs: the Hospital Value-Based Purchasing (HVBP) Program; the Hospital Readmission Reduction (HRR) Program; the Value Modifier (VM) Program (also called the Physician Value-Based Modifier [PVBM]); and the Hospital Acquired Conditions (HAC) Program. The goal of these programs is to link health care performance to payment. For the HVBP, hospitals are paid for inpatient acute care services based on the quality of care, not just quantity of the services they provide. Congress authorized Inpatient Hospital VBP in Section 3001(a) of the Affordable Care Act. The program uses the hospital quality data reporting infrastructure developed for the Hospital Inpatient Quality Reporting (IQR) Program, which was authorized by Section 501(b) of the Medicare Prescription Drug, Improvement, and Modernization Act of 2003. Measures used are based on evidence. For example, the inpatient quality measures for those with heart failure include discharge instructions to include activity, diet, follow-up, how to monitor and address signs and symptoms for worsening heart failure, and weight monitoring. These are important components for individuals with heart failure for managing their chronic illness following hospital discharge. A second example, catheter-associated urinary tract infection (CAUTI), is a quality measure because research demonstrates that the proper insertion and early removal of urinary catheters can reduce CAUTIs. Similarly, the unplanned hospital readmission for those with heart failure is based upon research demonstrating that effective coordination of care can lower the risk of readmission for patients with heart failure. Care coordination, home-based interventions, and exercise-based rehabilitation therapy among patients with heart failure all contribute to reducing the risk of hospitalization (www.cms.gov). These federal health policies are informed by evidence and impact health care delivery through payment incentives.

The Joint Commission for Accreditation of Healthcare Organizations

The JCAHO (now known simply as The Joint Commission) is a regulatory agency that sets standards of care for hospitals and other types of health care agencies. Standards are generally informed by a research base. For example, the recent Sentinel Event Alert about falls in hospitals notes that every year in the United States, hundreds of thousands of patients fall in hospitals, with 30% to 50% of those falls resulting in injury (Bagian et al., 2015). Injured patients require additional treatment and sometimes prolonged hospital stays. The average cost for a fall with injury is about $14,000. Successful strategies to reduce falls include the use of a standardized assessment tool to identify fall and injury risk factors, assessing an individual patient's risks that may not have been captured through the tool, and interventions tailored to an individual patient's identified risks. One of the JCAHO standards for reducing falls is in the Provision of Care, Treatment, and Services (PC) section—PC.01.02.08: The hospital assesses and manages the patient's risk for falls. EP 1: The hospital assesses the patient's risk for falls based on the patient population and setting. EP 2: The hospital implements interventions to reduce falls based on the patient's assessed risk.

Health Policies in Childhood Obesity

Examples of "small p" evidence-informed health policies are those adopted by local communities and school systems to reduce childhood obesity. The IOM has published several reports on prevention of childhood obesity that address increased physical activity; improving environments to include more parks, recreational spaces, and safe playgrounds; and types and amounts of foods and beverages provided in schools (IOM, 2009, 2011, 2013b, 2015). Schools are uniquely positioned to support physical activity and healthy eating and can serve as a focal point for obesity prevention among children and adolescents (IOM, 2012). Children spend up to half of their waking hours in school and therefore schools provide the best opportunity for a population-based approach to increase physical activity among the nation's youth. Similarly, children and adolescents consume one third to one half of their daily calories in schools, and therefore schools have an opportunity to influence their diets. School food–related policies have been shown to affect not only what students consume at school, but also what they and their parents perceive to be healthy choices (IOM, 2007). School-based interventions focused on increasing physical activities among children and adolescents have a positive impact on duration of physical activity, fitness, television viewing, and lifestyle patterns of regular physical activity that carry over to the adult years (IOM, 2012). School districts have enacted a variety of local policies to increase physical activity and create a healthy eating environment, such as requirements for physical education, increasing school-based physical activity outside of physical education, ensuring that school meals comply with the Dietary Guidelines for Americans (e.g., more fruits and vegetables; smaller portions; availability of low-fat and fat-free dairy products), and addressing the type and availability of foods and beverages sold outside the school meal programs (e.g., vending machines; snack bars; IOM, 2012).

In summary, these three examples illustrate the use of evidence in health policy formulation and decision making. Despite these examples, there are a number of barriers to use of research evidence in health policy.

BARRIERS TO EVIDENCE-INFORMED HEALTH POLICY

Studies have demonstrated multiple barriers to use of research evidence in health policy (Brownson, Chriqui, & Stamatakis, 2009; Jacobs et al., 2014; Hardwick, Anderson, & Cooper, 2015; Lavis, Moynihan, Oxman, & Paulsen, 2008; Naude et al., 2015; Tomm-Bonde et al., 2013; Tricco et al., 2016; Zardo & Collie, 2014). Common barriers include (a) beliefs and attitudes; (b) knowledge and skills; (c) relevance; and (d) organizational context.

Beliefs and Attitudes

Beliefs and attitudes include limited quantity, quality, and timeliness of research on topics of importance to policy makers (e.g., economic impact; use of emerging technologies); lack of value of research by the community; factors other than evidence being of higher importance in policy decisions (e.g., cost and equity); and perceived interference with autonomy of policy decision makers (Lavis et al., 2005; Tomm-Bonde et al., 2013; Tricco et al., 2016). Policy makers may disagree with the interpretation of research and systematic reviews and believe that the results are not valid. There may be a mismatch between the type of content in systematic reviews or other evidence sources and the information needs of policy makers. Communities may not value research findings for a variety of reasons, including trust with researchers, not being active participants in formulating and conducting the research, and important demographic characteristics that differ from populations in the original research. Policy makers want evidence that comes from a known, trusted, credible source that is timely and available at key points in the decision-making process. Tricco et al. (2016) found that policy makers who needed evidence in the prior 12 months often commissioned research or research reviews during this period, and then used the evidence to formulate the content of the health policy.

Knowledge and Skills

Knowledge and skills present common barriers to evidence-informed health policies. These barriers include a wide range of factors, such as (a) insufficient time, knowledge, and skills to search for evidence, critique research and systematic reviews, and synthesize the evidence for health policy; and (b) knowing how to interpret and use evidence to develop health policies and implement them. Furthermore, information overload leads to difficulty staying abreast of the research and may contribute to lack of awareness about research or systematic reviews on a particular topic. For people without research experience, it is difficult to evaluate and interpret original research and systematic reviews because the explanation of research methods and statistical analysis is long and complicated, with little attention given to policy implications of study findings. Policy makers report that they have a lack of time to find and discuss the evidence, as answers to policy issues are complex and often require attention within a short time frame (Hardwick et al., 2015; Lavis et al., 2005, 2008; Tricco et al., 2016). To improve use of evidence in health policy, capacity building for evidence-based decision making (EBDM) in health departments and public health agencies is needed (Brownson et al., 2014; Jacobs et al., 2014; Zardo & Collie, 2014).

Relevance

Perceived relevance includes (a) perceived usefulness and applicability of evidence sources, and (b) relevance of research to the role and day-to-day decision making of policy makers (Zardo & Collie, 2014). Systematic reviews are complex and not user-friendly. For example, it is difficult to identify the key messages in systematic reviews, and there is often a lack of detail on how to implement the recommendations (Lavis et al., 2011; Tricco et al., 2016). Public policy makers want a shorter and clearer presentation of the evidence with attention to the benefits, potential harms or risks, and costs, and a one-stop shop that provides high-quality reviews (Tricco et al., 2016). It is also a challenge for policy makers to interpret the applicability of findings for the local context (Lavis et al., 2005; Tricco et al., 2016).

Those who perceive research as relevant to their role are much more likely to use research as compared to those who perceive research of little or no relevance (Zardo & Collie, 2014). Relevance is complex and is influenced by utility; are research findings action-oriented, and do they challenge the status quo? Prior experience with research use is positive and may influence perceptions of relevance. Those who have used research in the past are likely to use it in future policy decision making (Zardo & Collie, 2014).

Research relevance also includes conceptual use of research to inform thinking, discussions, and debate, thereby influencing views on policy issues. This initial conceptual use of research by decision makers can lead to future action-oriented policy development or revisions, when the window of opportunity is created; that is, when the streams of policy, problems, and politics are aligned for new policy development or change (Zardo & Collie, 2014).

Context

Context is the setting or environment in which EBDM occurs, and policies and practices are delivered. Multiple context factors have been shown to influence knowledge use and uptake for application in practice, health care decision making, and policy formulation and implementation (Hardwick et al., 2015; Titler, 2010). A policy climate that is not receptive to research use is not likely to result in evidence-informed health policies.

Absorptive capacity for new knowledge affects research use. *Absorptive capacity* is the knowledge and skills to enact evidence-informed policies, remembering that the strength of evidence alone will not promote research use. An organization that is able to systematically identify, capture, interpret, share, reframe, and recodify new knowledge and put it to appropriate use will be better able to assimilate research findings. A learning organizational culture and proactive leadership that promotes knowledge sharing are important components of building absorptive capacity for new knowledge (Hardwick et al., 2015; Titler, 2010).

Components of a receptive context for use of research findings include strong leadership, clear strategic vision, good managerial relations, visionary staff in key positions, a climate conducive to experimentation and risk taking, and effective data capture systems. Leadership is critical in encouraging organizational members to break out of the convergent thinking and routines that are the norm in large, well-established organizations (Titler, 2010).

An organization may be generally amenable to innovations but not ready or willing to assimilate the evidence for a specified topic. Elements of system readiness include tension for change; assessment of implications, support and advocacy for research use; dedicated time and resources; and capacity to evaluate the impact of the evidence-informed policy during and following implementation. If there is tension around specific policy issues, and if staff perceive that the situation is intolerable, the evidence is likely to be assimilated if it can successfully address the issues and thereby reduce the tension (Hardwick et al., 2015; Titler, 2010).

STRATEGIES TO PROMOTE RESEARCH USE

Strategies to promote use of research findings and other types of evidence (e.g., local community data) for evidence-informed health policies include (a) capacity building; (b) provision of research findings for use by policy makers; (c) relationship building; and (d) models for knowledge translation in public policy. The research evidence for evidence-informed health policy implementation is not as robust as that available for research use in health care settings (Armstrong et al., 2013).

Capacity Building

Building capacity is one strategy to improve development and implementation of evidence-informed health policies (Brownson et al., 2014; Jacob et al., 2014; Jacobs et al., 2014; Litaker, Ruhe, Weyer, & Stange, 2008; Wilson, Rourke, Lavis, Bacon, & Travers, 2011). Competencies for EBDM have been developed and guide the organization of capacity-building programs (Brownson, Ballew, Kittur, et al., 2009;

Jacob et al., 2014). Content common across these programs includes understanding the basic concepts of EBDM; defining the problem or public health issue; locating and critiquing evidence sources; summarizing the scientific literature; prioritizing policy options; doing economic evaluation; developing an action plan and building a logic model; and implementing and evaluating the policy impact. The evidence-based public health training course developed by the Prevention Research Center in St. Louis has demonstrated improvements in participants' EBDM competencies following course completion (Baker, Brownson, Dreisinger, McIntosh, & Karamehic-Muratovic, 2009; Brownson, Chriqui, et al., 2009; Dreisinger et al., 2008). A quasi-experimental design, using a train-the-trainer approach, demonstrated the effectiveness of the program, with EBDM competencies improving more in the intervention than the control group (Jacobs et al., 2014). This is an excellent example of a capacity-building program designed for policy makers.

Provision of Research for Policy Makers

Provision of research findings for health policy makers is less than optimal. Hardwick et al. (2015) found that the way research is organized and presented does not lend itself to use by policy-making organizations and the way they work across communities, sectors, and settings. Policy makers have mixed views about the helpfulness of recommendations from systematic reviews. Lavis et al. (2005) found policy makers would benefit from systematic reviews that (a) highlight relevant information for decision making, such as contextual factors that affect local applicability, and information about the benefits, harms/risks, and costs of interventions; and (b) are presented in a way that allows rapid scanning for relevance, such as one page of take-home messages, and a three-page executive summary. Researchers could help to ensure that the future flow of systematic reviews will better inform policy making by involving policy makers in their production and better highlighting information that is relevant for decisions (Lavis et al., 2005). To ensure that the global stock of systematic reviews will better inform policy making, producers of systematic reviews should address local adaptation processes, such as developing and making available online more user-friendly "front ends" for systematic reviews.

Investigators should include a section on implications for policy makers in research manuscripts, and develop policy briefs that include impact statements on health and health outcomes. Examples of excellent policy briefs/snapshots are the Health Affairs Health Policy Briefs and those available from Robert Wood Johnson Foundation (RWJF). Health Affairs Health Policy Briefs provide clear, accessible overviews of timely and important health policy topics for policy makers, journalists, and others concerned about improving health care in the United States. The briefs explore competing arguments made on various sides of a policy proposal and point out wherever possible the relevant research behind each perspective. They are reviewed by distinguished *Health Affairs* authors and other outside experts (www.healthaffairs.org/healthpolicybriefs). An example of a Health

Affairs Policy Brief is "The Final 2015-20 Dietary Guidelines for Americans" based on the latest research.

The Health Policy Snapshots from the RWJF provide top takeaway messages, key facts on the public health issue, and recommendations for action (www.rwjf. org). For example, the health policy snapshot on "Schools Can Help Children Eat Healthy and Be Active" is an excellent example of a health policy brief for local policy makers. Every school district and local board of education in the United States has access to this research-based information for development and implementation of policies that address healthy eating and physical activities in schools.

Another approach to address availability of research evidence for policy makers is the development of a "one-stop shop" of research evidence for public health and health systems that are now available (Dobbins et al., 2010; Lavis et al., 2015; Moat & Lavis, 2014; www.healthsystemsevidence.org; www.health-evidence.ca; global.evi-pnet.org). For example, EVIPNet promotes the systematic use of research evidence in policy making, focusing on low- and middle-income countries, and promotes partnerships at the country level between policy makers, researchers, and civil society in order to facilitate both policy development and policy implementation using the best scientific evidence available (Moat & Lavis, 2014). The Centers for Disease Control and Prevention offers many resources for policy makers, including a guide to community preventive services to help policy makers choose programs and policies to improve health and prevent disease in communities (www.communityguide. org). Systematic reviews are used to answer these questions:

- Which program and policy interventions have been proven effective?
- Are there effective interventions that are right for a specific community?
- What might effective interventions cost; what is the likely return on investment?

Rapid reviews have emerged in response to the incompatibility between information needs of policy makers and the time requirements to complete systematic reviews. The rapid realist review (RRR) method is a knowledge synthesis process producing a product that is useful to policy makers in responding to time-sensitive and/or emerging issues where there is limited time and resources. The focus is on contextually relevant interventions/programs that are likely to be associated with specific outcomes within a specific set of parameters. RRRs include the policy makers in development of specific questions and other key decisions, and content experts to validate findings of the review. The time to perform these reviews has ranged from 2 to 6 months, in contrast to systematic reviews that may take 1 to 2 years. Examples include telehealth contributions to emergency department and discharge operations and evidence-informed public health policy and practice through a complexity lens (Saul, Willis, Bitz, & Best, 2013).

A second strategy used to assist policy makers in use of evidence is the rapid-response program (Mijumbi, Oxman, Panisset, & Sewankambo, 2014; Wilson, Lavis, & Gauvin, 2015). Products provided through such programs may include a listing of relevant research evidence, a brief synthesis of the evidence, and briefings with decision makers. Examples include improving leadership capacity in community care; active living for older adults; and optimal treatment for people with multiple comorbidities (www.mcmasterhealthforum.org).

Relationship Building

Building strong relationships between researchers and policy makers is a strategy to promote research use (Hardwick et al., 2015; Kislov, Harvey, & Walshe, 2011; Lavis et al., 2008; Shearer, Dion, & Lavis, 2014). Building and sustaining these relationships are not without challenges, such as managing tensions and conflicts of interests that can arise from differences in cultures, perceptions of research evidence, and the nature of decision making (Kislov, Harvey, & Walshe, 2011; Lavis et al., 2008).

Use of knowledge brokers or boundary spanners has been shown to be a helpful strategy in public health to facilitate bidirectional communication between researchers and users of evidence to promote mutual understanding of each other's languages, goals, and culture and to address barriers to the use of scientific knowledge in health policy (Dobbins et al., 2009). Knowledge brokers can be individuals, groups, and/or organizations, and in each case the knowledge broker focuses on promoting the integration of the best available evidence into policy and health care decision making. Knowledge brokers can play several roles, including: knowledge management, offering users valid information tailored to their settings and needs; liaison, facilitating direct contacts and collaboration between producers and users of scientific knowledge; and assessing user expectations and adjusting activities to better fit their work flow (Dagenais, Laurendeau, & Briand-Lamarche, 2015; Dobbins et al., 2009). The interpersonal dimension of knowledge brokers (interaction with the users) is a key factor in promoting knowledge use. Direct and frequent contacts (including face to face) between the broker and the intended users help build "relationship capital," trust, and understanding. It appears that settings with a weaker research culture (e.g., no academic connections; sporadic contacts with researchers) will need more intensive broker interaction to reduce the perceived "semantic distance" from the scientific knowledge and its use in policy development (Dagenais, Laurendeau, & Briand-Lamarche, 2015; Dobbins et al., 2010).

Last, understanding the social networks of policy decision makers and using those networks to spread evidence is another relationship strategy to consider (Shearer et al., 2014; Yousefi-Nooraie, Dobbins, Marin, Hanneman, & Lohfeld, 2015). Social network theory involves understanding the interpersonal exchange of information among members of a group. For example, engaging with policy makers who are centrally located (centrality) in a social network holds great promise for influencing others more peripheral in the network. Centrality in social networks should not be confused with those in organizational leadership positions (organizational structure), as their spheres of influence may differ. Shearer et al. (2014) demonstrated that network position—that is, connectedness to others—predicted use of knowledge by policy makers more than any other individual characteristic such as job position/ level, organizational affiliation, or experience as a researcher. Strategies for promoting use of evidence with policy makers should maximize deliberative dialogues with policy makers who are in strategic network positions to influence others, not just in strategic organizational positions.

Models

Various conceptual models of EBP and translation science are available. Hendriks et al. (2013) note several limitations of these models for use in public policy, including lack of a comprehensive approach; the fact that most are based on research in organizational settings; and the fact that many fail to take into account the factors that make policy development for complex public health problems difficult (e.g., childhood obesity). The conceptual model for policy integration, the Behavior Change Ball (Figure 3.1), adapted from Michie, van Stralen, and West's (2011) Behavior Change Wheel, addresses several important components of integrating knowledge into local policy development, including: 10 organizational behaviors (e.g., agenda setting; leadership); 3 categories of interrelated determinants of behavior (capability, opportunity, motivation [COM]); 9 strategies/interventions to improve suboptimal

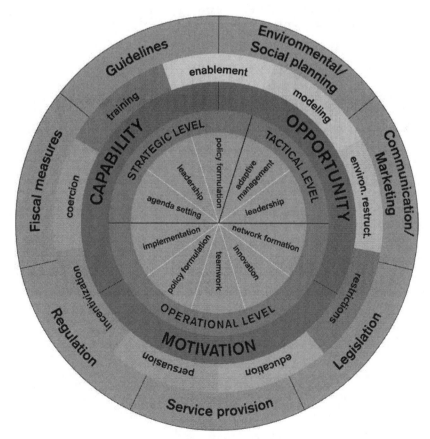

FIGURE 3.1 *Behavior* Change Ball.

Source: Hendriks et al. (2013).

determinants of behavior (COM) such as education, persuasion, incentivization, and modeling; and 7 factors that enable these 9 interventions, such as legislation, communication/marketing, and environment or social planning. The model is meant to illuminate the dynamic policy process. The authors of the model recommend application to case study designs or narrative inquiries to build research on policy development and implementation.

Armstrong et al. (2013) have developed a logic model for development and implementation of evidence-informed policies in local governments (Figure 3.2). It consists of three core components: tailored organizational support; group training; and targeted messages and evidence summaries. This logic model was developed from implementation science interventions; knowledge management and diffusion of innovation theories; and a qualitative study of evidence-informed decision making by local governments. The model is designed to address the lack of rigorous evidence to guide knowledge transfer in a public health decision-making context. This model holds great promise for designing knowledge translation interventions for local governments (Armstrong et al., 2013).

Scientists and experts in public health are recommending use of simulation models (based on systems science and nonlinear dynamics) to investigate and understand the nature of complex public health problems (Atkinson, Page, Wells, Milat, & Wilson, 2015; IOM, 2015). Simulation modeling allows virtual experimentation of policy

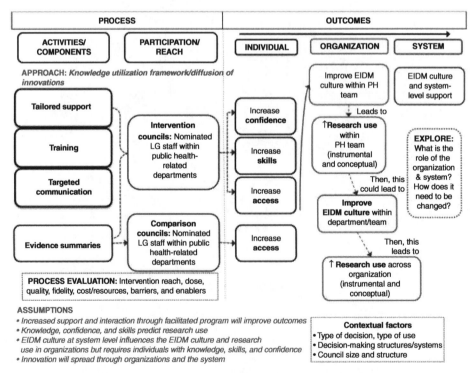

FIGURE 3.2 Knowledge translation model for local governments.

EIDM, evidence-informed decision making; LG, local government; PH, public health.

Source: Armstrong et al. (2013).

scenarios to test comparative impact and cost of various programs, interventions, and policies over various time frames. Simulation modeling is informed by reviews of research evidence, existing conceptual models, and expert opinions, and is able to incorporate the impact of contextual influences on policy making. Models are considered to be a theoretical representation of the problem and must undergo a validation process that includes how accurately the model can reproduce real-world historical data patterns (Anderson & Titler, 2014; Atkinson, Page, et al., 2015; IOM, 2015). In a systematic review to determine the effectiveness of system dynamics modeling for health policy and the nature of its application, only six papers were found comprising eight case studies. No analytic studies were found that examined the effectiveness of this type of modeling. The paucity of relevant papers indicates that, although the volume of descriptive literature advocating the value of system dynamics modeling is considerable, its practical application to inform health policy making is yet to be routinely applied and rigorously evaluated (Atkinson, Wells, et al., 2015). A recent report by the IOM (2015) discusses the use of agent-based models (a type of simulation model) to assess the effects of tobacco control policies. Although simulation models hold great promise, documenting and evaluating their applications will be vital to supporting uptake by policy makers (Atkinson, Wells, et al., 2015).

CHALLENGES

There are several challenges in implementation science. The first is that this field of inquiry has been referred to by numerous related, although not synonymous terms, including translational science, effectiveness science, dissemination science, implementation science, and knowledge translation (McKibbon et al., 2010; Newhouse, Bobay, Dykes, Stevens, & Titler, 2013; Table 3.1). Despite varying terminology, there is international agreement regarding the overall goal: to address the challenges associated with the use of research findings and EBP recommendations in health policy, care delivery, and decision making. This collective objective has led to the formation of academic journals like *Implementation Science* and *Translational Behavioral Medicine*, which are specifically interested in advancing the body of science in this field. However, the inconsistent terminology impedes theoretical formulation and scientific progress (Proctor, Powell, & McMillen, 2013; Smits & Denis, 2014). Differences in terminology are further complicated by the lack of mature taxonomies of implementation interventions (Lokker, McKibbon, Colquhoun, & Hempel, 2015; Mazza et al., 2013). Although standards are emerging for reporting implementation interventions in scientific journals, there is yet no agreement about these standards and the detail required about the implementation intervention included in published reports (Albrecht, Archibald, Arseneau, & Scott, 2013; Eccles, Foy, Sales, Wensing, & Mittman, 2012; Michie, Fixsen, Grimshaw, & Eccles, 2009; Mohler, Kopke, & Meyer, 2015; Pinnock et al., 2015; Proctor et al., 2013; Riley et al., 2008). Furthermore, fidelity to the implementation intervention is not always reported (Slaughter, Hill, & Snelgrove-Clarke, 2015). These challenges make it difficult to compare and contrast the effectiveness of implementation interventions across studies and their impact on health.

TABLE 3.1   *Related Terms Used in Implementation Science*

Term	Description
Translational research	Translational research exists along a dynamic continuum that connects basic research findings to decisions made within clinical settings and interventions that are applied in community and public health settings to improve health broadly. Translational research progresses across five phases, namely: Preclinical and animal studies (T0/Basic Science Research), Proof of concept/Phase I clinical trials (T1/Translation to Humans), Phase 2 and Phase 3 clinical trials (T3/Translation to Patients), Phase 4 clinical trials and clinical outcomes research (T4/Translation to Practice), and Phase 5 population-level outcomes research (T5/Translation to Community). The translational phases along this continuum are sometimes referred to as "bench-to-bedside" and "bedside-to-community" (IOM, 2013a).
Translation science	Translation of research findings into practice, communities, and policy to improve health and health outcomes. The focus is on T4 and T5 phases of the translational continuum. This term is used interchangeably with implementation science (Titler, 2010)
Implementation science	A field of science that focuses on testing implementation interventions to improve uptake and use of evidence to improve patient outcomes and population health, and explicate what implementation strategies work for whom, in what settings, and why (Eccles & Mittman, 2006; Titler, 2010; Titler, 2014b).
Dissemination research	The targeted distribution of information and intervention materials to a specific public health or clinical practice audience with the intent to spread, scale-up, and sustain knowledge use and evidence-based interventions.
Effectiveness science	Effectiveness research tests, in real world settings, the impact and value of interventions with demonstrated efficacy in controlled trials. The goal of effectiveness research is to test the generalizability of valid results achieved in efficacy studies across different populations and settings (Potempa, Daly, & Titler, 2012; Titler & Pressler, 2011).
Comparative effectiveness research (CER)	CER is the generation and synthesis of evidence that compares the benefits and harms of alternative methods to prevent, diagnose, treat, and monitor a clinical condition, or to improve the delivery of care. The purpose of CER is to assist consumers, clinicians, purchasers, and policy makers to make informed decisions that will improve health care at both the individual and population levels. This definition implies the direct comparison of two or more effective interventions in patients who are typical of day-to-day clinical care (IOM, 2009).
Knowledge translation	Knowledge translation is a term primarily used in Canadian implementation research and is defined by the Canadian Institute for Health Research (CIHR) as "a dynamic and iterative process that includes synthesis, dissemination, exchange and ethically-sound application of knowledge."
Knowledge transfer	"The process of getting knowledge from producers to potential users" (Graham et al., 2006). However, knowledge transfer has been criticized for its "unidirectional notion and its lack of concern with the implementation of transferred knowledge" (Graham et al., 2006).
Evidence-based practice	The conscientious and judicious use of current best evidence in conjunction with clinical expertise and patient values to guide health care decisions (Titler, 2014a).

(continued)

TABLE 3.1   *Related Terms Used in Implementation Science (continued)*

Term	Description
Evidence-based policy	Evidence-based policy is developed through a continuous process that uses the best available quantitative and qualitative evidence to improve public health outcomes (Brownson, Chriqui, & Stamatakis, 2009).
Evidence-informed decision making (EIDM)	EIDM is the process of combining a range of sources of evidence to inform a decision. In practice, this occurs within a political context that requires consideration of a range of other factors including research evidence, community views, budget constraints, and expert opinion (Armstrong et al., 2013).
Policy dissemination and implementation research	Policy dissemination and implementation research is focused on generating knowledge to effectively spread research evidence among policy makers and integrate evidence-based interventions into policy designs (Purtle, Peters, & Brownson, 2016)

The second challenge is the minimal cross-fertilization and knowledge exchange between implementation science and policy implementation research areas of inquiry (Nilsen et al., 2013). Research in both fields focuses on translating evidence into action, emphasizes the importance of interdisciplinary science, uses a variety of methods of inquiry, and is guided by a number of models and frameworks. Policy implementation research has given more attention to the context of implementation, whereas context appears to be a less understood mediator of change in implementation science (Nilsen et al., 2013). There are opportunities for investigators in these two fields of inquiry to learn from one another.

The third challenge is funding for implementation science, particularly for health policy. The program announcement (PAR) titled "Dissemination and Implementation Research in Health" (D&IRH) was issued in 2005 and reissued in 2013, with a greater emphasis on policy dissemination and implementation (D&I) research (Neta et al., 2015; Purtle, Peters, & Brownson, 2016; Tinkle, Kimball, Haozous, Shuster, & Meize-Grochowski, 2013). Tinkle et al. (2013) found that between 2005 and 2012, NIH had funded $79.2 million under the D&IRH PAR. The majority of projects (58%) were funded by the National Cancer Institute and the National Institute of Mental Health, which accounted for 61% of the total funding. The NINR awarded 6% of the projects totaling $4.9 million (3 R01s, 1 R21, 1 R03). The most commonly funded projects across institutes focused on cancer control and screening, substance abuse prevention and treatment, and mental health services. Topics funded by NINR included implementing evidence to prevent urinary infections and enhance patient safety; implementing interventions to reduce hospitalizations of nursing home residents; and dissemination of a theory-based bone health program (Tinkle et al., 2013). More recently, NIH funding (2007–2014) for policy D&I research, defined as generating knowledge to effectively spread research evidence among policy makers and integrate evidence into policy designs, was evaluated (Purtle et al., 2016). This analysis revealed that NINR funded seven D&I projects, comprising more than 1% of the institute's total grant spending—a proportion larger than any other institute.

Of the 146 projects funded during this period, only 8.2% were policy D&I research. Tobacco and cancer control were the most common topics funded.

D&I research has emerged as an important area of funding at NIH, which has advanced the science of implementation. The current D&I research PAR expires in May 2016. It will be important that NIH continues to fund D&I research by reissuance of this PAR or something similar. As noted by Purtle et al. (2016), the level of support for D&I policy research is probably not commensurate with the potential for evidence-based policy to impact human health.

The RWJF has committed significant funding to health policy research. The Policies for Action (P4A) program funds investigator-initiated research. For example, a recent call for proposals (CFP), *Policies for Action: Policy and Law Research to Build a Culture of Health* (P4A), was created to help build an evidence base for policies that can lead to a Culture of Health. P4A seeks to engage long-standing health researchers, as well as experts in fields like housing, education, transportation, and the built environment who have not worked in health before. The goal is to develop research that generates actionable evidence—the data and information that can guide legislators and other policy makers, public agencies, educators, advocates, community groups, and individuals. The research may examine established laws, regulations, and policies as well as potential new policies and approaches. The research funded under this CFP should inform the significant gaps in our knowledge regarding what policies can serve as levers to improve population health and well-being, and achieve greater levels of health equity.

RWJF has also funded three research hubs in health policy. The goal of a research hub is to provide a transdisciplinary setting to develop, implement, and manage a program of strategic policy research to explore how policies, laws, and regulations in both the public and private sectors can support building a Culture of Health. The Policies for Action Research Hub at the University of Michigan (UM), led by Dr. Paula Lance in the Ford School of Public Policy, will produce innovative, timely, and actionable transdisciplinary research in selected key policy areas to inform and strengthen the laws, policies, and initiatives necessary to accelerate progress toward population health improvement and health equity. The UM Hub is focused on a group of emergent policy innovations for which there is currently a fair amount of action and activity, yet existing efforts are fragmented and suffer from a nascent evidence base. This includes Pay-for-Success initiatives, "Health in All Policies" efforts, and interventions targeting superutilizers of health care. There is limited empirical evidence to determine what works and how initiatives/interventions are structured, implemented, and sustained over time. The UM Hub research projects aim to strengthen conceptual models, identify synergies, estimate potential impact, and inform best practices for future policy directions.

CONCLUSION

The future for implementation science and policy implementation research is bright. There are a number of factors, however, that we must consider.

First, nurse scientists are well positioned to make major contributions to evidence-informed health policy. Nurse scientists are contributing significantly to the science base for promoting health and preventing illness; self-care management; symptom science; end-of-life and palliative care; and development and use of innovative technologies to improve health. For these scientific investments to impact the health of the nation, however, findings from these fields of inquiry must be packaged for health policy and implementation. Providing funding streams that require partnerships among researchers investigating these phenomena and implementation scientists who promote knowledge use by health policy makers, communities, and health systems would advance the application of scientific findings in health policy and health care.

Second, final grant reports from federally funded agencies and foundations should require a section on policy implications and a health policy brief for policy makers.

Third, journal editors should standardize the reporting of implementation studies in scientific publications and come to some agreement about the details required regarding the implementation intervention. This is a large task, but an area of need to advance the science of implementation.

Fourth, we need to provide forums for implementation scientists and policy implementation researchers to discuss similarities and differences, as each of these scientific areas could learn from one another. Such forums could be hosted by federal and foundation funding agencies with invited papers presented and discussed, and with proceedings published in a scientific journal.

Last, we need to train the next generation of scientists in novel and innovative methodological approaches for addressing health in the context of complexity. Complexity is a dynamic and constantly emerging set of processes that interact with each other, but which also provoke change throughout the system (Cohn, Clinch, Bunn, & Stronge, 2013; Michie et al., 2009). The health of individuals and populations is affected by multiple complex factors, including the environment, lifestyles, personal factors (e.g., gender, ethnicity), and other social determinants of health. Consequently, studies must include consideration and/or modification of these multiple complex factors and testing complex health interventions to address them (Craig et al., 2008; Craig & Petticrew, 2013; Michie et al., 2009; Mohler, Bartoszek, & Meyer, 2013; Mohler et al., 2015). These complex interventions will vary in character and form due to the dynamic nature of the constituent parts and adaptations required for implementation in the local contexts (Cohn et al., 2013). Innovative scientific approaches to test interventions in the context of complexity include adaptive research designs, participatory action research, community-based participatory research, social network analysis, simulation and agent-based modeling, realist evaluation, sequential multiple assignment randomized trials, and adaptive interventions (Almirall, Nahum-Shani, Sherwood, & Murphy, 2014; Blackwood, 2006; Brown et al., 2009; Campbell, Mollison, Steen, Grimshaw, & Eccles, 2000; IOM, 2015; Kilbourne et al., 2014; Luke & Stamatakis, 2012; Nahum-Shani et al., 2012a, 2012b; Pawson & Tilley, 1997). Scientists of the future will need research training on the nature of complex systems and the well-established mathematical approaches of nonlinear dynamics to understand complex health problems and the range of interventions and policy solutions to address them (Atkinson, Wells, et al., 2015; Grant, Treweek, Dreischulte, Foy, & Guthrie, 2013; Luoto, Shekelle, Maglione, Johnsen, & Perry, 2014; Wilson, Grimshaw, et al., 2015).

REFERENCES

Agency for Healthcare Research and Quality. (2015). *2014 National healthcare quality and disparities report.* Rockville, MD: U.S. Department of Health and Human Services. Retrieved from http://www.ahrq.gov/research/findings/nhqrdr/nhqdr14/index.html

Albrecht, L., Archibald, M., Arseneau, D., & Scott, S. D. (2013). Development of a checklist to assess the quality of reporting of knowledge translation interventions using the Workgroup for Intervention Development and Evaluation Research (WIDER) recommendations. *Implementation Science, 8,* 52–57.

Almirall, D., Nahum-Shani, I., Sherwood, N. E., & Murphy, S. A. (2014). Introduction to SMART designs for the development of adaptive interventions: With application to weight loss research. *Translational Behavioral Medicine, 4*(3), 260–274.

Anderson, C. A., & Titler, M. G. (2014). Development and verification of an agent-based model of opinion leadership. *Implementation Science, 9,* 136–149.

Armstrong, R., Waters, E., Dobbins, M., Anderson, L., Moore, L., Petticrew, M., . . . Swinburn, B. (2013). Knowledge transition strategies to improve the use of evidence in public health decision making in local government: Intervention design and implementation plan. *Implementation Science, 8,* 121–131.

Atkinson, J.-A., Page, A., Wells, R., Milat, A., & Wilson, A. (2015). A modelling tool for policy analysis to support the design of efficient and effective policy responses for complex public health problems. *Implementation Science, 10,* 26–35.

Atkinson, J.-A., Wells, R., Page, A., Dominello, A., Haines, M., & Wilson, A. (2015). Applications of system dynamics modelling to support health policy. *Public Health Research & Practice, 25*(3), 1–8.

Bagian, J. P., Federico, F., Barnsteiner, J. H., Battles, J. B., Beeson, W. H., Benjamin, B. E., . . . Swenson, D. (2015). Preventing falls and fall-related injuries in health care facilities. *Sentinel Event Alert/The Joint Commission, 55,* 1–5. Retrieved from http://www.jointcommission.org/sea_issue_55

Baker, E. A., Brownson, R. C., Dreisinger, M., McIntosh, L. D., & Karamehic-Muratovic, A. (2009). Examining the role of training in evidence-based public health: A qualitative study. *Health Promotion Practice, 10*(3), 342–348.

Blackwood, B. (2006). Methodological issues in evaluating complex healthcare interventions. *Journal of Advanced Nursing, 54*(5), 612–622.

Brown, C. H., Ten Have, T. R., Booil, J., Dagne, G., Wyman, P. A., Muthén, B., & Gibbons, R. D. (2009). Adaptive designs for randomized trials in public health. *Annual Review of Public Health, 30,* 1–25.

Brownson, R. C., Ballew, P., Kittur, N. D., Elliott, M. B., Haire-Joshu, D., Krebill, H., & Kreuter, M. W. (2009). Developing competencies for training practitioners in evidence-based cancer control. *Journal of Cancer Education, 24,* 186–193.

Brownson, R. C., Chriqui, J. F., & Stamatakis, K. A. (2009). Understanding the evidence-based public health policy. *American Journal of Public Health, 99*(9), 1576–1583.

Brownson, R. C., Reis, R. S., Allen, P., Duggan, K., Fields, R., Stamatakis, K. A., & Erwin, P. C. (2014). Understanding administrative evidence-based practices: Findings from a survey of local health department leaders. *American Journal of Preventative Medicine, 46*(1), 49–57.

Campbell, M. K., Mollison, J., Steen, N., Grimshaw, J. M., & Eccles, M. (2000). Analysis of cluster randomized trials in primary care: A practical approach. *Family Practice, 17*(2), 192–196.

Centers for Disease Control and Prevention. (2016, May 2). Retrieved from http://www.cdc.gov

Centers for Medicare and Medicaid Services. (2016). *CMS quality strategy 2016.* Baltimore, MD: Author. Retrieved from https://www.cms.gov/Medicare/Quality-Initiatives-Patient -Assessment-Instruments/QualityInitiativesGenInfo/Downloads/CMS-Quality-Strategy.pdf

Cohn, S., Clinch, M., Bunn, C., & Stronge, P. (2013). Entangled complexity: Why complex interventions are just not complicated enough. *Journal of Health Services Research & Policy, 18*(1), 40–43.

Conway, L. J., Pogorzelska, M., Larson, E., & Stone, P. W. (2012). Adoption of policies to prevent catheter-associated urinary tract infections in United States intensive care units. *American Journal of Infection Control, 40*(8), 705–710.

Craig, P., Dieppe, P., Macintyre, S., Michie, S., Nazareth, I., & Petticrew, M. (2008). Developing and evaluating complex interventions: The new medical research council guidance. *British Medical Journal, 337*, a1655–a1661.

Craig, P., & Petticrew, M. (2013). Developing and evaluating complex interventions: Reflections on the 2008 MRC guidance. *International Journal of Nursing Studies, 50*(5), 585–587.

Dagenais, C., Laurendeau, M. C., & Briand-Lamarche, M. (2015). Knowledge brokering in public health: A critical analysis of the results of a qualitative evaluation. *Evaluation and Program Planning, 53*, 10–17.

Dobbins, M., DeCorby, K., Robeson, P., Husson, H., Tirilis, D., & Greco, L. (2010). A knowledge management tool for public health: Health-evidence.ca. *BioMed Central Public Health, 10*, 496–512.

Dobbins, M., Hanna, S. E., Ciliska, D., Manske, S., Cameron, R., Mercer, S. L., . . . Robeson, P. (2009). A randomized controlled trial evaluating the impact of knowledge translation and exchange strategies. *Implementation Science, 4*, 61–77.

Dreisinger, M., Leet, T. L., Baker, E. A., Gillespie, K. N., Haas, B., & Brownson, R. C. (2008). Improving the public health workforce: Evaluation of a training course to enhance evidence-based decision making. *Journal of Public Health Management Practice, 14*(2), 128–143.

Eccles, M. P., Foy, R., Sales, A., Wensing, M., & Mittman, B. (2012). Our evolving scope and common reasons for rejection without review. *Implementation Science, 7*, 71–77.

Eccles, M. P., & Mittman, B. S. (2006). Welcome to implementation science. *Implementation Science, 1*, 1–3.

Graham, I. D., Logan, J., Harrison, M. B., Straus, S. E., Tetroe, J., Caswell, W., & Robinson, N. (2006). Lost in knowledge translation: Time for a map? *Journal of Continuing Education in the Health Professions, 26*(1), 13–24.

Grant, A., Treweek, S., Dreischulte, T., Foy, R., & Guthrie, B. (2013). Process evaluations for cluster-randomised trials of complex interventions: A proposed framework for design and reporting. *Trials, 14*(15), 1–10.

Hardwick, R., Anderson, R., & Cooper, C. (2015). How do third sector organisations use research and other knowledge? A systematic scoping review. *Implementation Science, 10*, 84–96.

Hendriks, A.-M., Jansen, M. W. J., Gubbels, J. S., De Vries, N. K., Paulussen, T., & Kremers, S. P. J. (2013). Proposing a conceptual framework for integrated local public health policy, applied to childhood obesity—The behavior change ball. *Implementation Science, 8*, 46–62.

Henly, S. J., McCarthy, D. O., Wyman, J. F., Heitkemper, M. M., Redeker, N. S., Titler, M. G., . . . Dunbar-Jacob, J. (2015). Emerging areas of science: Recommendations for nursing science education from the Council for the Advancement of Nursing Science Idea Festival. *Nursing Outlook, 63*(4), 398–407.

Institute of Medicine. (2007). *Nutrition standards for foods in schools: Leading the way toward healthier youth.* Washington, DC: National Academies Press.

Institute of Medicine. (2009). *Local government actions to prevent childhood obesity.* Washington, DC: National Academies Press.

Institute of Medicine. (2011). *Early childhood obesity prevention policies.* Washington, DC: National Academies Press.

Institute of Medicine. (2012). *Accelerating progress in obesity prevention: Solving the weight of the nation.* Washington, DC: National Academies Press.

Institute of Medicine. (2013a). *The CTSA program at NIH: Opportunities for advancing clinical and translational research.* Washington, DC: National Academies Press.

Institute of Medicine. (2013b). *Educating the student body: Taking physical activity and physical education to school.* Washington, DC: National Academies Press.

Institute of Medicine. (2015). *The current state of obesity solutions in the United States: Workshop in brief.* Washington, DC: National Academies Press.

Jacob, R. R., Baker, E. A., Allen, P., Dodson, E. A., Duggan, K., Fields, R., . . . Brownson, R. C. (2014). Training needs and supports for evidence-based decision making among the public health workforce in the United States. *BMC Health Services Research, 14,* 564–566.

Jacobs, J. A., Duggan, K., Erwin, P., Smith, C., Borawski, E., Compton, J., . . . Brownson, R. C. (2014). Capacity building for evidence-based decision making in local health departments: Scaling up an effective training approach. *Implementation Science, 9,* 124–135.

Kilbourne, A. M., Bramlet, M., Barbaresso, M. M., Nord, K. M., Goodrich, D. E., Lai, Z., . . . Bauer, M. S. (2014). SMI life goals: Description of a randomized trial of a collaborative care model to improve outcomes for persons with serious mental illness. *Contemporary Clinical Trials, 39*(1), 74–85.

Kislov, R., Harvey, G., & Walshe, K. (2011). Collaborations for leadership in applied health research and care: Lessons from the theory of communities of practice. *Implementation Science, 6,* 64–74.

Lavis, J., Davies, H., Oxman, A., Denis, J.-L., Golden-Biddle, K., & Ferlie, E. (2005). Towards systematic reviews that inform health care management and policy-making. *Journal of Health Services Research & Policy, 10*(S1), 35–48.

Lavis, J. N., Moynihan, R., Oxman, A. D., & Paulsen, E. J. (2008). Evidence-informed health policy 4—Case descriptions of organizations that support the use of research evidence. *Implementation Science, 3,* 56–65.

Lavis, J. N., Wilson, M. G., Grimshaw, J. M., Haynes, R. B., Hanna, S., Raina, P., . . . Ouimet, M. (2011). Effects of an evidence service on health-system policy makers' use of research evidence: A protocol for a randomized controlled trial. *Implementation Science, 6,* 51–59.

Lavis, J. N., Wilson, M. G., Moat, K. A., Hammill, A. C., Boyko, J. A., Grimshaw, J. M., & Flottorp, S. (2015). Developing and refining the methods for a "one-stop shop" for research evidence about health systems. *Health Research Policy and Systems, 13*(10), 1–10.

Litaker, D., Ruhe, M., Weyer, S., & Stange, K. C. (2008). Association of intervention outcomes with practice capacity for change: Subgroup analysis from a group randomized trial. *Implementation Science, 3,* 25–31.

Lokker, C., McKibbon, K. A., Colquhoun, H., & Hempel, S. (2015). A scoping review of classification schemes of interventions to promote and integrate evidence into practice in healthcare. *Implementation Science, 10,* 27–39.

Luke, D. A., & Stamatakis, K. A. (2012). Systems science methods in public health: Dynamics, networks, and agents. *Annual Review of Public Health, 33,* 357–376.

Luoto, J., Shekelle, P. G., Maglione, M. A., Johnsen, B., & Perry, T. (2014). Reporting of context and implementation in studies of global health interventions: A pilot study. *Implementation Science, 9,* 57–66.

Mark, D. B., Titler, M. G., & Latimer, R. W. (Eds.). (2014). Integrating evidence into practice for impact (edited issue). *Nursing Clinics of North America, 49*(3), 269–452.

Mazza, D., Bairstow, P., Buchan, H., Chakraborty, S. P., Van Hecke, O., Grech, C., & Kunnamo, I. (2013). Refining a taxonomy for guideline implementation: Results of an exercise in abstract classification. *Implementation Science, 8,* 32–42.

McKibbon, K. A., Lokker, C., Wilczynski, N. L., Ciliska, D., Dobbins, M., Davis, D. A., . . . Straus, S. E. (2010). A cross-sectional study of the number and frequency of terms used to refer to knowledge translation in a body of health literature in 2006: A tower of Babel? *Implementation Science, 5,* 16–27.

Michie, S., Fixsen, D., Grimshaw, J. M., & Eccles, M. P. (2009). Specifying and reporting complex behaviour change interventions: The need for a scientific method. *Implementation Science, 4*, 40–46.

Michie, S., van Stralen, M. M., & West, R. (2011). The behaviour change wheel: A new method for characterizing and designing behaviour change interventions. *Implementation Science, 6*, 42–54.

Mijumbi, R. M., Oxman, A. D., Panisset, U., & Sewankambo, N. K. (2014). Feasibility of a rapid response mechanism to meet policymakers' urgent needs for research evidence about health systems in a low income country: A case study. *Implementation Science, 9*, 114–124.

Moat, K. A., & Lavis, J. N. (2014). Supporting the use of research evidence in the Americas through an online "one-stop shop": The EVIPNet VHL. *Cadernos de Saúde Pública, 30*(12), 2697–2701.

Mohler, R., Bartoszek, G., & Meyer, G. (2013). Quality of reporting of complex healthcare interventions and applicability of the CReDECI list—A survey of publications indexed in PubMed. *BMC Medical Research Methodology, 13*(125), 1–8.

Mohler, R., Kopke, S., & Meyer, G. (2015). Criteria for reporting the development and evaluation of complex interventions in healthcare: Revised guideline (CReDECI 2). *Trials, 16*(204), 1–9.

Nahum-Shani, I., Qian, M., Almirall, D., Pelham, W. E., Gnagy, B., Fabiano, G. A., . . . Murphy, S. A. (2012a). Experimental design and primary data analysis methods for comparing adaptive interventions. *Psychological Methods, 17*(4), 457–477.

Nahum-Shani, I., Qian, M., Almirall, D., Pelham, W. E., Gnagy, B., Fabiano, G. A., . . . Murphy, S. A. (2012b). Q-learning: A data analysis method for constructing adaptive interventions. *Psychological Methods, 17*(14), 478–494.

National Institute of Nursing Research. (2016). Strategic plan 2016. Retrieved from National Institute of Nursing Research website: https://www.ninr.nih.gov/newsandinformation/newsandnotes/stratplan2016#.Vyef_vkrJph

Naude, C. E., Zani, B., Ongolo-Zogo, P., Wiysonge, C. S., Dudley, L., Kredo, T., . . . Young, T. (2015). Research evidence and policy: Qualitative study in selected provinces in South Africa and Cameroon. *Implementation Science, 10*, 126–136.

Neta, G., Sanchez, M. A., Chambers, D. A., Phillips, S. M., Leyva, B., Cynkin, L., . . . Vinson, C. (2015). Implementation science in cancer prevention and control: A decade of grant funding by the National Cancer Institute and future directions. *Implementation Science, 10*, 4–14.

Newhouse, R., Bobay, K., Dykes, P. C., Stevens, K. R., & Titler, M. G. (2013). Methodology issues in implementation science. *Medical Care, 51*(4), S32–S40.

Nilsen, P., Stahl, C., Roback, K., & Cairney, P. (2013). Never the twain shall meet? A comparison of implementation science and policy implementation research. *Implementation Science, 8*, 63–75.

Pawson, R., & Tilley, N. (1997). An introduction to realist evaluation. In E. Chelimsky & W. R. Shadish (Eds.), *Evaluation for the 21st century: A handbook* (pp. 405–418). Thousand Oaks, CA: Sage Publications.

Pinnock, H., Epiphaniou, E., Sheikh, A., Griffiths, C., Eldridge, S., Craig, P., & Taylor, S. J. C. (2015). Developing standards for reporting implementation studies of complex interventions (StaRI): A systematic review and e-Delphi. *Implementation Science, 10*, 42–51.

Potempa, K., Daly, J., & Titler, M. G. (2012). Building the clinical bridge to support nursing effectiveness science. *Nursing Research and Practice, 2012*, 1–3.

Proctor, E. K., Powell, B. J., & McMillen, J. C. (2013). Implementation strategies: Recommendations for specifying and reporting. *Implementation Science, 8*, 139–150.

Project HOPE: The People-to-People Health Foundation, Inc. (2016). Health policy briefs. Retrieved from http://www.healthaffairs.org/healthpolicybriefs

Purtle, J., Peters, R., & Brownson, R. C. (2016). A review of policy dissemination and implementation research funded by the National Institutes of Health, 2007–2014. *Implementation Science, 11*, 1–8.

Riley, B. L., MacDonald, J., Mansi, O., Kothari, A., Kurtz, D., vonTettenborn, L. I., & Edwards, N. C. (2008). Is reporting on interventions a weak link in understanding how and why they work? A preliminary exploration using community heart health exemplars. *Implementation Science, 3*, 27–39.

Saul, J. E., Willis, C. D., Bitz, J., & Best, A. (2013). A time-responsive tool for informing policy making: Rapid realist review. *Implementation Science, 8*(103), 103–118.

Shearer, J. C., Dion, M., & Lavis, J. N. (2014). Exchanging and using research evidence in health policy networks: A statistical network analysis. *Implementation Science, 9,* 126–138.

Shever, L. L., Titler, M. G., Mackin, M. L., & Kueny, A. (2010). Fall prevention practices in adult medical-surgical nursing units described by nurse managers. *Western Journal of Nursing Research, 33*(3), 385–397.

Slaughter, S. E., Hill, J. N., & Snelgrove-Clarke, E. (2015). What is the extent and quality of documentation and reporting of fidelity to implementation strategies: A scoping review. *Implementation Science, 109,* 129–141.

Smits, P. A., & Denis, J.-L. (2014). How research funding agencies support science integration into policy and practice: An international overview. *Implementation Science, 9,* 28–40.

Sving, E., Gunningberg, L., Högman, M., & Mamhidir, A.-G. (2012). Registered nurses' attention to and perceptions of pressure ulcer prevention in hospital settings. *Journal of Clinical Nursing, 21*(9–10), 1293–1303.

Tinkle, M., Kimball, R., Haozous, E. A., Shuster, G., & Meize-Grochowski, R. (2013). Dissemination and implementation research funded by the U.S. National Institutes of Health, 2005–2012. *Nursing Research and Practice, 2013,* 1–15.

Titler, M. G. (2010). Translation science and context. *Research and Theory for Nursing Practice, 24*(1), 35–55.

Titler, M. G. (Guest Ed.). (2011). Nursing science and evidence-based practice. *Western Journal of Nursing Research, 33*(3), 291–295.

Titler, M. G. (2014a). Developing an evidence-based practice. In G. LoBiondo-Wood & J. Haber (Eds.), *Nursing research: Methods and critical appraisal for evidence-based practice* (8th ed., pp. 418–441). St. Louis, MO: Elsevier Mosby.

Titler, M. G. (2014b). Overview of evidence-based practice and translation science. *Nursing Clinics of North America, 49*(3), 269–274.

Titler, M. G., & Pressler, S. J. (2011). Advancing effectiveness science: An opportunity for nursing. *Research and Theory for Nursing Practice, 25*(2), 75–79.

Tomm-Bonde, L., Schreiber, R. S., Allan, D. E., MacDonald, M., Pauly, B., & Hancock, T. (2013). Fading vision: Knowledge translation in the implementation of a public health policy intervention. *Implementation Science, 8,* 59–70.

Tricco, A. C., Cardoso, R., Thomas, S. M., Motiwala, S., Sullivan, S., Kealey, M. R., . . . Straus, S. E. (2016). Barriers and facilitators to uptake of systematic reviews by policy makers and health care managers: A scoping review. *Implementation Science, 11,* 4–24.

Wilson, M. G., Grimshaw, J. M., Haynes, R. B., Hanna, S. E., Raina, P., Gruen, R., . . . Lavis, J. N. (2015). A process evaluation accompanying an attempted randomized controlled trial of an evidence service for health system policymakers. *Health Research Policy and Systems, 13*(78), 1–8.

Wilson, M. G., Lavis, J. N., & Gauvin, F.-P. (2015). Developing a rapid-response program for health system decision-makers in Canada: Findings from an issue brief and stakeholder dialogue. *Systematic Reviews, 4*(25), 1–11.

Wilson, M. G., Rourke, S. B., Lavis, J. N., Bacon, J., & Travers, R. (2011). Community capacity to acquire, assess, adapt, and apply research evidence: A survey of Ontario's HIV/AIDS sector. *Implementation Science, 6,* 54–60.

Yousefi-Nooraie, R., Dobbins, M., Marin, A., Hanneman, R., & Lohfeld, L. (2015). The evolution of social networks through the implementation of evidence-informed decision-making interventions: A longitudinal analysis of three public health units in Canada. *Implementation Science, 10,* 166–178.

Zardo, P., & Collie, A. (2014). Predicting research use in a public health policy environment: Results of a logistic regression analysis. *Implementation Science, 9,* 142–152.

4

Integration of Genomics in Nursing Research

Janet K. Williams

The integration of genomics into nursing has a long history encompassing basic and applied research, clinical practice, and health care professional training. Genomic nursing research addressing health of individuals and populations provides evidence that can contribute to health policy decisions to guide actions. As noted in a recently completed bibliometric review of genomic nursing research from 2010 to 2014 (Williams, Tripp-Reimer, Daack-Hirsch, & DeBerg, 2016), genetic aspects of health were recognized in the 1990s as an essential component of nursing science, training, and practice (Lashley, 1997; Pesut, 1999). The emphasis on genomics continues to the present. In this chapter, the term *genetic* refers to characteristics of a gene, the basic physical unit of inheritance, while the term *genomic* refers to the entire set of genetic instructions found within a cell (National Human Genome Research Institute [NHGRI], 2016, www.genome.gov/glossary). The term *policy* refers to governmental, organizational, and institutional policies, guidelines, and statements that guide actions.

The National Institute of Nursing Research (NINR) strategic plan (NINR, 2011) focuses on investigation of multiple health determinants, including genomic aspects of health. From 2010 to 2014, the purpose of the majority of genomic nursing science studies was the discovery of biological aspects of diseases and symptoms, and describing clinical implications of genetic or genomic variations on health (Williams, Tripp-Reimer et al., 2016). This is consistent with the trajectory of genomic research, beginning with discovery science and moving through several stages toward improving effectiveness of health care (E. D. Green, Guyer, & NHGRI, 2011). Factors facilitating the influence of nursing research on health policy include genomic nurse researchers partnering with multiple disciplines, conducting research that informs major current health issues, and establishing strong visibility of researchers' work (Hinshaw, 2010).

Three national documents, the Affordable Care Act (ACA; HealthCare.gov, 2010), *The Future of Nursing* report (Institute of Medicine [IOM], 2011), and the genomic nursing science blueprint (Calzone et al., 2013) identify national health priorities that can be informed by genomic nursing research. Additional opportunities to shape genomic health policies by nursing research exist at the state level through informing health department policies, and in local health care institutions where results of genomic nursing research contribute to development and evaluation of practice policies or guidelines. Recent attention on the concept of personalized medicine includes goals highlighted in the Precision Medicine Initiative (White House, 2015). This initiative focuses on targeted treatment of individuals, and on discovery of factors contributing to common diseases, and may launch new opportunities for genomic nursing science to inform health policy across all settings.

This chapter describes integration of genomics into nursing research, and provides examples of genomic nursing research that have relevance to local, state, and national policies. In some cases, the policy relevance is identified from the researchers' grants and publications, and in other cases it is articulated through interviews with the researchers. The examples selected for this chapter have links with health policies, but are not inclusive of all policy-related activities by genomic nurse researchers. Many of the studies highlighted in this chapter are ongoing, and the impact on policies is in process. These examples illustrate the importance of research training for inquiry into genomic aspects of health and interdisciplinary collaboration, and highlight nurse researchers who are responding to or creating opportunities to influence health policy through genomic nursing research.

POLICY-RELEVANT GENOMIC NURSING FOCI

A large proportion of nursing research investigating genomic aspects of health, which may have relevance to health policies, is not conducted to address specific policy topics. Priorities for future genomic nursing research are examined in the blueprint. This document identifies gaps in genomic nursing science and identifies strategies to support the capacity of nurses to implement genomics into health care to improve patient outcomes. The blueprint, developed by a panel of experts, organized topics into five major areas: health promotion and disease prevention, advancing quality of life, innovation, training, and cross-cutting themes (Calzone et al., 2013). A bibliometric review of 5 years of data-based publications reported that genomic nursing science is developing a foundational body of knowledge in three of the five blueprint areas: health promotion and disease prevention, advancing quality of life, and training. However, nursing science activities are at the very early stages of development in the remaining areas of innovation and cross-cutting themes, specifically policy and costs (Williams, Tripp-Reimer, et al., 2016).

Biological Plausibility and Quality of Life

The problems most commonly investigated by genomic nurse researchers from 2010 to 2014 are biological aspects of clinical diagnoses, phenotypes, symptoms, or symptom management; and quality of life. Although these studies may answer basic and applied research questions, and will advance scientific knowledge, many findings are not yet developed to the point of informing health policy. Further, the direction of biological inquiry and subsequent clinical implications can change rapidly when new analytic methods are developed. This is illustrated by the introduction of tumor profiling into oncology practice, adding to prior clinical use of genetic testing of individuals to identify risk for disease, and family history analysis in oncology practice. Several nurse researchers who are conducting investigations that address biological and quality-of-life questions also identify policy implications of these topics.

One example is the ongoing work by Sue Gardner in which genomic aspects of severe pain and pain control during wound care are examined. This program of research investigates patient biomarkers and the wound microbial population, each of which may contribute to severe pain during wound care. Nonadherent dressings used to protect wounds are costly, and there is currently no evidence to guide decisions on which patients would benefit from the selection of which wound dressing that would be most effective for reducing pain. The significance of this research includes not only advancing scientific and clinical knowledge, but also the potential to determine the effect of targeted selection of wound dressings in decreasing wound care costs (Gardner, 2016; S. Gardner, personal communication, February 16, 2016).

A second example of the potential for genomic nursing research to influence policy from biological plausibility and quality-of-life research is illustrated by an investigation of genomics and negative lifestyle factors (cigarette smoking) that are statistically significantly associated with risk for hypertension in African American populations (Klebaner et al., 2016). Additionally, Jacquelyn Taylor has examined attitudes toward genetic testing for risk for hypertension that includes perceived barriers or benefits of genetic testing for risk for hypertension in African American women and girls (Taylor, Peternell, & Smith, 2013). Finally, Dr. Taylor is currently funded by the NINR to examine intergenerational impact of psychosocial and genetic factors on blood pressure among African American mother–child dyads. The findings will contribute to moving clinical care into a more precision-driven model as championed by the White House Precision Medicine Initiative (Crusto, Barcelona de Mendoza, Connell, Sun, & Taylor, 2006; Taylor, Wright, Crusto, & Sun, 2016). Recognition of the potential utility of these findings for improving health, and reducing costs for management of hypertension in this population, is reflected in commendations received by Dr. Taylor from leaders who influence policy at the local, state, and federal levels: three mayors, the governor of Connecticut, and a congresswoman from Connecticut (http://intergen.yale.edu/gallery/professional-award-dr-taylor; J. Taylor, personal communication, February 4, 2016).

A third example of policy implications of genomic nursing research bridging biological and quality-of-life inquiry is a program of research by Angela Starkweather regarding phenotyping and management of low back pain (Baumbauer et al., 2016; Starkweather et al., 2016). This research program was planned with recognition that the results would be relevant to clinical policies and guidelines. The link with policy pertains to using results to predict who will be at higher risk for pain, and the recognition that treatment options for this group should include strategies that reduce the potential for opioid abuse. Findings from this program of research have the potential not only to influence policies regarding a range of effective pain management choices and avoiding the misuse of opioids for pain management, but also to influence health care insurance decisions regarding payment for these pain management options (A. Starkweather, personal communication, January 26, 2016).

Genomic aspects of health are experienced and managed within the context of an individual's, a family's, and a community's day-to-day experiences, environment, culture, challenges, and resources. Ongoing research by Suzanne Ameringer addresses one of these challenges, which is the absence of guidelines for exercise as a self-management strategy by people with sickle cell hemoglobinopathies. Findings of her program of research have the potential to inform guidelines regarding how to improve fitness, as well as improve pain and fatigue in the short term, and to decrease cardiopulmonary complications in the long term (Ameringer, 2016).

Genomic nursing research also addresses the fit of existing policies with unique populations. The examination of feeding practices by mothers of infants with phenylketonuria (PKU) was conducted by Banta-Wright, Shelton, Lowe, Knafl, and Houck (2012). This study documented that feeding practices of infants with PKU were consistent with national and worldwide recommendations that breast milk is the nutrition of choice for infants, and that phenylalanine levels in breastfed infants in her study were within the normal range. This study provides evidence of actions directed by policy that promote health of infants with PKU.

Genomic nursing research also informs the development of new clinical guidelines. This is illustrated by findings from Kathleen Hickey's research documenting the need for genomic aspects of risk assessment, diagnosis, and treatment plans for those at risk for sudden cardiac death to be in a language that is understandable to each clinical population. Her research documented that not only does the language have to be appropriate, but also that the information is likely to be most effective when it addresses the concerns of the patient and family (Hickey et al., 2014). Results of this work inform policy in the clinical setting where she practices. It is also reflected in contributions by Dr. Hickey and genomic nurse researcher Dr. Lorraine Frazier to the American Heart Association's Scientific Statement on genomics for cardiovascular and stroke clinicians (Musunuru et al., 2015). Examples in this section highlight contributions of genomic nurse researchers to health policy through the conduct of research with interdisciplinary colleagues, and recognition of the relevance of their research to existing or future policies.

Researcher and Health Care Provider Education and Training

Health Care Provider Education

The Future of Nursing report, ACA, and genomic nursing science blueprint all emphasize the importance of increasing the number of doctoral prepared nurse researchers, educators, and advanced practice nurses (APNs). A recommendation in *The Future of Nursing* report (IOM, 2011) is that the number of nurses with a doctorate should double by 2020 to add to the cadre of nurse faculty and researchers. A review of the progress on increasing the number of doctorally prepared nurses since the 2010 report indicated that enrollment in Doctor of Nursing Practice (DNP) has doubled and enrollment in PhD programs rose by 15%. However, this assessment concluded that more emphasis on PhD program expansion and scholarships for baccalaureate-PhD programs is warranted (National Academies of Sciences, Engineering, and Medicine, 2016). The blueprint (Calzone et al., 2013) addresses training to build capacity of nursing scientists in genomics as well as methods to train the existing workforce. The ACA (HealthCare.gov, 2010) includes training of new primary care providers, including APNs. A component of this primary care is preventive services for women at increased risk for breast cancer (Wakefield, 2015).

Policies addressing health care education reflect recognition that application of genomic research findings into clinical practice requires a prepared workforce and one that has access to appropriate resources for use in day-to-day clinical practice (Williams & Cashion, 2015). Mechanisms for certification for advanced genetic nursing are available through the American Nurses Credentialing Center (2016a).

One clinical area where nurse researchers contribute basic and applied research findings that influence practice is oncology. The Oncology Nursing Society (ONS) position policy on oncology nurses specifies expectations for competencies, continuing education, and practice. First issued in 2012, it is updated each year (ONS, 2012).

An example of clinical implementation of genomic nursing education to improve patient outcomes is the assessment of wait time and adherence to national guidelines for genomic profiling for treatment decisions in breast cancer patients. In a quality improvement project, improved process outcomes were documented when a nurse navigator using an APN–RN model was responsible for timely access to the genetic testing for each patient. Using this guideline, the turnaround time for reporting results was reduced from 38 to 20 days, and the need for a follow-up appointment was eliminated (McAllister & Schmitt, 2015).

Genomic nurse researchers document gaps in nursing education, and examine strategies to fill these gaps. One example is the documentation of genomic literacy among faculty and students providing data and introduction of an instrument useful for curriculum evaluation and revision. This research led to a workshop funded by a regional genetic collaborative, resulting in development and implementation of tailored curriculum plans in five nursing programs in the region (Daack-Hirsch, Driessnack, Perkhounkova, Furukawa, & Ramirez, 2012).

Policies addressing doctoral education for advanced nursing practice specifically identify genomics, among other bodies of knowledge, as a component of the scientific underpinnings for practice. Genomic education is essential for adherence to each essential, including Essential VIII: advanced nursing practice where the DNP program prepares the graduate to design, implement, and evaluate therapeutic interventions based on nursing science and other sciences; and in the description of advanced pharmacology, which includes knowledge and skills to analyze the relationship between pharmacologic agents and physiologic/pathologic responses (American Association of Colleges of Nursing [AACN], 2006). Capacities of advanced nurse practitioners to participate in genomic health care also rest on prior education. The integration of genetics and genomics into the AACN Essentials of Baccalaureate Education for Professional Nursing Practice (AACN, 2008) reflects essential competencies for practicing RNs (Consensus Panel on Genetic/Genomic Nursing Competencies, 2009).

Nurse Researcher Education

The genomic nursing science blueprint (Calzone et al., 2013) examines training of future nurse scientists in genomics. This includes preparation of nurse scientists to lead interprofessional teams, employ innovative uses of biorepositories, and incorporate bioethics in generating knowledge regarding critical genomic problems. The review of genomic nursing research from 2010 to 2014 noted that genomic nursing research is most often interdisciplinary, with 71.5% of studies being conducted by interdisciplinary teams (Williams, Tripp-Reimer, et al., 2016). With regard to educational preparation of nurse researchers, genomics was included in the recommendations for researcher preparation by the Council for the Advancement of Nursing Science idea festival (Henly et al., 2015). However, Wyman and Henly (2015) document that fewer than 8% of 120 U.S. PhD programs in nursing mention genetics or genomics on their websites. Training that enables nurse researchers to investigate genomic aspects of health is an essential component of generating evidence that is useful in developing guidelines and health policies.

NURSING IMPLICATIONS OF GENOMIC POLICIES

Health policies at the institutional, state, or national level may involve use of an individual's genomic data. In some cases, nurse researchers participate in the examination of implementation of existing policies. Contributions to health policies by genomic nurse researchers are illustrated by examples at individual health care institutions, state health departments, and the national level.

Local Institution Policies

The Magnet Recognition Program® recognizes health care organizations for quality patient outcomes and nursing excellence (ANCC, 2016b). Jean Jenkins, Kathleen

Calzone, and Laurie Badzek examined genomic education, and nursing capacity to apply genomics in nursing practice, in 23 Magnet Recognition Program hospitals. The purpose of this study was to develop, implement, and evaluate a year-long genomic education intervention. However, one component of the study was to examine existing institutional guidelines or policies that would influence integration of genomics in that setting. Policies and guidelines can define and support expectations within the clinical environment. Although the educators and administrators representing nursing at the majority of the Magnet hospitals did not identify specific policies that applied to genomics, in several hospitals, investigators found components of genomic health care such as family history, genetic testing, and pharmacogenetic guidance, in the existing institutional procedures. Participation by the institutional representatives in the study led to identification of gaps with designation of interdisciplinary representatives (including APNs) for further policy or guideline development to delineate expectations for genomic health care within their clinical settings (Jenkins et al., 2015).

Statewide Disease Risk or Early Diagnosis Screening

Newborn screening is a public health program that seeks to identify conditions, most of which are genetic, that can affect health or survival of infants and for which early detection, diagnosis, and intervention can prevent death or disability (www .cdc.gov/newbornscreening). Policies for the best practice for notifying parents of newborn screening results in one state reflect the contribution of research findings by Audrey Tluczek. Her research documented problems experienced by parents during the waiting time between the screening test and communication of results (Tluczek et al., 2006). Her work contributed to changing the standard for the initial telephone communication with parents about test results for infants who are found to be carriers of sickle cell hemoglobinopathy or positive screens for cystic fibrosis (CF; Tluczek et al., 2011). Tluczek's work led to reducing the wait time between parent notification of abnormal screening results for CF and follow-up diagnostic testing, as well as implementation of a family-centered approach to genetic counseling for parents (Tluczek et al., 2011; Tluczek, Koscik, Farrell, & Rock, 2005). Dr. Tluczek also identified concerns of parent users of the CF Foundation (CFF) website who need timely and easy access to research and treatment resource information. She analyzed how parents prefer to locate and use information on the foundation's website. Through her work with the CFF, policies governing the format and operation of the website were revised to be responsive to parent preferences. Dr. Tluczek also contributed to CFF national guidelines for newborn screening and procedures for CF, to be used in the United States and as a basis for guideline development in Europe. Her service on the taskforce that developed the guidelines included inviting a genetic counselor to contribute, and providing evidence from her research on how, when, and by whom parents prefer to be notified about abnormal test results (A. Tluczek, personal communication, February 16, 2016).

Maternal serum screening is one of many options for identifying if a fetus is at risk for or has a genetic condition or birth defect. In one state, samples are processed by a central laboratory. However, the number of specimens received by the laboratory was dropping and the reasons were unknown. This led to a request to Sandra Daack-Hirsch (S. Daack-Hirsch, personal communication, January 27, 2016) to obtain evidence to determine barriers to screening practices across the state, leading to a survey of providers, a review of claims data, and interviews with women receiving prenatal care. This study is ongoing and results will inform state-level policies to maintain affordable and comprehensive prenatal care for women.

Screening for breast cancer is a health concern for women, their families, clinicians, professional and lay organizations, and governmental bodies. The ACA (Health-Care.gov, 2010) requires health insurance plans to cover health care for women at higher risk for breast cancer, and there are to be no out-of-pocket costs for wellness visits and genetic counseling for women at increased risk of breast cancer (Wakefield, 2015). State and community health departments, and faculty in health sciences in one state, implemented a 3-year project to increase awareness of breast cancer genetics and cancer surveillance among young breast cancer survivors and their at-risk female relatives in their state. Approached by members of the department of health, nurse researchers led an interdisciplinary team to implement a study using the state health department's cancer registry to identify participants, document screening activities, and test interventions to increase use of cancer genetic services and cancer surveillance in these high-risk families. This research contributes to the knowledge base regarding health care needs and use of genetic services in families at increased risk for hereditary breast cancer. It uses nontraditional methods for obtaining family history at a public health level; new methods to advance family-based and minority recruitment in research studies; new methods to assess access to genetic services and locate women who moved out of state, including family members at risk for hereditary forms of breast and related cancers; and tests public health interventions to promote use of cancer genetic services (Jones et al., 2016; Katapodi, 2015). Findings of this study informed policies regarding how to ensure that young breast cancer survivors—a growing clinical population for which little is known—and their at-risk relatives have access to the wellness visits and genetic counseling that are included in the ACA. Evidence from this study may also contribute to new policies to address disparities due to limited availability, accessibility, and acceptability of cancer genetic services.

Federal Protection Against Discrimination

The Genetic Information Nondiscrimination Act (GINA) of 2008 was designed to protect individuals from health insurance or employment discrimination based on their genetic information. Numerous bodies, including researchers and patient advocacy groups, provided data, and continue to gather data to identify the nature and extent of genetic discrimination, and the potential impact of changes to the Act that could restrict participant privacy. Prior to the passage of GINA, an interdisciplinary research group, led by an ethicist, nurse, and psychologist, conducted research documenting perceptions and experiences of discrimination by people with or at risk for Huntington disease (HD), a hereditary neurodegenerative disorder. Participants were from the United States, Canada, and Australia. This research provided evidence regarding discrimination among healthy people at risk for HD, not only in employment and insurance situations, but also in relationships and other transactions in their communities (Erwin et al., 2010).

These examples all illustrate how nurse researchers inform genomic health policies. These examples also illustrate the importance of external factors that supported their work at the local institution, state, organization, or federal levels (Hinshaw, 2010). The researchers highlighted are in university or government environments that support genomic nursing science. The researchers led investigative teams with members from multiple disciplines, including researchers, clinicians, and health department representatives. The topics reflected current health care issues, and the nurse researchers were asked to contribute data to solve a problem, leading to policies that would direct actions. Finally, these researchers were visible, and many were sought out by the public health, scientific, or genomic health care organizations because of their engagement on committees or working groups, and the quality of their peer-reviewed presentations and publications on genomic health topics.

FUTURE GENOMIC NURSING RESEARCH AND POLICY OPPORTUNITIES

Health policies based on evidence will be needed to facilitate implementation of genomic discoveries into health care (IOM, 2014). Nursing science is positioned to contribute evidence that fits opportunities created through the ACA, *The Future of Nursing* report, and the Precision Medicine Initiative; and inform policies addressing symptom science, wellness, self-management, and end-of-life and palliative care (NINR, 2011). Implementation of genomic discoveries into health care will require systems and a workforce with the capacity to access and use these discoveries for individual patient care. This is an opportunity for genomic nurse researchers to provide evidence that reflects the perspective of those involved in direct patient care, to document patient outcomes of genomic aspects of health care, and to identify barriers to implementation of innovations—all necessary components to inform ongoing development of guidelines and policies that incorporate new innovations. The potential for genomic nursing research to inform new policies in several emerging areas is illustrated in this section.

Informatics and Electronic Health Records

One source for clinical decisions, electronic health records (EHRs), can support use of genomic health information in clinical decisions. However, the EHR can also be useful in generating new discoveries about the meaning of specific genetic variants regarding disease risk, and treatment choices and outcomes (Williams, Cashion, Shekar, & Ginsburg, 2015). A nursing informatics research agenda emphasizes the importance of fairness, privacy, and confidentiality of genomic information, among other topics; all these support the integration and use of genomic data for nursing care and nursing research (Bakken, Stone, & Larsen, 2012). These research directions have the potential to inform guidelines and policies at all levels regarding collection, management, analysis, and sharing of genomic data across databases.

Big Data Science

Sharing of data has potential benefits through enabling new models for conducting science (Collins & Varmus, 2015), as well as the undesired potential for reluctance of patients to share their own genomic health data due to fears of discrimination (R. C. Green, Lautenbach, & McGuire, 2015). Experiences from the ENCyclopedia Of DNA Elements (ENCODE) consortium to build an encyclopedia of functional DNA elements generated insights into the need for all participants to agree to a structure, code of conduct, and common goal of high-quality data that are accessible to all (Birney, 2012). The development of big data science initiatives opens opportunities for genomic nurse researchers to generate evidence that will both inform new policies regarding use of big data in research, but also contribute nursing's advocacy role in health care (Brennan & Bakken, 2015).

Return of Unanticipated or Incidental Genomic Test Results

Genomic analysis methods, including whole genome and whole exome sequencing, create the need for policies regarding disclosure of unanticipated or incidental findings to individuals. Genomic nurse researchers and bioethics colleagues contribute evidence through documentation of preferences of the public regarding incidental findings (Daack-Hirsch et al., 2013) and perspectives of researchers and Institutional Review Board chairs (Williams et al., 2012). Numerous professional organizations and policy-making bodies continue to debate the issues essential for policies regarding return and management of incidental findings from genomic research. Evidence documenting patient preferences and impact of policies will be needed and can be generated by nurse researchers in partnership with APNs and other colleagues (Williams, Katapodi, et al., 2016).

Pharmacogenomics

Policies regarding selection and administration of medications that reflect individual genomic aspects of drug response will be developed as these drugs become available in health care. In 2015, 28% of new drugs approved by the Food and Drug

Administration (FDA) were "personalized medicine," that is, a product with a label referring to specific biological markers to be used in guiding clinical decisions for patients (Personalized Medicine Coalition, 2016). Nurse researchers and advanced practice clinicians are positioned to contribute to the discovery and implementation research to reach the goal of minimized drug reactions and optimized drug doses (Cheek, Bashore, & Brazeau, 2015). One example of interdisciplinary collaboration by a nurse researcher is Cindy Prows's participation on the Electronic Medical Records and Genomics-Pharmacogenomics (eMERGE-PGx) Project. Based in a multicenter network of health systems with biorepositories linked with EHRs, the purpose of the project is to identify novel genetic associations with disease using EHR data and develop mechanisms for integrating genotyping and sequencing results into clinical practice (Rasmussen-Torvik et al., 2014). One component of the project addresses pharmacogenetic tests that can reveal genetic variants influencing adverse drug reactions as well as variation in drug response.

Prows led the development of pharmacogenomic test result reports that were put into the EHR at one participating site for children enrolled in the study who were undergoing painful procedures such as tonsillectomy and adenoidectomy (Kullo et al., 2014; Prows et al., 2014). She also is leading a separate project to document and analyze parental understanding and preferences for receiving results of pharmacogenomic testing on their child (C. Prows, personal communication, February 11, 2016).

Biobanks and Representation

Among essential components of a precision medicine approach to health care is the importance of representation of people from different ancestries in studies and investigations of genetic variations associated with diseases and treatments (Kohane, 2015). Representation is also critical in studies that evaluate the most promising discoveries when implemented into clinical practice and then evaluated over longer periods of time. Here, larger numbers of participants will be necessary, all of whom may be asked to provide permission for analysis of biological, clinical, and other health-related data (Collins & Varmus, 2015). Issues of protection of privacy, access to opportunities to participate, and representativeness of resulting findings will all require solutions and policies that are consistent with the profession of nursing's emphasis on advocacy as well as equitable delivery and access to care for all (Williams, Katapodi, et al., 2016).

Nurse researchers identify aspects of biobank information, recruitment, and enrollment important to members of underserved and underrepresented groups (Cohn, Husamudenn, Larson, & Williams, 2015). Nurse researchers document the key components of research practice related to DNA biobanking that are critical for members of the new Black African immigrant community (Buseh, Underwood, Stevens, Townsend, & Kelber, 2013). Taken together, the findings of these studies, and engagement by members of the community throughout the entire process, guide decisions and actions regarding documenting ancestry in genomic research and clinical projects.

Equitable Genomic Health Care Delivery

Access to genomic health care services continues to be a problem for which policies are inequitable or missing. Genomic nurse researchers investigate the genomic variations among populations, and the relationships among genomics, environment, and illness, in understanding health disparities among disadvantaged populations (Spruill et al., 2014). Genomic nursing researchers are seeking evidence, such as documenting endorsement by 380 members of the National Coalition of Ethnic Minority Organizations (NCEMO) where the majority endorsed the importance of basic and continuing genomic education for nurses as a component of preparing these nurses to implement genomic discoveries into practice (Coleman et al., 2014). Insights from these studies may be useful in policy development that reflects clinician and minority population concerns.

Precision Medicine and Health

The terms *precision* and *personalized medicine* both address maximizing health of the individual. The concept of precision medicine is the tailoring of prevention and treatment strategies to the individual characteristics of each person (Collins & Varmus, 2015), rather than making clinical decisions based on evidence of what works for the average person. A closely related older term is *personalized medicine*, which can be misinterpreted as suggesting that a unique treatment can be designed for each person, rather than selection of a treatment being based on the person's characteristics (IOM, 2011). The realization of the goals of precision medicine will rely on many factors, including development of an accurate body of knowledge regarding meaning and interpretation of genomic variants, and their relevance to health, when considered within the entire set of an individual's pertinent clinical and life history data. This has direct relevance to all health care providers and especially for nurses. Nursing science is connected to precision medicine through development of personalized strategies to prevent and manage adverse symptoms of illness across diverse populations and settings and the clinical application of genomic science (NINR, 2016), as well as nursing research on personalized strategies for health promotion and disease prevention to improve quality of life throughout the life span.

Precision medicine is in its early stages. However, this concept is not unfamiliar to nurse researchers. An example of an innovative program of research based on personal characteristics is an ongoing research led by Bernice Coleman. This research began when she noted, at the annual holiday parties for cardiac transplant patients, African Americans were not returning in subsequent years because they appeared to be dying at a proportionally higher rate. This led to an investigation where she ruled out potential explanations for mortality due to medication regimens, lack of access to care, or variations in posttransplant patient education or treatment protocols. Her inquiries led to a series of studies with interdisciplinary colleagues identifying genetic variants among African American and Caucasian heart transplant recipients that are associated with differences in survival rates. Findings from this work are relevant for future development of clinical guidelines regarding genomic factors increasing risk for death following cardiac transplant in African Americans (B. Coleman, personal communication, February 2, 2016).

CONCLUSION

Genomic nursing research focuses on topics relevant to the science of health. Characteristics of nursing research that shape health policy, and are pertinent to genomic nursing research, are: addresses major public health issues; is relevant to multiple disciplines and audiences; is conducted by interdisciplinary teams; focuses on clients, patients, families, and communities; and integrates complex health issues (Hinshaw, 2010). The examples cited in this chapter illustrate genomic nursing research conducted by investigators who recognized the relevance of their work to health policy. However, this is not apparent in the majority of data-based research reports published in the previous 5 years, where policy implications were seldom addressed in the introduction or implications of the studies (Williams, Tripp-Reimer, et al., 2016). Early consideration of actions that are needed, which would be guided by policies and guidelines in response to identification of a solution to a problem, may help principal investigators shape their research projects' purposes and designs, as well as increase awareness of the research generated by the genomic nursing research community by those who develop and implement policy.

Examples in this chapter illustrated effective engagement by genomic nurse researchers with policy makers at institutional, state, and national levels throughout the research and policy-making processes. Some collaborated with policy makers to solve existing problems, others generated research that is necessary to lead to solutions to problems that are emerging, and still others are producing knowledge that will be needed to inform policies for new health care challenges in the future. Engagement by genomic nurse researchers with policy makers facilitates the incorporation of pertinent genomic nursing research results into health policies at all levels.

ACKNOWLEDGMENTS

The author thanks researchers Calzone, Cohn, Coleman, Daack-Hirsch, Gardner, Hickey, Jenkins, Katapodi, Prows, Starkweather, Taylor, and Tluczek for providing information regarding policy implications of their research; The University of Iowa Clinical Education Librarian Jen DeBerg for her assistance with the scan of published and NINR funded genomic nursing research; and Dr. Sandra Daack-Hirsch and Dr. Toni Tripp-Reimer for their thoughtful reviews of the chapter.

REFERENCES

American Association of Colleges of Nursing. (2006). *The essentials of doctoral education for advanced nursing practice.* Retrieved from www.aacn.nche.edu/dnp/Essentials.pdf

American Association of Colleges of Nursing. (2008). The essentials of baccalaureate education for professional nursing practice. Retrieved from http://www.aacn.nche.edu/education -resources/BaccEssentials08.pdf

American Nurses Credentialing Center. (2016a). Advanced genetics nursing certification eligibility criteria. Retrieved from http://nursecredentialing.org/Advanced-Genetics -Eligibility

American Nurses Credentialing Center. (2016b). ANCC Magnet Recognition Program®. Retrieved from http://www.nursecredentialing.org/Magnet

Ameringer, S. W. (2016). Subjective responses and metabolic state during exercise in sickle cell anemia. Retrieved from https//projectreporter.nih.gov/reporter.cfm

Bakken, S., Stone, P. W., & Larsen, E. L. (2012). A nursing informatics research agenda for 2008–18: Contextual influences and key components 2008. *Nursing Outlook, 60*(5), 2280–2288. doi:10.1016/j.outlook.2012.06.001

Banta-Wright, S. A., Shelton, K. C., Lowe, N. D., Knafl, K. A., & Houck, G. M. (2012). Breast-feeding success among infants with phenylketonuria. *Journal of Pediatric Nursing, 27*(4), 319–327. doi:10.1016/j.pedn.2011.03.015

Baumbauer, K. M., Young, E. E., Starkweather, A. R., Guite, J. W., Russell, B. S., & Manworren, R. C. (2016). Managing chronic pain in special populations with emphasis on pediatric, geriatric, and drug abuser populations. *Medical Clinics of North America, 100*(1), 183–197. doi:10.1016/j .mcna.2015.08.013

Birney, E. (2012). The making of ENCODE: Lessons for big-data projects. *Nature, 489*(7414), 49–51. doi:10.1038/489049a

Brennan, P. F., & Bakken, S. (2015). Nursing needs big data and big data needs nursing. *Journal of Nursing Scholarship, 47*(5), 477–484. doi:10.1111/jnu.12159

Buseh, A. G., Underwood, S. M., Stevens, P. E., Townsend, L., & Kelber, S. T. (2013). Black African immigrant community leaders' views on participation in genomics research and DNA bio-banking. *Nursing Outlook, 61*(4), 196–204. doi:10.1016/j.outlook.2012.10.004

Calzone, K. A., Jenkins, J., Bakos, A. D., Cashion, A. K., Donaldson, N., Ferro, W. G., . . . Webb, J. A. (2013). A blueprint for genomic nursing science. *Journal of Nursing Scholarship, 45*(1), 96–104. doi:10.1111/jnu.12007

Cheek, D. J., Bashore, L., & Brazeau, D. A. (2015). Pharmacogenomics and implications for nursing practice. *Journal of Nursing Scholarship, 47*(6), 496–504. doi:10.1111/jnu.12168

Cohn, E. G., Husamudenn, M., Larson, E. L., & Williams, J. K. (2015). Increasing participation in genomic research and biobanking through community-based capacity building. *Journal of Genetic Counseling, 24*(3), 491–502. doi:10.1007/s10897-014-9768-6

Coleman, B., Calzone, K. A., Jenkins, J., Paniagua, C., Rivera, R., Hong, O. S., . . . Bonham, V. (2014). Multi-ethnic minority nurses' knowledge and practice of genetics and genomics. *Journal of Nursing Scholarship, 46*(4), 235–244. doi:10.1111/jnu.12083

Collins, F. S., & Varmus, H. (2015). A new initiative on precision medicine. *New England Journal of Medicine, 372*(9), 793–795. doi:10.1056/NEJMp1500523

Consensus Panel on Genetic/Genomic Nursing Competencies. (2009). *Essentials of genetic and genomic nursing: Competencies, curricula guidelines, and outcome indicators* (2nd ed.). Silver Spring, MD: American Nurses Association. Retrieved from http://www.genome.gov/ Pages/Careers/HealthProfessionalEducation/geneticscompetency.pdf

Crusto, C. A., Barcelona de Mendoza, V., Connell, C., Sun, Y. V., & Taylor, J. Y. (2016). The intergenerational impact of genetic and psychological factors on blood pressure study (InterGEN): Design and methods for recruitment and psychological measures. *Nursing Research, 65*(4), 331–338.

Daack-Hirsch, S., Driessnack, M., Hanish, A., Johnson, V. A., Shah, L. L., Simon, C. M., & Williams, J. K. (2013). Information is information: A public perspective on incidental findings in clinical and research genome-based testing. *Clinical Genetics, 84*(1), 11–18. doi:10.1111/cge.12167

Daack-Hirsch, S., Driessnack, M., Perkhounkova, Y., Furukawa, R., & Ramirez, A. (2012). A practical first step to integrating genetics into the curriculum. *Journal of Nursing Education, 41*(5), 294–298. doi:10.3928/01484834-20120309-02

Erwin, C., Williams, J. K., Juhl, A. R., Mengling, M., Mills, J.A., Bombard, Y., . . . Paulsen, J. S. (2010). Perception, experience, and response to genetic discrimination in Huntington disease: The international RESPOND-HD study. *American Journal of Medical Genetics, Part B: Neuropsychiatric Genetics,* 153B(5), 1081–1093. doi:10.1002/ajmg.b.31079

Gardner, S. E. (2016). Severe pain during wound care procedures: Model and mechanisms. Retrieved from www.projectreporter.nih.gov/reporter.cfm

The Genetic Information Nondiscrimination Act. (2008). Retrieved from http://ghr.nlm.nih.gov/spotlight=thegeneticinformationnondiscriminationactgina

Green, E. D., Guyer, M. S., & National Human Genome Research Institute. (2011). Charting a course for genomic medicine from base pairs to bedside. *Nature, 470*(7333), 204–213. doi:10.1038/nature09764

Green, R. C., Lautenbach, D., & McGuire, A. L. (2015). GINA, genetic discrimination, and genomic medicine. *New England Journal of Medicine, 372*(5), 397–399. doi:10.1056/NEJMp1404776

HealthCare.gov. (2010). The Affordable Care Act: Rights and protections. Retrieved from https://www.healthcare.gov/health-care-law-protections

Henly, S. J., McCarthy, D. O., Wyman, J. F., Heitkemper, M., Redeker, N. S., Titler, M. G., . . . Dunbar-Jacob, J. (2015). Emerging areas of science: Recommendations for nursing science education from the Council for the Advancement of Nursing Science idea festival. *Nursing Outlook, 63*(4), 398–407. doi:10.1016/j.outlook.2015.04.007

Hickey, K. T., Taylor, J. Y., Sciacca, R. R., Aboelela, S., Gonzale, P., Castillo, C., . . . Frulla, A. P. (2014). Cardiac genetic testing: A single-center pilot study of a Dominican population. *Hispanic Health Care International, 12*(4), 183–188. doi:10.1891/1540-4153.12.4.183

Hinshaw, A. S. (2010). Science shaping health policy. In A. S. Hinshaw & P. A. Grady (Eds.), *Shaping health policy through nursing research* (pp. 1–16). New York, NY: Springer Publishing.

Institute of Medicine. (2011). *The future of nursing: Leading change, advancing health.* Washington, DC: National Academies Press.

Institute of Medicine. (2014). *Assessing genomic sequencing information for health care decision making—Workshop summary.* Washington, DC: National Academies Press.

Jenkins, J., Calzone, K. A., Caskey, S., Culp, C., Weiner, M., & Badzek, L. (2015). Methods of genomic competency integration into practice. *Journal of Nursing Scholarship, 47*(3), 200–210. doi:10.1111/jnu.12131

Jones, T., Lockhart, J. S., Mendelsohn-Victor, K., Duquette, D., Northouse, L. L., Duffy, S., . . . Katapodi, M. C. (2016). Use of cancer genetic services in African American young breast cancer survivors. *American Journal of Preventive Medicine, 51*(4), 427–436.

Katapodi, M. C. (2015, November 6–8). *Preliminary findings from an efficacy statewide trial aiming to increase use of cancer genetic services in families at risk for hereditary breast cancer.* International Society of Nurses in Genomics, Annual Congress, Pittsburg, PA.

Klebaner, D., Huang, Y., Hui, Q., Taylor, J. Y., Goldberg, J., Vaccarino, V., & Sun, Y. V. (2016). X chromosome-wide analysis identifies DNA methylation sites influenced by cigarette smoking. *Clinical Epigenetics, 8,* 20. doi:10.1186/s13148-016-0189-2

Kohane, I. S. (2015). Ten things we have to do to achieve precision medicine. *Science, 349*(6243), 37–38. doi:10.1126/science.aab1328

Kullo, I. J., Haddad, R., Prows, C. A., Holm, I., Sanderson, S. C., Garrison, N. A., . . . Jarvik, G. P. (2014). Return of results in the genomic medicine projects of the eMERGE network. *Frontiers in Genetics, 5,* 50. doi:10.3389/fgene.2014.00050

Lashley, F. (Ed.). (1997). *The genetics revolution: Implications for nursing*. Washington, DC: American Academy of Nursing.

McAllister, K. A., & Schmitt, M. L. (2015). Impact of a nurse navigator on genomic testing and timely treatment decision making in patients with breast cancer. *Clinical Journal of Oncology Nursing, 19*(5), 510–512. doi:10.1188/15.CJON.510-512

Musunuru, K., Hickey, K. T., al-Khatib, S. M., Delles, C., Fornage, M., Fox, C. S., . . . Rosand, J. (2015). Basic concepts and potential applications of genetics and genomics for cardiovascular and stroke clinicians: A scientific statement from the American Heart Association. *Circulation: Cardiovascular Genetics, 8*, 216–242. doi:10.1161/HCG.0000000000000020

National Academies of Sciences, Engineering, and Medicine. (2016). *Assessing progress on the Institute of Medicine report*, The Future of Nursing. Washington, DC: National Academies Press.

National Human Genome Research Institute. (2016). Talking glossary of genetic terms. Retrieved from https://www.genome.gov/glossary

National Institute of Nursing Research. (2011). *Bringing science to life: NINR strategic plan*. Bethesda, MD: Author.

National Institute of Nursing Research. (2016). Precision medicine and NINR-supported nursing science. Retrieved from https://www.ninr.nih.gov/researchandfunding/precisionmedicine #.VrjuO8sUWUk

Oncology Nursing Society. (2012). Oncology nursing: The application of cancer genetics and genomics throughout the oncology care continuum. Retrieved from https://www.ons.org/ advocacy-policy/positions/education/genetics

Personalized Medicine Coalition. (2016). PMC press releases: More than 1 in 4 novel new drugs approved by FDA in 2015 are personalized medicines. Retrieved from http://www .personalizedmedicinecoalition.org

Pesut, D. J. (1999). Health genetics. *Nursing Outlook, 47*(2), 55.

Prows, C. A., Zhang, X., Huth, M. M., Zhang, K., Saldaña, S. N., Daraiseh, N. M., . . . Sadhasivam, S. (2014). Codeine-related adverse drug reactions in children following tonsillectomy: A prospective study. *Laryngoscope, 124*(5), 1242–1250. doi:10.1002/lary.24455

Rasmussen-Torvik, L. J., Stallings, S. C., Gordon, A. S., Almoguera, B., Basford, M. A., Bielinski, S. J., . . . Denny, J. C. (2014). Design and anticipated outcomes of the eMERGE-PGx project: A multicenter pilot for preemptive pharmacogenomics in electronic health record systems. *Clinical Pharmacology & Therapeutics, 96*(4), 482–488. doi:10.1038/clpt.2014.137

Spruill, I. J., Taylor, J., Ancheta, I. B., Adeyemo, A. A., Powell-Young, Y., & Doswell, W. (2014). Health disparities in genomics and genetics. *Nursing Research and Practice, 2014*, 1–2. doi:10.1155/2014/324327

Starkweather, A. R., Ramesh, D., Lyon, D. E., Siangphorn, U., Deng, X., Sturgill, J., . . . Greenspan, J. (2016). Acute low back pain: Differential somatosensory function and gene expression compared to healthy no-pain controls. *Clinical Journal of Pain, 32*(11), 933–939. doi:10.1097/ AJP.0000000000000347

Taylor, J. Y., Peternell, B., & Smith, J. A. (2013). Attitudes toward genetic testing for hypertension among African American women and girls. *Nursing Research & Practice, 2013*, 1–10. doi:10.1155/2013/341374

Taylor, J. Y., Wright, M., Crusto, C., & Sun, Y. V. (2016). The intergenerational impact of genetic and psychological factors on blood pressure study (InterGEN): Design and methods for complex DNA analysis. *Biological Research for Nursing, 18*(5), 521–530.

Tluczek, A., Koscik, R. L., Farrell, P. M., & Rock, M. J. (2005). Psychosocial risk associated with newborn screening for cystic fibrosis: Parents' experience while awaiting the sweat-test appointment. *Pediatrics, 115*(6), 1692–1703.

Tluczek, A., Koscik, R. L., Modaff, P., Pfeil, D., Rock, M. J., Farrell, P. M., . . . Sullivan, B. (2006). Newborn screening for cystic fibrosis: Parents' preferences regarding counseling at the time of infants' sweat test. *Journal of Genetic Counseling, 15*, 277–291.

Tluczek, A., Zaleski, C., Stachiw-Hietpas, D., Modaff, P., Adamski, C. R., Nelson, M. R., & Josephson, K. D. (2011). A tailored approach to family-centered genetic counseling for cystic fibrosis newborn screening: The Wisconsin model. *Journal of Genetic Counseling, 20*(2), 115–28. doi:10.1007/s10897-010-9332-y

Wakefield, M. K. (2015). Beating breast cancer with coverage, prevention and precision medicine. Retrieved from http://www.hhs.gov/blog/2015/10/16/beating-breast-cancer-coverage-prevention.html#

The White House. (2015). Fact sheet: President Obama's precision medicine initiative. Retrieved from https://www.whitehouse.gov/the-press-office/2015/01/30/fact-sheet-president-obama-s-precision-medicine-initiative

Williams, J. K., & Cashion, A. K. (2015). Using clinical genomics in health care: Strategies to create a prepared workforce. *Nursing Outlook, 63*(5), 607–609. doi:10.1016/j.outlook.2015.04.001

Williams, J. K., Cashion, A. K., Shekar, S., & Ginsburg, G. S. (2015). Genomics, clinical research, and learning health care systems: Strategies to improve patient care. *Nursing Outlook, 64*(3), 225–228. doi:10.1016/j.outlook.2015.12.006

Williams, J. K., Daack-Hirsch, S., Driessnack, M., Downing, N., Shinkunas, L., Brandt, D., & Simon, C. (2012). Researcher and institutional review board chair perspectives on incidental findings in genomic research. *Genetic Testing and Molecular Biomarkers, 16*(6), 508–513. doi:10.1089/gtmb.2011.0248

Williams, J. K., Katapodi, M., Starkweather, A., Badzek, L., Cashion, A., Coleman, B., . . . Hickey, K. (2016). Genetics expert panel call to action: Advanced nursing practice and research contributions to precision medicine. *Nursing Outlook, 64*(2), 117–123.

Williams, J. K., Tripp-Reimer, T., Daack-Hirsch, S., & DeBerg, J. (2016). Five-year bibliometric review of genomic nursing science. *Journal of Nursing Scholarship, 48*(2), 179–186. doi:10.1111/jnu.12196

Wyman, J. F., & Henly, S. J. (2015). PhD programs in nursing in the United States: Visibility of American Association of Colleges of Nursing core curricular elements and emerging areas of science. *Nursing Outlook, 63*(4), 390–397. doi:10.1016/j.outlook.2014.11.003

5

Team Science: Challenges and Opportunities in the 21st Century

Alma Vega and Mary D. Naylor

[Enhancing our] ability to work across disciplines and professions may well be the hallmark of the 21st century.

—Grady (2010, p. 165)

The sheer complexity of the phenomenon "health" provides the most compelling argument in support of team science. Health is influenced by a vast interplay of individual factors such as genetics, as well as environmental influences such as socioeconomic status and neighborhood safety. Thus, it follows that substantive advances in knowledge about health will require the engagement of scholars representing multiple disciplines and perspectives. Epistemological arguments reinforce the critical nature of a team approach to generating and translating knowledge designed to inform and positively impact the health of individuals, families, communities, and societies. The exponential growth in the pool of available knowledge, coupled with the rapid proliferation of information sources, demands the participation of a diverse group of scientists who are on top of their respective areas of inquiry and can position others to meaningfully build upon extant research (Institute of Medicine, 2013).

In this chapter, scholars from demography and nursing join forces to explore the current state of team science in the area of health and offer recommendations designed to accelerate this critically important orientation to knowledge development and translation. Particular attention is paid to teams in which nurse scholars play a key role. To frame our recommendations, we suggest a definition of team science, provide examples of initiatives to strengthen collaboration among scholars from multiple disciplines, describe selected contributions of teams in advancing knowledge about health, and identify barriers to foster successful scholarly teams within academic environments and potential strategies to address these challenges.

DEFINITION OF TEAM SCIENCE

Cooke and Hilton (2015) defined *team science* as "scientific collaboration, that is, research conducted by more than one individual in an interdependent fashion, including research conducted by small teams and larger groups" (Cooke & Hilton, 2015, p. 22). These and other scholars also have been explicit about the need for teams to include representatives from a range of disciplines (referred to as *multidisciplinarity*; e.g., Cooke & Hilton, 2015; Disis & Slattery, 2010). In their analysis of 28 innovative teams at 14 Industrial Research Institute member companies, Post, De Lia, DiTomaso, Tirpak, and Borwankar (2009) provided insight regarding the value of multidisciplinary teams. Their findings suggest that teams with diverse membership engage in more connective thinking (joining previously unconnected ideas) than sequential thinking (i.e., using logical thinking), with the former resulting in bolder ideas.

Increasingly, the unique contributions of scholars who cross traditional boundaries and share perspectives to address significant research questions (referred to as *interdisciplinarity*) have been stressed (e.g., Aboelela et al., 2007; Fuqua, Stokols, Gress, Phillips, & Harvey, 2004). Indeed, Rosenfield (1992) argued that true interdisciplinarity involves more than juxtaposing the independent results of a group of scientists from different disciplines, but rather requires a true melding of perspectives. The National Academy of Sciences (2005) echoes this sentiment with the statement that "[r]esearch is truly interdisciplinary when it is not just pasting two disciplines together to create one product but rather an integration and synthesis of ideas and methods" (p. 27). In this chapter, we use the phrase "team science" to reflect the generation and translation of knowledge related to health that is grounded in interdisciplinarity.

INITIATIVES TO STRENGTHEN TEAM SCIENCE

A growing appreciation of the value of team science has led to a number of public and private initiatives designed to stimulate interdisciplinary research (IR) in the area of health. The *National Institutes of Health (NIH) Roadmap for Medical Research's Interdisciplinary Research* program is a prime example of a federally supported effort. Over an 8-year period (2004–2012), the IR focused on four major initiatives: (a) the establishment of nine consortia comprising multidisciplinary experts to address complex health problems; (b) an interdisciplinary training initiative, which included postdoctoral training in a new interdisciplinary field; (c) a program that fostered innovation in interdisciplinary methodologies using technology; and (d) the introduction of the multiple principal investigator policy. Collectively, the IR contributed to many changes in research-intensive environments, such as the creation of departments with an explicit IR focus and statistical packages that better accommodated the participation of multiple disciplines (NIH, 2015). The program also enabled the investigators' home institutions to recognize the leadership of researchers from more than one discipline in federally funded projects.

A number of other NIH-funded efforts established to foster team science have yielded similar positive results. For example, K. L. Hall et al. (2012) compared the number of publications produced by National Cancer Institute (NCI)-funded Transdisciplinary Tobacco Use Research Centers (TTURCs) grants to similar investigator-initiated tobacco studies that relied on the traditional R01 grant mechanism. The authors found that the 10-year TTURC grantees produced 100% more publications than the investigator-initiated R01 grants during this same period. The National Institute of Nursing Research (NINR)-funded Training in Interdisciplinary Research to Reduce Antimicrobial Resistance (TIRAR) initiative was developed to prepare pre- and postdoctoral scholars who would effectively engage in team science related to antimicrobial resistance. Among a number of metrics to assess TIRAR's success, the number of trainees who completed the program and maintained interdisciplinary collaborations was calculated. Larson, Cohen, Gebbie, Clock, and Saiman (2011) reported that all of the 11 scholars trained between 2007 and 2011 continued to pursue interdisciplinary scholarship.

The *Interdisciplinary Nursing Quality Research Initiative (INQRI)* program, funded by the Robert Wood Johnson Foundation (RWJF) from 2005 to 2013, is illustrative of a major commitment by selected private foundations to advance team science. INQRI was designed to stimulate rigorous IR that would uncover nursing's contributions to the quality of patient care. Equally important, the program also was focused on promoting the use of such evidence by a diverse range of stakeholders, including health system leaders and policy makers. Led by a nurse scientist (Mary Naylor, co-author) and a health care economist, the INQRI program funded 48 multidisciplinary teams, each with scholars from nursing and another discipline as principal investigators, who developed and implemented innovative research in targeted areas such as measurement of the value of nurses to high-quality health care and the impact of nurse-led interventions designed to enhance patient outcomes (Naylor, Lustig, et al., 2013). Early findings from an analysis of peer-reviewed papers suggested that the evidence linking nursing to the quality of patient care had grown since the launch of INQRI, as demonstrated by increased numbers of reported studies in this line of inquiry, higher quality of publications, enhanced methodological rigor, and stronger interdisciplinary reach (Naylor, Volpe, et al., 2013). INQRI teams also were successful in using their findings to advance the measurement of outcomes important to patients, including pain management (Beck et al., 2013) and increased use of evidence-based interventions in areas such as fall prevention (Titler, Wilson, Resnick, & Shever, 2013).

While we describe the core elements of successful team science, we must acknowledge the limitations of current measurement efforts. Unquestionably, commonly used metrics of team science used by current programs such as publications in prestigious interdisciplinary journals are important. Yet, multiple challenges associated with a comprehensive assessment of the short- and long-term impact of team science remain. Such measurement requires not only navigating diverse research agendas, but also obtaining agreement on desired outcomes (Feller, 2006). Klein (2008) offers parameters to consider in assessing the effects of team science, including the extent to which the various goals of team members are accomplished, the degree to which integration of knowledge is achieved and leveraged, and the impact of the science. Mâsse et al. (2008) developed a set of scales that capture multiple dimensions of team science, including satisfaction with the collaborative process; the impact of collaboration on knowledge production; trust and respect in the team science setting; and cross-disciplinary integration (Mâsse et al., 2008).

From our perspectives, the hallmarks of successful team science are the findings produced through rigorous research conducted by interdisciplinary scholars and the effects of their findings on the health of individuals and the public. In the following section, we offer a few examples of the impact of team science.

ADVANCES IN KNOWLEDGE ABOUT HEALTH

There are numerous examples of major advances in the science of health that have been contributed through interdisciplinary teams. As highlighted in the NIH *Roadmap for Medical Research* (NIH, 2015), team science has led to an increased understanding of the association between genes and behavioral inflexibility (Laughlin, Grant, Williams, & Jentsch, 2011) and the role of brain cells in mediating antidiabetic actions of the brain (Xu et al., 2010). Advances in the treatment of patients with cancer also have resulted from interdisciplinary science (Raj et al., 2011). Nurse scholars have played a key role in teams that have increased our understanding of the relationship between genetics and chemotherapy-induced mucositis (Coleman et al., 2015), the role of high-sensitivity C-reactive protein (hsCRP) in determining cardiac events (Frazier, Vaughn, Willerson, Ballantyne, & Boerwinkle, 2009), and the neuropsychological patterns of patients with ventricle dysfunction in heart failure (Bratzke-Bauer, Pozehl, Paul, & Johnson, 2012).

In addition to their contributions to basic science research, nurse scholars in collaboration with colleagues from other disciplines have contributed strong evidence to address significant and complex health care issues through clinical and translational research. Findings derived from rigorous designs, including large-scale randomized controlled trials and longitudinal analyses of nationally representative health care databases, have been reported in high-impact journals that reach multiple disciplines, such as the *Journal of the American Medical Association* and *Health Affairs*. Consequently, the body of evidence in support of nurses' central role as partners in redesigning health care is stronger and increasingly used to inform changes in health care practices and policies. The following are a few examples of such research contributions.

The Nurse-Family Partnership (NFP) is a community-based program that includes prenatal and infancy/toddler home visits by public health nurses to economically disadvantaged mothers and young children. The first clinical trial demonstrating its effectiveness was conducted by individuals representing the fields of pediatrics, obstetrics, gynecology, human development, and family studies, among others (Olds, Henderson, Tatelbaum, & Chamberlin, 1986). The NFP was initially funded by a federal grant (U.S. Public Health Service), which was followed by private foundation support (RWJF); subsequent support has been provided by numerous private and public sources (Goodman, 2006), including an NINR grant to assess the effects of an intimate partner violence component to the program.

For decades, the NFP has been recognized as being highly effective in improving maternal and child outcomes. Since 2010, NFP has been a flagship community program under provision H.R. 3590 of the Affordable Care Act (H.R. 3590), which established a $1.5 billion federal funding stream to help expand home visitation programs. Currently, the program serves the needs of more than 31,000 families in more than 550 economically disadvantaged communities across the United States. Recent studies reveal that the NFP has demonstrated significant improvements in a range of longer term outcomes for economically disadvantaged mothers and infants, including reduced mortality, better mental health, and enhanced socioeconomic outcomes. Economic analyses demonstrate that the NFP also was cost-effective over a 20-year period in reducing welfare dependency by more than the NFP program costs. The following are among the more recent NFP outcomes:

- Participation in the NFP was associated with a significant reduction in all-cause mortality for mothers and preventable mortality for infants throughout the 20-year follow-up period (Olds et al., 2014).
- Infants participating in the NFP had lower rates of being arrested or convicted of criminal acts as adults; had more stable partner relationships (Olds et al., 2010); were less likely to be welfare-dependent (Eckenrode et al., 2010; Olds et al., 2010), or to use tobacco, alcohol, and illegal drugs (Kitzman et al., 2010; Olds et al., 2010); had a lower incidence of mental health disorders; and scored higher on academic achievement tests (Kitzman et al., 2010; Olds et al., 2014).
- From infancy to age 12, the NFP was cost-effective, with $12,300 in discounted savings compared with a program cost of $11,511 for 594 urban economically disadvantaged, primarily African American families (Olds et al., 2010).

For more than two decades, the Transitional Care Model (TCM), an advanced practice nurse coordinated, team-based model, has been rigorously tested among at-risk, chronically ill older adults via multiple NINR-funded, multisite randomized clinical trials. From initial conceptualization and testing through ongoing expansion to different patient populations and contexts and subsequent efforts to study implementation of TCM by local health systems across the United States, the TCM has been grounded in interdisciplinarity. Ideas and perspectives from scholars representing nursing, medicine, social work, health care economics, social science, and biostatistics, among others, have influenced advances in this body of knowledge.

The TCM has consistently demonstrated improved health and quality of life outcomes and reduced rehospitalizations and total health care costs for this at-risk population when compared to standard care (Naylor et al., 1999; Naylor et al., 2004; Naylor, Aiken, Kurtzman, Olds, & Hirschman, 2011). For example, all-cause reductions in rehospitalizations were demonstrated through 1-year postindex hospital discharge among older adults hospitalized with heart failure. After accounting for program costs, the cost savings per Medicare beneficiary were estimated at $5,000 per year (Naylor et al., 2011). Initially, the TCM focused on the transitions of older adults from hospitals to home. More recently, the team has extended application of this model to prevent avoidable hospitalizations among older adults living in their communities (Naylor, Hirschman, O'Connor, Barg, & Pauly, 2013).

Multiple provisions of the Affordable Care Act incorporated the core components and research findings generated from the TCM as the basis to advance evidence-based transitional care services in emerging models of health care delivery, including accountable care organizations and patient-centered medical homes (Naylor et al., 2011). A 2015 survey funded by the RWJF revealed that approximately 60% of 582 responding health systems or communities in the United States have adopted or adapted the TCM (M. Naylor, personal communication, May 25, 2016). The Coalition for Evidence-Based Policy has recognized the TCM as a "top-tiered" evidence-based approach that, if scaled, could have a positive impact on the health and well-being of chronically ill adults, while ensuring wiser use of societal resources.

In recent years, the effects of the TCM, when compared to other evidence-based approaches and when translated into health systems and communities, have been reported. The following are among key findings reported during this period:

- A National Institute of Aging (NIA)-funded comparative effectiveness study revealed that hospitalized cognitively impaired older adults who transition to home experienced a significantly longer time to first rehospitalization and fewer all-cause rehospitalizations through 6 months postindex hospitalization when compared to other evidence-based approaches (Naylor et al., 2014).
- In partnership with the University of Pennsylvania Health System and a major payer, a study of the effects of translating the TCM in the mid-Atlantic region revealed significant decreases in the total number of rehospitalizations, total days hospitalized, and total health care costs per member per month (Naylor, Bowles, et al., 2013).

A number of intervention studies conducted by multidisciplinary teams have focused on nursing's central role in improving a range of important patient outcomes. Common themes emerging from this work that are relevant to the importance of interdisciplinarity in both the conduct of science and the nature of interventions studied are as follows:

- *Nurses contribute unique knowledge and skills to share with other disciplines* (Balas et al., 2012; Dykes et al., 2010; Hamilton, Mathur, Gemeinhardt, Eschiti, & Campbell, 2010; Kennerly, Yap, & Miller, 2012; Marshall, Edmonson, Gemeinhardt, & Hamilton, 2012; Marsteller et al., 2012; Newhouse et al., 2011; Nosbusch, Weiss, & Bobay, 2011; Setter, Corbett, & Neumiller, 2012; Shever, Titler, Mackin, & Kueny, 2010; Yap & Kennerly, 2011). The research conducted by

Dykes et al. (2010) is illustrative of this theme. The most common safety issue associated with the hospitalization of adult patients is falls. Dykes and members of her multidisciplinary team designed and tested the effects of a web-based fall prevention toolkit (FPTK) in four urban, acute care hospitals. The FPTK provides nurses and other team members with the tools and strategies to prevent falls. Findings demonstrated that intervention units had a significantly lower adjusted fall rate than control units (Dykes et al., 2010).

- *Nursing's collaborations with other disciplines are essential to ensuring safe and effective health care* (Balas et al., 2012; Feldman et al., 2012; Happ et al., 2010; Kennerly et al., 2012; Marsteller et al., 2012; Nosbusch et al., 2011; Setter et al., 2012). For example, Feldman et al. (2012) reported the effects of a nurse–pharmacist-led medication reconciliation process to prevent potential adverse drug events (ADEs). Baccalaureate-prepared nurses delivered the primary intervention by developing a home medication list, tracking changes and discrepancies, and conducting a review of these findings in collaboration with a hospital-based pharmacist at hospital admission and at discharge. The nurse then initiated contact with the prescriber(s) to determine if a discrepancy was unintended. This collaborative effort was efficient, potentially "averting 81 ADEs for every 290 patients" (Feldman et al., 2012). The team estimated the projected cost of each prevented ADE to be $9,300.

- *Nurse leadership of interdisciplinary teams is associated with improved safety and higher quality outcomes* (Kennerly et al., 2012; Marsteller et al., 2012; Needleman, Buerhaus, Vanderboom, & Harris, 2013; Yap & Kennerly, 2011). For example, prior studies on reducing central line-associated bloodstream infections (CLABSIs) did not explore the role of the nursing environment, nor did quality improvement studies provide causal evidence that these infections are largely preventable. Marsteller et al. (2012) refined and evaluated a nursing-driven intervention to successfully reduce CLABSIs. This study was conducted with 45 intensive care units (ICUs) from 35 hospitals participating in the multicenter, cluster-randomized controlled trial (Marsteller et al., 2012). CLABSI rates were reduced by 81% in the intervention group compared to the control group.

- *Nurse team leadership is associated with greater team interdependence which, in turn, fosters increased respect among team members and positively contributes to the organizational culture of interprofessional learning* (Balas et al., 2012; Wholey et al., 2014). An example of this theme can be found in the work of Balas et al. (2012). Approximately two thirds of ICU patients develop delirium, which is associated with longer hospital stays and tremendous human and economic consequences. The *Awakening and Breathing Coordination, Delirium Monitoring and Management, and Early Mobility (ABCDE)* bundle incorporates available evidence on delirium, immobility, sedation and analgesia, and ventilator management in the ICU that has been tested in clinical trials and has been adapted for everyday use in the ICU (Balas et al., 2012). This innovative effort to improve care for ICU patients reveals that a bundle of practices, delivered by a nurse-led interprofessional team of health care providers, helps ICU patients avoid delirium and weakness.

As reflected in the aforementioned studies, nursing is assuming an increasingly prominent role in redesigning health care due, in large part, to the rigorous interdisciplinary science that is the foundation for their work and that of other team members. As suggested by these examples, team science can create synergistic relationships, which produce outcomes greater than those possible by single disciplines. Scholars who have been fortunate to experience interdisciplinarity throughout their careers understand the value that the "integration and synthesis of ideas and methods" (National Academy of Sciences, 2005, p. 27) has on their body of research and its capacity to have maximal impact.

While a team orientation to knowledge development and translation in the area of health is growing, this approach is far from the norm. Indeed, we are in the midst of a transformation throughout the research enterprise related to team science. In the following section, we describe major challenges to achieving this transformation and suggest strategies to address them.

ACCELERATING TEAM SCIENCE

In its current stage of development, achieving the promise of team science in the foreseeable future will require a substantial investment by multiple stakeholders. Foundational to accelerating a movement toward team science as the dominant orientation to knowledge generation related to health is the recognition of the scope and dimensions of the desired change as well as the challenges leaders will need to address in successfully navigating this transformation. In the following section, we examine these key dimensions to accelerating team science.

Scope of Desired Change

Most current researchers have been socialized in environments that nurture and reward the contributions of individual scientists or teams from single disciplines. Thus, it is not surprising that these scientists have a bias toward unidisciplinary research. Moving from such an orientation to one that places a premium on interdisciplinary scholarship often requires questioning disciplinary beliefs, navigating perceived and actual threats to disciplinary integrity, and recognizing power differentials (Reich & Reich, 2006). Post, De Lia, DiTomaso, Tirpak, and Borwankar (2009) suggest that these challenges can be addressed in psychologically safe environments where team members believe that expressing differing perspectives will not result in negative consequences.

To foster such an environment, all team members must learn to demonstrate respect for others' viewpoints. As Levinson and Thornton (2003) noted, "[a]ll investigators need to park their egos at the door" (p. 677). Similar to ethnic diversity, team science can be thought of as a melding of different cultures that requires new competencies (Reich & Reich, 2006). Tervalon and Murray-Garcia (1998) suggest that one such competency is cultural humility, which they define as a lifelong process of continually questioning one's own beliefs. To train in cultural humility, researchers may adapt strategies proven successful in diminishing ethnic biases (Juarez et al., 2006). Translated into research contexts, these strategies could include sessions where the same research question is addressed from the perspectives of multiple disciplines or research proposal reviews that include oral and written critiques by members of other disciplines.

Interacting with diverse scholars through activities such as interdepartmental colloquia and even informal lunches can help dislodge cultural beliefs and enhance one's willingness to accept alternative viewpoints. Personal relationships cultivated during these interactions are especially important in navigating disciplinary boundaries. As one author stated, "You collaborate with the people you have lunch with" (Disis & Slattery, 2010, p. 3).

All team members must be willing to invest the time needed to understand diverse communication styles (R. Hall, Stevens, & Torralba, 2002; Levinson & Thornton, 2003), develop a common language (National Academy of Sciences, 2005), and, ultimately, achieve consensus (Leipzig et al., 2002; National Academy of Sciences, 2005). For example, team members who participated in the Water and Watersheds Program, a federally supported effort, initially disagreed on the best research strategy to test the efficacy of this initiative. Arguments, largely driven by disciplinary norms, centered on the use of qualitative versus quantitative methods, experimental versus survey designs, and analytical plans (Levinson & Thornton, 2003). The team's willingness to invest in working through these differences eventually led to agreement on a more robust research design that incorporated multiple datasets and methods. This example, as well as others (e.g., Corbett et al., 2013; R. Hall et al., 2002), reinforces that high-quality communication is essential to successful team science.

Leadership

Central to accelerating team science is leadership. Scholars will only be able and willing to utilize a team-based approach to knowledge development when they perceive that such an orientation is highly valued by the stakeholders who influence their work. Key stakeholders include leaders of their home institutions, public and private funders, heads of health systems, policy makers, and consumers, among others. In this paper, we limit our attention to leaders of the research environments in which scholars work and, to a more limited extent, to leaders of funding organizations. There are multiple ways in which leadership of researchers' home institutions demonstrates support, or lack thereof, for team science. We focus on recruitment and retention strategies and programmatic initiatives.

Recruitment and Retention of Scholars

A huge opportunity for research environments to accelerate team science is to recruit individual scholars who have demonstrated their commitment to IR. Often, these are senior scientists who are seeking the potential to expand their collaborative network. Leaders of research-intensive environments make their interest in such scientists abundantly clear by offering incentives such as enabling the scholars to bring members of their team to their new positions and/or appointing them to major roles such as heads of IR centers. Faculty appointment to more than one discipline and role titles also reflect the leaders' intentions. At the University of Pennsylvania, for example, distinguished faculty with strong background in team science are recruited as Penn Integrates Knowledge (PIK) professors with appointments in two schools and the expectation that they will be visible leaders in advancing IR (Office of the President: University of Pennsylvania, 2014). Importantly, institutions are better positioned to recruit junior faculty committed to team science when these faculty observe examples of the university's overall commitment. Similarly, universities will be most interested in junior faculty members who have been socialized to the values of team science through training programs such as NINR's TIRAR (described earlier).

Retention of highly productive investigators also is of great importance. Many of these scientists are successful in their independent lines of inquiry but may not sufficiently understand, or value, IR. Even if they choose not to participate in team science, getting these scholars to appreciate this approach to knowledge development is essential so that they can support their colleagues in their roles as mentors and members of personnel committees.

Another issue of great importance for leaders of academic institutions is alignment of the promotion and tenure system with the goals of team science in order to better recognize and reward the contributions of individual team members. This remains a particular challenge for junior faculty (Feller, 2006). Junior scholars whose contributions to the team are not explicit or who publish in interdisciplinary journals run the risk of having their research viewed as of lesser impact and quality than those with a unidisciplinary line of inquiry and publications in discipline-specific journals (Feller, 2006). In addition to modifying promotion and tenure guidelines to reflect this new cultural orientation, mentorship teams, preferably comprising multidisciplinary members, are needed to ensure that junior faculty members clearly demonstrate their unique lines of inquiry and the relationships of their findings to overall team contributions. There are multiple other mechanisms leaders can use to highlight the contributions of interdisciplinary researchers. For example, the creation of awards for teams of science in addition to those for single investigators would help to signal institutional commitment.

Programmatic Efforts

Leaders should assess where each of their current faculty and staff is on the continuum spanning from unidisciplinary to interdisciplinary research. They can then employ a variety of programmatic efforts tailored to individual's or groups' needs, each designed to accelerate the movement of faculty and staff along this continuum. For those interested in but new to IR, for example, leaders need to provide them with the time and resources required to build new teams. Fuqua et al. (2004) also advise that new teams will work more fluidly if members are in close physical proximity, represent narrower set of disciplines, and have some prior working relationships. Other scholars recommend that new teams start with a well-defined goal that can be achieved in the shorter term, which can better position them for future, larger interdisciplinary collaborations (Arbaje et al., 2010). Thus, leaders need to facilitate the environmental conditions and provide newer teams with the knowledge and opportunities for success.

A range of programmatic initiatives have evolved for scholars actively involved in team science. Most research-intensive environments have institutes or research centers whose membership includes scholars from a range of disciplines and who frequently host visiting scholars, colloquia, or symposia, and thus promote access to the research conducted by diverse scientists. Some schools have majors or departments that are specifically designed to foster a culture of team science. Programs also have emerged with built-in allowances for the time demands of team science. One example is a "think tank" funded by the Mellon Foundation in the College of the Environment at Wesleyan University. This program provides faculty with one semester of teaching relief to pursue research in another department (Poulos et al., 2012).

Regardless of where faculty and students are on the continuum, leaders of existing programs need to continue their efforts to implement the aforementioned strategies and others aimed at developing new competencies among all members specific to fostering a culture of team science. Leaders in environments without such resources should consider partnering with funders to establish such programs.

All academic leaders with research enterprises should increase their efforts to partner directly with private and public funders to advance team science. As Feller (2006) observes, "Federal funding, in short, represents an explicit pro-active effort to catalyze institutional and cultural change in the way academic research is conducted" (p. 9). Thus, federal and private program priorities heavily influence knowledge production. Partnerships between academic leaders and funders can affect the direction of changes. Academic leaders contributed to changes in federal policies, including the Multiple Principal Investigator Policy (NIH, 2015) and the use of specific panels by NIH and the National Science Foundation (NSF; Feller, 2006), that benefit interdisciplinary scholars.

Similarly, academic leaders need to partner with private funders to promote team science and their support of innovative structures and mechanisms to advance this agenda. In doing so, academic leaders should capitalize on the opportunities to engage other key stakeholders in the design and implementation of new programs and in the uptake and spread of key findings. Teams funded under the RWJF-funded INQRI invited health system leaders, policy makers, consumers, and others to be actively engaged throughout the research process (Corbett et al., 2013). Their engagement tremendously facilitated the conduct of the teams' research and its impact.

A strong partnership model is one in which each party contributes and each benefits. Leaders of academic institutions not only need to cultivate a culture of team science among their faculty and students, but also to advance this orientation by encouraging their members to be fully engaged in efforts that spread this culture, including participating in peer review or advisory panels sponsored by the funders. Additionally, faculty members should be encouraged to critique research publications and meaningfully contribute to reviews of candidates for appointment and promotion at other institutions. Each of these opportunities can be used to spread the value of team science.

CONCLUSION

As information becomes more abundant and health becomes more complex, scholars are more and more dependent on each other as we work toward advancing health. It is only by pooling our collective knowledge and experiences that we can generate and translate important research findings into improved population health. As the 20th century was marked by tremendous advances in the reduction of infectious disease, we hope the 21st century sees even greater strides in prevention and management of complex chronic conditions. This can only be achieved if we step out of our disciplinary silos, cross the aisle, and work together.

ACKNOWLEDGMENT

The authors are grateful to Dr. Olga Yakusheva, associate professor in the Department of Systems, Populations and Leadership at the University of Michigan School of Nursing, for her review of selected studies on the contributions of nurses to team interventions and science highlighted in this chapter.

REFERENCES

Aboelela, S. W., Larson, E., Bakken, S., Carrasquillo, O., Formicola, A., Glied, S. A., . . . Gebbie, K. M. (2007). Defining interdisciplinary research: Conclusions from a critical review of the literature. *Health Services Research*, 42(1 Pt. 1), 329–346.

Arbaje, A. I., Maron, D. D., Yu, Q., Wendel, V. I., Tanner, E., Boult, C., . . . Durso, S. C. (2010). The geriatric floating interdisciplinary transition team. *Journal of the American Geriatrics Society*, 58(2), 364–370.

Balas, M. C., Vasilevskis, E. E., Burke, W. J., Boehm, L., Pun, B. T., Olsen, K. M., . . . Ely, E. W. (2012). Critical care nurses' role in implementing the "ABCDE bundle" into practice. *Critical Care Nurse*, 32(2), 35–47.

Beck, S. L., Weiss, M. E., Ryan-Wenger, N., Donaldson, N. E., Aydin, C., Towsley, G. L., & Gardner, W. (2013). Measuring nurses' impact on health care quality: Progress, challenges, and future directions. *Medical Care*, 51, S15–S22.

Bratzke-Bauer, L. C., Pozehl, B. J., Paul, S. M., & Johnson, J. K. (2012). Neuropsychological patterns differ by type of left ventricle dysfunction in heart failure. *Archives of Clinical Neuropsychology*, 28, 114–124.

Coleman, E. A., Lee, J. Y., Erickson, S. W., Goodwin, J. A., Sanathkumar, N., Raj, V. R., . . . Stephens, O. (2015). GWAS of 972 autologous stem cell recipients with multiple myeloma identifies 11 genetic variants associated with chemotherapy-induced oral mucositis. *Supportive Care in Cancer*, 23(3), 841–849.

Cooke, N. J., & Hilton, M. L (Eds.). (2015). *Enhancing the effectiveness of team science*. Washington, DC: National Academies Press. Retrieved from https://www.nap.edu/catalog/19007/enhancing-the-effectiveness-of-team-science

Corbett, C. F., Costa, L. L., Balas, M. C., Burke, W. J., Feroli, E. R., & Daratha, K. B. (2013). Facilitators and challenges to conducting interdisciplinary research. *Medical Care*, 51(4 Suppl. 2), S23–S31.

Disis, M. L., & Slattery, J. T. (2010). The road we must take: Multidisciplinary team science. *Science Translational Medicine*, 2(22), 1–4.

Dykes, P. C., Carroll, D. L., Hurley, A., Lipsitz, S., Benoit, A., Chang, F., . . . Middleton, B. (2010). Fall prevention in acute care hospitals: A randomized trial. *JAMA*, 304(17), 1912–1918.

Eckenrode, J., Campa, M., Luckey, D. W., Henderson, C. R., Cole, R., Kitzman, H., . . . Olds, D. (2010). Long-term effects of prenatal and infancy nurse home visitation on the life course of youths: 19-year follow-up of a randomized trial. *Archives of Pediatrics & Adolescent Medicine*, 164(1), 9–15.

Feldman, L. S., Costa, L. L., Feroli, E. R., Nelson, T., Poe, S. S., Frick, K. D., . . . Miller, R. G. (2012). Nurse-pharmacist collaboration on medication reconciliation prevents potential harm. *Journal of Hospital Medicine*, 7(5), 396–401.

Feller, I. (2006). Multiple actors, multiple settings, multiple criteria: Issues in assessing interdisciplinary research. *Research Evaluation*, 15(1), 5–15.

Frazier, L., Vaughn, W. K., Willerson, J. T., Ballantyne, C. M., & Boerwinkle, E. (2009). Inflammatory protein levels and depression screening after coronary stenting predict major adverse coronary events. *Biological Research for Nursing*, 11(2), 163–173.

Fuqua, J., Stokols, D., Gress, J., Phillips, K., & Harvey, R. (2004). Transdisciplinary collaboration as a basis for enhancing the science and prevention of substance use and "abuse." *Substance Use & Misuse*, 39(10–12), 1457–1514.

Goodman, A. (2006). The story of David Olds and the nurse home visiting program. Retrieved from http://www.rwjf.org/content/dam/farm/reports/program_results_reports/2006/rwjf13780

Grady, P. A. (2010). Translational research and nursing science. *Nursing Outlook*, 58(3), 164–166.

Hall, K. L., Stokols, D., Stipelman, B. A., Vogel, A. L., Feng, A., Masimore, B., . . . Berrigan, D. (2012). Assessing the value of team science: A study comparing center- and investigator-initiated grants. *American Journal of Preventive Medicine*, 42(2), 157–163.

Hall, R., Stevens, R., & Torralba, T. (2002). Disrupting representational infrastructure in conversations across disciplines. *Mind, Culture, and Activity*, 9(3), 179–210.

Hamilton, P., Mathur, S., Gemeinhardt, G., Eschiti, V., & Campbell, M. (2010). Expanding what we know about off-peak mortality in hospitals. *Journal of Nursing Administration*, 40(3), 124–128.

Happ, M. B., Baumann, B. M., Sawicki, J., Tate, J. A., George, E. L., & Barnato, A. E. (2010). SPEACS-2: Intensive care unit "communication rounds" with speech language pathology. *Geriatric Nursing*, 31(3), 170–177.

Institute of Medicine. (2013). *Best care at lower cost: The path to continuously learning health care in America*. Washington, DC: National Academies Press. Retrieved from https://www.nap.edu/catalog/13444/best-care-at-lower-cost-the-path-to-continuously-learning

Juarez, J. A., Marvel, K., Brezinski, K. L., Glazner, C., Towbin, M. M., & Lawton, S. (2006). Bridging the gap: A curriculum to teach residents cultural humility. *Family Medicine*, 38(2), 97–102.

Kennerly, S. M., Yap, T., & Miller, E. (2012). A nurse-led interdisciplinary leadership approach targeting pressure ulcer prevention in long-term care. *The Health Care Manager*, 31(3), 268–275.

Kitzman, H. J., Olds, D. L., Cole, R. E., Hanks, C. A., Anson, E. A., Arcoleo, K. J., . . . Holmberg, J. R. (2010). Enduring effects of prenatal and infancy home visiting by nurses on children: Follow-up of a randomized trial among children at age 12. *Archives of Pediatrics & Adolescent Medicine*, 164(5), 412–418.

Klein, J. T. (2008). Evaluation of interdisciplinary and transdisciplinary research: A literature review. *American Journal of Preventive Medicine, 35*(2 Suppl.), S116–S123.

Larson, E. L., Cohen, B., Gebbie, K., Clock, S., & Saiman, L. (2011). Interdisciplinary research training in a school of nursing. *Nursing Outlook, 59,* 29–36.

Laughlin, R. E., Grant, T. L., Williams, R. W., & Jentsch, J. D. (2011). Genetic dissection of behavioral flexibility: Reversal learning in mice. *Biological Psychiatry, 69*(11), 1109–1116.

Leipzig, R. M., Hyer, K., Ek, K., Wallenstein, S., Vezina, M. L., Fairchild, S., . . . Howe, J. L. (2002). Attitudes toward working on interdisciplinary healthcare teams: A comparison by discipline. *Journal of the American Geriatrics Society, 50*(6), 1141–1148.

Levinson, B., & Thornton, K. (2003). *Managing interdisciplinary research: Lessons learned from the EPA-STAR/NSF/USDA Water and Watersheds Research Program.* Paper presented at First Interagency Conference on Research in the Watersheds, Benson, AZ. Retrieved from http://www .tucson.ars.ag.gov/icrw/proceedings/levinson.pdf

Marshall, J., Edmonson, C., Gemeinhardt, G., & Hamilton, P. (2012). Balancing interests of hospitals and nurse researchers: Lessons learned. *Applied Nursing Research, 25*(3), 205–211.

Marsteller, J. A., Sexton, J. B., Hsu, Y.-J., Hsiao, C.-J., Holzmueller, C. G., Pronovost, P. J., & Thompson, D. A. (2012). A multicenter, phased, cluster-randomized controlled trial to reduce central line-associated bloodstream infections in intensive care units. *Critical Care Medicine, 40*(11), 2933–2939.

Mâsse, L. C., Moser, R. P., Stokols, D., Taylor, B. K., Marcus, S. E., Morgan, G. D., . . . Trochim, W. M. (2008). Measuring collaboration and transdisciplinary integration in team science. *American Journal of Preventive Medicine, 35*(2 Suppl.), S151–S160.

National Academy of Sciences. (2005). Facilitating interdisciplinary research. Retrieved from https://www.nap.edu/catalog/11153/facilitating-interdisciplinary-research

National Institutes of Health, Office of Strategic Coordination—The Common Fund. (2015). A decade of discovery: The NIH roadmap and common fund (NIH Pub No. 14-8013). Retrieved from https://commonfund.nih.gov/sites/default/files/ADecadeofDiscoveryNIHRoadmap CF.pdf

Naylor, M. D., Aiken, L. H., Kurtzman, E. T., Olds, D. M., & Hirschman, K. B. (2011). The importance of transitional care in achieving health reform. *Health Affairs, 30*(4), 746–754.

Naylor, M. D., Bowles, K. H., McCauley, K. M., Maccoy, M. C., Maislin, G., Pauly, M. V., & Krakauer, R. (2013). High-value transitional care: Translation of research into practice. *Journal of Evaluation in Clinical Practice, 19*(5), 727–733.

Naylor, M. D., Brooten, D., Campbell, R., Jacobsen, B. S., Mezey, M. D., Pauly, M. V., & Schwartz, J. S. (1999). Comprehensive discharge planning and home follow-up of hospitalized elders: A randomized clinical trial. *JAMA, 281*(7), 613–620.

Naylor, M. D., Brooten, D. A., Campbell, R. L., Maislin, G., McCauley, K. M., & Schwartz, J. S. (2004). Transitional care of older adults hospitalized with heart failure: A randomized, controlled trial. *Journal of the American Geriatrics Society, 52*(5), 675–684.

Naylor, M. D., Hirschman, K. B., Hanlon, A. L., Bowles, K. H., Bradway, C., McCauley, K. M., & Pauly, M. V. (2014). Comparison of evidence-based interventions on outcomes of hospitalized, cognitively impaired older adults. *Journal of Comparative Effectiveness Research, 3*(3), 245–257.

Naylor, M. D., Hirschman, K. B., O'Connor, M., Barg, R., & Pauly, M. V. (2013). Engaging older adults in their transitional care: What more needs to be done? *Journal of Comparative Effectiveness Research, 2*(5), 457–468.

Naylor, M. D., Lustig, A., Kelley, H. J., Volpe, E. M., Melichar, L., & Pauly, M. V. (2013). Introduction: The interdisciplinary nursing quality research initiative. *Medical Care, 51*(4 Suppl. 2), S1–S5.

Naylor, M. D., Volpe, E. M., Lustig, A., Kelley, H. J., Melichar, L., & Pauly, M. V. (2013). Linkages between nursing and the quality of patient care: A 2-year comparison. *Medical Care, 51*(4 Suppl. 2), S6–S14.

Needleman, J., Buerhaus, P. I., Vanderboom, C., & Harris, M. (2013). Using present-on-admission coding to improve exclusion rules for quality metrics: The case of failure-to-rescue. *Medical Care, 51*(8), 722–730.

Newhouse, R., Dennison, C., Liang, Y., Morlock, L., Frick, K., & Pronovost, P. (2011). Smoking-cessation counseling by registered nurses: Description and predictors in rural hospitals. *American Nurse Today Online, 6*(6). Retrieved from https://americannursetoday.com/smoking-cessation-counseling-by-nurses-description-and-predictors-in-rural-hospitals

Nosbusch, J. M., Weiss, M. E., & Bobay, K. L. (2011). An integrated review of the literature on challenges confronting the acute care staff nurse in discharge planning. *Journal of Clinical Nursing, 20*(5–6), 754–774.

Office of the President: University of Pennsylvania. (2014). Penn integrates knowledge interdisciplinary university professors: About the program. Retrieved from https://pikprofessors.upenn.edu/about-pik

Olds, D. L., Henderson, C. R., Tatelbaum, R., & Chamberlin, R. (1986). Improving the delivery of prenatal care and outcomes of pregnancy: A randomized trial of nurse home visitation. *Pediatrics, 77*(1), 16–28. Retrieved from http://pediatrics.aappublications.org/content/77/1/16

Olds, D. L., Holmberg, J. R., Donelan-McCall, N., Luckey, D. W., Knudtson, M. D., & Robinson, J. (2014). Effects of home visits by paraprofessionals and by nurses on children: Follow-up of a randomized trial at ages 6 and 9 years. *JAMA Pediatrics, 168*(2), 114–121.

Olds, D. L., Kitzman, H. J., Cole, R. E., Hanks, C. A., Arcoleo, K. J., Anson, E. A., . . . Bondy, J. (2010). Enduring effects of prenatal and infancy home visiting by nurses on maternal life course and government spending: Follow-up of a randomized trial among children at age 12 years. *Archives of Pediatrics & Adolescent Medicine, 164*(5), 419–424.

Post, C., De Lia, E., DiTomaso, N., Tirpak, T. M., & Borwankar, R. (2009). Capitalizing on thought diversity for innovation. *Research-Technology Management, 52*(6), 14–25.

Poulos, H., Bannon, B., Isard, J., Stonebarker, P., Royer, D., Yohe, G., & Chernoff, B. (2012). The world through an interdisciplinary lense: A new college at Wesleyan University breaks down departmental divisions. *Academe.* Retrieved from http://www.aaup.org/article/world-through-interdisciplinary-lens#.WCL_n9R95iw

Raj, L., Ide, T., Gurkar, A. U., Foley, M., Schenone, M., Li, X., . . . Shamji, A. F. (2011). Selective killing of cancer cells by a small molecule targeting the stress response to ROS. *Nature, 475*(7355), 231–234.

Reich, S. M., & Reich, J. A. (2006). Cultural competence in interdisciplinary collaborations: A method for respecting diversity in research partnerships. *American Journal of Community Psychology, 38*(1–2), 1–7.

Rosenfield, P. L. (1992). The potential of transdisciplinary research for sustaining and extending linkages between the health and social sciences. *Social Science and Medicine, 35*(11), 1343–1357.

Setter, S. M., Corbett, C. F., & Neumiller, J. J. (2012). Transitional care: Exploring the home healthcare nurse's role in medication management. *Home Healthcare Now, 30*(1), 19–26.

Shever, L. L., Titler, M. G., Mackin, M. L., & Kueny, A. (2010). Fall prevention practices in adult medical-surgical nursing units described by nurse managers. *Western Journal of Nursing Research, 33*(3), 385–397.

Tervalon, M., & Murray-Garcia, J. (1998). Cultural humility versus cultural competence: A critical distinction in defining physician training outcomes in multicultural education. *Journal of Health Care for the Poor and Underserved, 9*(2), 117–125.

Titler, M. G., Wilson, D. S., Resnick, B., & Shever, L. L. (2013). Dissemination and implementation: INQRI's potential impact. *Medical Care, 51*(4 Suppl. 2), S41–S46.

Wholey, D. R., Disch, J., White, K. M., Powell, A., Rector, T. S., Sahay, A., & Heidenreich, P. A. (2014). Differential effects of professional leaders on health care teams in chronic disease management groups. *Health Care Management Review, 39*(3), 186–197.

Xu, Y., Berglund, E. D., Sohn, J.-W., Holland, W. L., Chuang, J.-C., Fukuda, M., . . . Zigman, J. M. (2010). 5-HT2CRs expressed by pro-opiomelanocortin neurons regulate insulin sensitivity in liver. *Nature Neuroscience, 13*(12), 1457–1459.

Yap, T. L., & Kennerly, S. M. (2011). A nurse-led approach to preventing pressure ulcers. *Rehabilitation Nursing, 36*(3), 106–110.

6

Data Science

Suzanne Bakken

OVERVIEW

Data Science and Big Data

The National Consortium for Data Science defined *data science* "as the systematic study of the organization and use of digital data in order to accelerate discovery, improve critical decision-making processes, and enable a data-driven economy" (p. iii; Ahalt et al., 2014). Data science draws upon theories and techniques from multiple fields, including mathematics, statistics, and information technology, and includes methods such as probability models, machine learning, statistical learning, computer programming, pattern recognition and learning, visualization, predictive analytics, uncertainty modeling, data warehousing, and high performance computing. Data science methods are applied to what is commonly called "big data" that are typically conceptualized in terms of volume, variety, and velocity (e.g., sensor or streaming data) and more recently, veracity, which refers to the level of uncertainty associated with the collection of data sources (IBM, 2015). These multiple attributes of big data reflect an additional complexity beyond that of simple volume (e.g., Medicare claims data may be considered voluminous, but do not necessarily meet other aspects of the data science definition due to their well-structured nature).

The Big Data to Knowledge (BD2K) initiative at the National Institutes of Health (NIH) reinforces this in their definition of biomedical big data as "more than just very large data or a large number of data sources" and "comprising the diverse, complex, disorganized, massive, and multimodal data being generated by researchers, hospitals, and mobile devices around the world," including "imaging, phenotypic, molecular, exposure, health, behavioral, and many other types of data" (NIH, 2016b).

In a panel at the Council for the Advancement of Nursing Science, Meeker (2014) offered an operational perspective by contrasting properties of big data and associated processing in distributed research networks versus traditional outcomes research in federated research networks:

- Analysis questions: patterns, predictions, classification versus causal inference, and hypothesis testing
- Data distribution: randomly distributed across process versus tied to a site
- Number of network nodes: 100s versus 10s
- Common analytic platforms: R-Volution/R-Hadoop, Apache Mahout, Spark Machine Learning Library, Spark Graph X Library versus SAS, R, STATA

Some authors also consider a fifth "V" in data science attributes—value (Marr, 2015). The attribute of value also highlights the significance of domain expertise in data science to ensure that appropriate questions are asked of relevant data sources and that results are interpreted accurately through the stages of data science inquiry: obtain, scrub, explore, model, and interpret (Mason & Wiggins, 2010).

Drivers for Data Science in Nursing and Other Health and Biomedical Research

There are multiple drivers for data science in nursing and other health and biomedical research. First, electronic health-related data have increased in volume and variety. This is particularly relevant to several aspects of the National Institute of Nursing Research (NINR) Strategic Plan, including symptom science, self-management, and precision medicine (NINR, 2016a). For example, consumer-generated data from mobile apps, wearables, medical devices, and sensors, along with multiple sources of environmental and "omic" data, complement traditional electronic sources of research data such as surveys, clinical data warehouses, and transaction data (Bakken & Reame, 2016). In addition, the Patient-Centered Outcomes Research Institute (PCORI) development of PCORnet has increased the availability of data from a variety of data sources through its Clinical Research Data Networks and Patient Powered Research Networks (Fleurence et al., 2014). The inclusion of the strong patient voice in the latter broadens the available data types and ensures their relevance to patient centeredness. Moreover, through the U.S. government's Health Data Initiative and the open data portal (NIH, 2016c), thousands of datasets are accessible for linking with big data streams. These include datasets from federal agencies such as the Centers for Medicare and Medicaid Services, Centers for Disease Control and Prevention, Department of Health and Human Services, Food and Drug Administration, Health Resources and Services Administration, and NIH as well as states (e.g., Hawaii, Michigan, New York) and cities (e.g., Boston, San Francisco).

Second, through the BD2K initiative (NIH, 2016b), the NIH has acknowledged the role of big data to advance scientific knowledge and launched a set of funding opportunities designed to develop new approaches, methods, software tools, and related resources and increase the competency of the biomedical workforce in data science in three core areas: computer science, biostatistics, and biomedical science. The BD2K Centers program has funded 11 centers of excellence for big data computing and two additional centers, the LINCS-BD2K Perturbation Data Coordination and Integration Center, and the Broad Institute LINCS Center for Transcriptomics, which are collaborative projects with the NIH Common Fund LINCS program (NIH, 2016b). The centers also provide training to advance big data science in the context of biomedical research as part of the overall BD2K investments in training (NIH, 2016a). Training goals include increasing the data science skills of all biomedical scientists as well as preparing specialists in data science. Consequently, the training-related awards use a variety of funding mechanisms to support course development, including massive open online courses (MOOCs) on data management for biomedical big data and training resource development and coordination, as well as supplements to existing T32 and T15 predoctoral training programs. To foster the development of new teams consisting of biomedical scientists and data scientists, BD2K is also supporting the Quantitative Approaches to Biomedical Big Data Program along with the National Science Foundation.

Third, initiatives related to precision medicine and biobanking are growing, including the recent launch of President Obama's Precision Medicine Initiative (PMI; Collins & Varmus, 2015). The NIH defined *precision medicine* as an emerging approach for disease treatment and prevention that takes into account individual variability in genes, environment, and lifestyle for each person. Consequently, there is no doubt that data science methods are essential to implementing the vision of more than a million persons' PMI cohort and other aspects of precision medicine, because PMI takes advantage of increased connectivity through social media and mobile devices as well as "omic" and traditional data sources such as electronic health record (EHR) data and surveys.

NURSING SCIENCE FOUNDATIONS FOR DATA SCIENCE

In "Nursing Needs Big Data and Big Data Needs Nursing," Brennan and Bakken (2015) argue that nursing's role in data science is motivated by the American Nurses Association's Social Policy Statement, which specifically delineates the role of nurses in the generation and application of knowledge and technology to health care outcomes and planning for health policy and regulation that is responsive to consumer needs and provides for best resource use in the provision of health care for all (American Nurses Association, 2010). Nursing science has resulted in critical foundation for data science in nursing and other health and biomedical research in multiple areas. Four key aspects are (a) health care standards that facilitate semantic interoperability; (b) common data elements (CDEs); (c) theories, models, and frameworks; and (d) ethical, legal, and social implications (ELSI). Moreover, nurse scientists have demonstrated application of analytic techniques relevant to data science to datasets that do not meet the definitions of biomedical big data, but are reflective of approach competencies that can be applied to big data.

Health Care Standards That Facilitate Semantic Interoperability

Documentation of patient status, nursing interventions, and patient outcomes in EHRs extends the patient phenotypes beyond demographics, medical diagnoses, medical procedures, and laboratory values and the care processes and outcomes beyond those attributable to physician practice. This includes data such as assessments related to fall risk (Dykes et al., 2010), high risk for readmission (Bowles et al., 2015), and nursing-sensitive patient outcomes (Brown, Donaldson, Burnes Bolton, & Aydin, 2010). Although aggregation of well-structured phenotypic data in large volumes and application of traditional analytic methods do not meet the definition of data science, these data are a critical data source that complements other less structured EHR (e.g., progress notes) and high volume and velocity data such as that from continuous physiological monitoring or environmental data.

Nurse scientists have led efforts to establish the necessary standards to support inclusion of nursing data in a variety of EHRs and establish comparability across sites and settings at the national (Harris et al., 2015; Henry, Holzemer, Reilly, & Campbell, 1994; Westra et al., 2015) and international levels (Hardiker, 2003; Hardiker & Coenen, 2007; Matney et al., 2012). As part of interdisciplinary teams, nurse scientists have also contributed to integration of genomic data and knowledge into EHRs (Jing, Kay, Marley, Hardiker, & Cimino, 2012). Complementing the data standardization efforts, nurse scientists have also focused efforts on other aspects of semantic interoperability, including information models (Danko et al., 2003) and document representation standards (Hyun et al., 2009; Hyun & Bakken, 2006; Matney, Dolin, Buhl, & Sheide, 2016). These structures enhance the application and performance of natural language processing, a data science method for extracting nursing-relevant data from narrative documents such as progress notes or reports (Hyun, Johnson, & Bakken, 2009; Johnson et al., 2008).

Although nurses have been working in interdisciplinary standards development organizations for several decades, there are still knowledge and implementation gaps. To address these gaps, the University of Minnesota School of Nursing has convened a series of conferences and related activities to promote a national action plan for sharable and comparable nursing data to support practice and research (Westra et al., 2015).

Common Data Elements

Complementary to the efforts in semantic interoperability, the NIH has significantly invested in the creation of CDEs, including standardized measures. Use of CDEs— variables conceptually defined, operationalized, and measured in identical ways across studies and clinical practice—improves data quality and opportunities for data sharing (Redeker et al., 2015). In addition, CDEs enable comparison of outcomes across multiple studies and also support analysis of important subsamples, which is typically not possible due to inadequate statistical power (National Library of Medicine, 2015).

An important source of CDEs, the Patient Reported Outcome Measure Information System (PROMIS®), includes a collection of highly reliable, precise measures of patient-reported health status for physical, mental, and social well-being. The measures are supplemented by web-based tools for administration including computer adaptive testing. A CDE effort specific to nursing science that occurred within the context of the NINR Centers of Excellence program built upon the PROMIS work to select a set of symptom CDEs (Redeker et al., 2015). The recommended CDEs for six of seven symptoms were PROMIS measures: pain (PROMIS Pain), fatigue (PROMIS Fatigue), sleep disturbance (PROMIS Sleep Disturbance plus additional duration question), affective mood disturbance (PROMIS Positive Affect and PROMIS Depression), affective well-being (Medical Outcomes Study Short Form-36 Psychological Well-being Scale), and Cognitive Disturbance (PROMIS Applied Cognition and General Concerns).

As with structured EHR data, a large volume of CDEs alone does not constitute data science. However, these data represent important variables that can be combined with other data to conduct analyses and discover insights for hypothesis generation. For example, in the area of symptom science, consumer-facing technologies such as mobile devices and sensors provide an important source of high volume and velocity data related to the symptom experience, including the environmental conditions under which the symptoms exacerbate (Bakken & Reame, 2016).

Theories, Models, and Frameworks

Brennan and Bakken note that "nursing's long tradition of theory-driven science provides the frameworks that can guide explorations towards promising phenomena and leverage insights into new knowledge, thereby avoiding the distractions of opportunistic exploration" (Brennan & Bakken, 2015, p. 481). Nurse theorists have generated grand theories that address the metaparadigm concepts of person, environment, and health. For example, the Roy Adaptation Model has influenced nursing science and education for more than 40 years (Roy, 2011). In addition, middle range theories have been developed that can be used to frame data science-based inquiry to advance nurse science. For instance, Riegel developed a middle range theory of self-care that addresses the process of maintaining health with health promoting practices within the context of chronic illness management and includes major concepts of self-care maintenance, self-care monitoring, and self-care management (Riegel, Jaarsma, & Stromberg, 2012). Another study tested a middle range theory of adaptation of chronic pain in community-dwelling older adults, and found that contextual stimuli should be considered when developing plans of care for older adults experiencing chronic pain (Dunn, 2005). The increasing availability

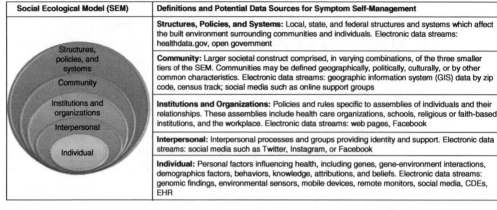

FIGURE 6.1   Social Ecological Model definitions and potential electronic data streams for symptom self-management.

CDE, common data element; EHR, electronic health record.

of electronic data streams will enable further development and testing of such middle range theories.

Moreover, nurse scientists have applied theories, models, or frameworks from other disciplines to advance nursing science. For example, the Precision in Symptom Self-Management (PriSSM) Center uses data science approaches to advance the science of symptom self-management for Latinos through a social ecological lens that takes into account variability in individual, interpersonal, organizational, and environmental factors across the life course. The Social Ecological Model (SEM) was chosen as the theoretical model for the center (Centers for Disease Control and Prevention, 2015). Definitions and potential electronic data streams are summarized in Figure 6.1 to illustrate the intersection of data science and theoretical approaches.

Ethical, Legal, and Social Implications

Bakken and Reame (2016) explicated the potential ethical perils related to data science, using the three principles for the ethical conduct of research subjects as articulated in the historic Belmont Report: respect for persons (i.e., autonomy), beneficence, and justice (The National Commission for the Protection of Human Subjects of Biomedical and Behavioral Research, 1979).

The primary mechanism for protection of autonomy, which relates to the principle of respect for persons, is informed consent that includes adequate information—understandable in lay terms—to make an informed decision about participation. Some big data sources have explicit opt-in or opt-out consent processes, and use of protected health information for research receives ethical and regulatory oversight from institutional review boards and the Health Insurance Portability and Accountability Act (HIPAA). However, this is not true of data streams that are generated from sources such as social network sites and mobile health devices, because terms of service are usually lengthy and although an individual may technically consent by clicking "I agree," the consent does not meet typical research criteria. Moreover, commercial uses may not be highlighted or described in a health-literate manner. Kahn, Vayena, and Mastroianni (2014) recommend that "approaches to informed consent must be reconceived for research in the social-computing environment, taking advantage of the technologies available and developing creative solutions that will empower users who participate in research, yield better results, and foster greater trust" (p. 13678).

Methodological rigor is an ethical requirement, not just a scientific one, to ensure that scarce resources are used wisely and decisions are not made based on unsound findings. This requirement, which relates to the principle of beneficence (i.e., optimizing benefits while minimizing risks), remains critical in data science, although the methods vary from traditional research designs (Vayena, Salathe, Madoff, & Brownstein, 2015). Beyond poor methodological rigor, other important perils to beneficence relate to risks associated with loss of confidentiality and commodification of patient/consumer-generated data. Through prosumption, digital exhaust is produced as digital content (e.g., websites, mobile health applications, tweets) and is consumed. In some instances, these data are commodified and used for commercial purposes in which the data producer does not reap the benefit.

The principle of justice gives rise to moral requirements that there be fair procedures and equitable outcomes in the selection of research participants. In regard to big data, the investigator may be using existing data sources that may result in biases against underrepresented groups such as racial and ethnic minorities. For example, Latinos are less likely than Whites or Blacks to use an app for health tracking, and racial and ethnic minorities are less likely to participate in biobanks (Dang et al., 2014; Shaibi, Coletta, Vital, & Mandarino, 2013), thus hindering discoveries that may be of particular relevance to race or ethnicity.

Application of Data Science Analytics

The application of data science analytics to datasets that do not meet the definition of biomedical big data, typically due to lack of diversity and complexity in data types, demonstrates the promise and relevance of these analytics to advance nursing science. For example, using Outcome and Assessment Information Set (OASIS) data from a convenience sample of 270,634 home health care patient records, Dey et al. (2015) applied association analysis to identify sets of variables (patterns) associated with each other and also with mobility outcomes (i.e., improvement versus no improvement as compared to baseline). They found that the patterns of factors discovered through association mining typically comprised combinations of functional and cognitive status and the type and amount of help required at home and provided the foundation for tailored intervention development.

Clancy (Clancy, 2004; Clancy, Effken, & Pesut, 2008) pioneered the application of computational modeling and simulation to examine complex systems related to nursing and health care systems. For example, Clancy et al. (2007) used a variety of electronic data sources, observation of physician work patterns, and computational modeling and simulation to predict the impact of an EHR that integrated heart failure guidelines on practice patterns of physicians of nurses. The results indicated that such an implementation would decrease nursing workload, but increase physician workload in the community hospital setting. Predictive analytics are ubiquitous in the business world and are increasingly being used in the health care setting.

HOW HAVE RESEARCHERS USED DATA SCIENCE TO ADVANCE NURSING SCIENCE?

Although the drivers for data science have only increased in intensity in recent years and continue to do so, there are some examples of application of data science to big data to advance nursing science. The following nurse-scientist-led examples were selected to reflect a variety of settings, data sources, and analytic methods.

Embedded Home Sensor Technology

Rantz and colleagues have conducted a series of studies about the use of sensor technology to enable aging in place (Rantz, Lane, et al., 2015; Rantz, Skubic, et al., 2015). Working collaboratively with engineering and other interdisciplinary scientists, Rantz has led the development and evaluation of environmentally embedded sensor technology in elder housing along with associated nursing interventions (e.g., care coordination). Sensors continuously monitor functional status, including: (a) respiration, pulse, and restlessness during sleep; (b) gait speed, stride length, and stride time for calculation of fall risk; and (c) fall detection. Algorithms are applied to large volumes of sensor data and generate automated health alerts to health care staff who are then able to assess and intervene as necessary. Significant innovation and iteration was necessary in algorithm creation and refinement. For example, in the instance of fall detection, a framework was developed that fused Doppler radar sensor data with a motion sensor network in order to identify and disregard false alarms generated by visitors (Liu, Popescu, Skubic, & Rantz, 2014). A recent evaluation indicated that residents living with sensors were able to live in the elder housing for 1.7 years longer than elders without sensors (Rantz, Lane, et al., 2015). Moreover, costs of sensor technology and nursing care coordination were significantly lower than the costs that would be associated with nursing home care.

Virtualizing Home Environments

Motivated by vizHOME, a multiyear program to examine personal health information management in the home environment in a way that minimizes repeated, intrusive, and potentially disruptive in vivo assessments, Brennan and colleagues (Brennan, Ponto, Casper, Tredinnick, & Broecker, 2015) reported proof of concept for two methodological advances for studying interior health care environments. In terms of data capture, they implemented Light Detection and Ranging (LiDAR) scanning methods to create point cloud datasets (i.e., high-fidelity, three-dimensional spatial and color depictions) of home environments that included the location of physical boundaries and object perimeters, color, and light. To display the large (more than 1 billion data points) point cloud datasets in an immersive environment, the research team implemented custom visualization software and a VR CAVE—an immersive virtual reality environment in which data were displayed on six sides of a room-sized cube. They have also demonstrated visualization of the datasets in two-dimensional desktop viewers and three different virtual reality immersive environments. The point cloud datasets of home environments provide the foundation for a variety of purposes, including understanding personal health information management in context, designing interventions, and characterizing home environment for use in clinical practice including discharge planning.

Public Health Systems

Merrill and colleagues collected data from 11 local public health departments and used organizational network analysis, a computational method derived from social network analysis, to examine the linkage between network structure and performance on essential public health services (Merrill, Keeling, & Carley, 2010). They found that local public health departments exhibited compound organizational structures in which centralized hierarchies were coupled with distributed networks at the point of service. These departments were distinguished from random networks by a pattern of high centralization and clustering. Network measurements were positively associated with performance for three of ten essential public health services.

In a subsequent study, the researchers conducted a longitudinal organizational network analysis at three points in time for one local public health department to examine the influence of management and environment on local health department organizational structure and adaptation (Keeling, Pryde, & Merrill, 2013). The baseline organizational network analysis was presented to managers as an intervention with information on evidence-based management strategies to address the findings. At times 2 and 3, the organizational network analysis was complemented by interviews with managers to document decision making and events in the task environment. Screening and case identification increased for chlamydia and for gonorrhea. These specific population health outcomes were traced directly to management decisions based on network evidence.

Mining Social Media

Social media provide a unique source for understanding phenomena of interest to nurse researchers, for discovery of intervention targets, and for the delivery of interventions. Researchers at the Columbia University School of Nursing have conducted a series of NINR-funded studies (P30NR010677, T32NR007969, R01NR014430-03S1) related to structure and content mining of tweets related to physical activity and to caregiving for those with Alzheimer's disease or other dementias. They summarized methods for content mining applied to physical activity tweets and illustrated differences in sentiments associated with physical activities such as biking and hiking (positive sentiments) as compared to wood chopping and running (negative sentiments; Yoon, Elhadad, & Bakken, 2013). Structure mining of the same tweet corpus examined macronetwork structures and identified 65 communities associated with individual professionals (e.g., Harvard psychiatrist), researchers (e.g., obesity and physical activity), and organizations (e.g., Young Men's Christian Association [YMCA] free summer programs for families and children), among others (Yoon & Bakken, 2010). Also in the area of physical activity, another study assessed the extent to which tweet contents reflected two concepts (motivation, psychological needs) related to social determination theory, which has been shown to be particularly relevant in intervention research aimed at increasing physical activity levels (Yoon, Shaffer, Momberg, & Bakken, 2013). In terms of discovering insights regarding dementia caregiving, Yoon, Hunter, and Bakken (under review) applied topic modeling and visualization approaches to compare the contents of a random sample of tweets mentioning "dementia" (n = 73,564) or "demencia" (n = 2,501) with human-coded focus group data from Hispanic caregivers of dementia patients.

In the application domain of public health outbreak surveillance, Odlum and Yoon (2015) analyzed tweets mentioning Ebola in the early stages of the outbreak using content analysis, geographic visualization, and time series analysis. They found that tweets in Nigeria started to rise 3 to 7 days before the official announcement of the first probable Ebola case and included topics related to risk factors, prevention education, disease trends, and compassion. The authors concluded that Twitter mining can provide the foundation for public health education in terms of understanding sources of misconception, dispelling myths, and disseminating accurate information.

Combining Phenotypic and Genotypic Data to Advance Symptom Science

The NIH Symptom Science Model, which was developed by NINR, has four components: (a) complex symptom or cluster identification, (b) phenotypic characterization including standardization of measurements across groups and/or conditions, (c) biomarker discovery across populations and conditions, and (d) clinical application (i.e., symptom management interventions; Cashion & Grady, 2015). Big data streams are relevant to instantiating the model for a particular symptom or symptom cluster including electronic clinical data such as narrative text, imaging, physiologic monitoring; "omics" data (e.g., genomics, microbiomics, proteomics, metabolomics); and self-tracking data on aspects of a person's daily life (e.g., vegetables consumed, local air quality), states (e.g., anxiety, blood pressure [BP]), and performance (e.g., mental functioning and physical activity; Bakken & Reame, 2016). Each of these requires data science query and analytic processes matched to the data streams as a prerequisite for integration to address research questions (for example, bioinformatics tools for genomic analyses).

In addition, some nurse scientists combine traditional data sources such as standardized surveys and structured clinical data with big data such as genomic data to advance symptom science (Alfaro et al., 2014; Kohen et al., 2016; Koleck & Conley, 2016). For example, Alfaro et al. (2014) combined standardized measures of functional status and sleep disturbance, clinical data, and genomic analyses to identify associations between distinct latent classes of those with higher and lower levels of sleep disturbance and genetic variations. Variations in three cytokine genes predicted latent class membership, suggesting that cytokine genes may partially explain interindividual variability in sleep disturbance in breast cancer and provide the foundation for targeted interventions.

MOVING FROM TRADITIONAL DATA SOURCES AND RESEARCH METHODS TO DATA SCIENCE: A CASE STUDY

Although some examples of application of data science to nursing have been published, a case study is used to illustrate how one project is evolving from traditional data sources and research methods to data science, to stimulate other nurse scientists to think about how their research could be enhanced through data science. The Washington Heights Inwood Informatics Infrastructure for Comparative Effectiveness Research (WICER, R01HS019853) project and the study that followed, WICER 4 U (R01HS022961), had the overall goal of understanding and improving the health of the community (A. Wilcox et al., 2011). Focused on the clinically significant problem of hypertension in the primarily Latino community of Washington Heights Inwood, WICER combined existing electronic health data from NewYork-Presbyterian Columbia University Medical Center, ColumbiaDoctors, Visiting Nurse Service of New York, and Isabella Senior Center with primary survey data collection and physical measurements (height, weight, BP) of almost 6,000 Latinos (Lee, Boden-Albala, Jia, Wilcox, & Bakken, 2015; A. Wilcox et al., 2011; A. B. Wilcox, Gallagher, & Bakken, 2013). An analysis of these data sources according to the indicators of the County Health Rankings Framework demonstrated that the WICER data sources alone populated the majority of the indicators for the categories in the framework and if complemented by the Behavioral Research Surveillance Survey and New York City Community Health Survey would populate all indicators (Yoon, Wilcox, & Bakken, 2013).

While the volume of data points for each person was relatively large because of electronic health data, the data sources were varied, and the efforts to create an integrated dataset were significant, these data would not meet the big data definition related to velocity and veracity. Moreover, applying traditional analytic methods to these data (Figure 6.2A, 6.2B, & 6.2C) generated research insights and questions that would benefit from data science approaches.

The high frequency of systolic BPs in the hypertensive range (Figure 6.2A) for those who answered either yes or no to "Have you ever been told by a health care professional that you have high blood pressure?" generates multiple research questions. These include: (a) What patterns of BP measurements would be revealed by 3 days of ambulatory BP measurement (i.e., improved BP phenotype through multimodal data)?; (b) Are those who have been told that they had high BP uncontrolled on an ineffective regimen, nonadherent to their existing regimen, or not receiving hypertension treatment?; and (c) In the instance of ineffectiveness or nonadherence, would N-of-1 trials result in a regimen that maximizes effectiveness and minimizes side effects?

Some individuals with hypertension in the WICER sample reported stopping their antihypertensive medication because of side effects (Figure 6.2B); this also

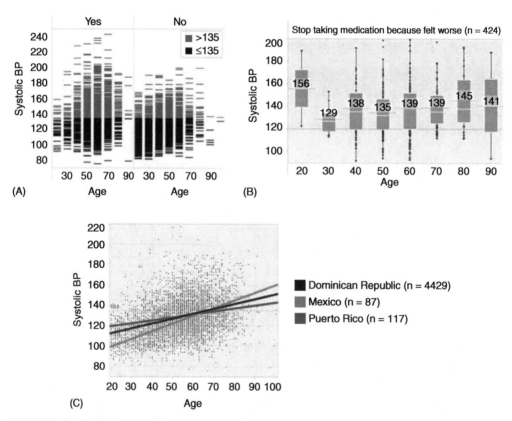

FIGURE 6.2 (A) Systolic BP by age of individuals reporting whether or not they had been told by a health care professional that they had high BP; (B) systolic BP of those reporting that they stopped taking their hypertension medicine because they felt worse; (C) comparison of systolic BP by age and self-reported Latino subgroup.

BP, blood pressure.

generates research questions such as the previously mentioned N-of-1 trial, and also: (a) Would ecological momentary assessment methods on a mobile device offer insights regarding the context of side effects in terms of time, activity, and location?; and (b) Is there a relationship between genomic variation and symptom side effect variability in those with hypertension?

In terms of the patterns of BP differences among Dominican Americans, Mexican Americans, and Puerto Ricans (Figure 6.2C), it must first be determined if the patterns are due to small samples of Mexican Americans and Puerto Ricans as compared with Dominican Americans. If the patterns are valid in larger samples, then several potential questions arise, among them: (a) Are the differences in BP due to genomics, culture, environment, behavior (e.g., adherence, diet, exercise), or some combination of relationships?; and (b) What is the contribution of ancestry informative markers to understanding the patterns of differences in BP?

To transition from WICER and WICER 4 U to WICER/precision medicine in order to address questions such as those posed previously requires new data sources and analytic platforms. Potential relevant data sources are:

- Environment: socioeconomic, physical, and built (e.g., geographic information system data related to healthy food supply or places to exercise)
- Genetics: ancestry informative markers for admixed population and single nucleotide polymorphisms (SNPs) related to sodium
- Mobile devices: physical activity, sleep, symptom status
- Social media: social networks, behaviors (e.g., nutrition, exercise)
- Physiological: 24-hour ambulatory BP monitoring, sodium load

These additional data sources and their integration to address new research questions will require transition from the traditional statistical packages used (e.g., SAS, SPSS, and R) to new analytic platforms (e.g., R-Volution, R-Hadoop, Apache Mahout, Spark Machine Learning Library), as well as an additional storage and computational process such as that available in distributed processing. As the program of research transitions to increased integration of data science, the research team must also evolve, given the interdisciplinary nature of data science and the criticality of team approaches.

MOVING FROM TRADITIONAL DATA SOURCES AND RESEARCH METHODS TO DATA SCIENCE: COMPETENCIES REQUIRED

The breadth and depth of required data science competencies and the manner in which the competencies are achieved will vary by role. BD2K conceptualizes expertise as three broad areas: computational (e.g., cloud computing, workflow automation, visual analytics), mathematical and statistical (e.g., research design, traditional and machine learning analytic techniques), and domain (e.g., nursing, genomics, public health). Published Venn diagrams of data science competencies emphasize the interdisciplinary and team science aspects of data science by naming the intersection of all the competencies "the unicorn"—that is, nonexistent.

Educational pathways for nurse scientists should reflect their primary areas of knowledge development. Nurses who wish to focus on creating computational methods and tools should pursue graduate training in a computational field such as computer science, data science, or biomedical informatics. Their nursing perspective will influence the types of methods and tools that are developed.

However, most nurse scientists will seek education in nursing PhD programs, so these programs must evolve to include data science. Every nurse scientist should have a general understanding of data science just as they have for methods such as qualitative inquiry, experimental and quasi-experimental designs, and health services research. Because data science reflects a different way of knowing and generates potential threats to bioethical principles, it is vital that data science be threaded throughout the PhD curriculum (e.g., social and intellectual foundations, bioethics) rather than simply integrated into research method courses.

In addition, to meet the goal of advancing nursing science through data science, some nurse scientists must be prepared as specialists who have data science as their major method of inquiry. NINR has made significant efforts to meet these needs for existing nurse scientists through the provision of week-long boot camps in data science and precision health (NINR, 2016b). These efforts must be complemented by pre- and postdoctoral nurse scientist training for individuals who wish to have data science as their primary research method. Given the breadth of data science, such training programs should include interaction with interdisciplinary colleagues and designate a particular area of excellence in data science that is relevant to the four science areas of the NINR strategic plan: symptom science, wellness, self-management, and end-of-life and palliative care. For example, a training program might focus on data science methods to support symptom self-management and augment the data-science-enriched core PhD curriculum with specialty courses in data science as well as practical research experience in applying data science methods such as machine learning, information visualization, and visual analytics.

DATA SCIENCE AND NURSING SCIENCE SYNERGY TO INFLUENCE POLICY

The synergy of data science and nursing science will enhance policy influence at multiple levels. Data science can support the ability of nursing science to influence policy through providing the technical foundation for making its datasets findable, accessible, interoperable, and reusable (FAIR; Wilkinson et al., 2016) and linkable with associated publications. A key strategy for achieving this at the federal level is the NIH Commons Framework (NIH, 2015). NIH Commons is conceptualized as a three-layered system. The bottom level is a computational platform comprising high performance and cloud computing. The middle layer includes reference datasets and user-defined data. The top level is composed of services (e.g., application programming interfaces [APIs], containers, indexing such as PubMed and DataMed) and tools (e.g., scientific analysis, workflows). There are plans for extending the top layer to include an app store and user interface, which will make the Commons more accessible for those without technical backgrounds. Although document object identifiers are now attached to publications in journals indexed in Medline and available through PubMed, unique identifiers for other resources are still evolving. For example, the research resource identifier (RRID) is designed to provide unique identifiers for resources such as reagents, tools, data, software, and materials used in a study; RRIDs are intended to be reported in the methods section of a paper to enhance reproducibility of the results.

There are several other activities associated with the BD2K initiative and its Centers of Excellence program that will improve the ability of nursing science to advance policy. First, annotating the dataset (i.e., creating metadata for the dataset) is essential for reuse for policy as well as other purposes. To meet this need, the Center for Expanded Data Annotation and Retrieval (CEDAR) at Stanford University is generating community-based metadata standards and a metadata repository for training learning algorithms to develop metadata templates that customize themselves as the user enters data about the dataset (Musen et al., 2015). Second, as illustrated in the fall detection example (Rantz, Skubic, et al., 2015), sensors can provide important data for surveillance and intervention. Researchers at the Center of Excellence for Mobile Sensor Data-to-Knowledge are developing innovative tools to make it easier to gather, analyze, and interpret data from mobile sensors (Kumar et al., 2015). Its test cases for the tools reflect two outcomes of relevance to nursing science: reducing hospital readmissions for patients with congestive heart failure and preventing relapse in those who have quit smoking. Third, nursing science that has the potential to influence policy will increasingly be based upon multiple data streams. The Patient-Center Information Commons: Standardized Unification of Research Elements (PIC-SURE, 2016) at Harvard Medical School is focusing on the challenge of linking biomedical data (Weber, Mandl, & Kohane, 2014) and developing systems to combine genetic, environmental, imaging, behavioral, and clinical data on individual patients from multiple sources into integrated sets.

The promise of these data science efforts as a foundation for advancing policy through nursing science can only be achieved if they are informed by the diverse needs of nurse scientists. Consequently, it is important for nurse scientists to get involved with BD2K at the federal or more local level through the BD2K centers. In addition, since data science is interdisciplinary and there is much to be learned from initiatives outside of health and biomedicine, participation in university-level data science initiatives has the potential to lay the foundation for advancing policy through nursing science.

Lessons from the participation of nurse scientists in the Clinical and Translational Science Award program (Knafl & Grey, 2008; Sampselle, Knafl, Jacob, & McCloskey, 2013) suggest not only that nursing science will benefit from the BD2K and other data science infrastructure, but also that data science will benefit from the participation of nurse scientists, including in the area of data science policy. Given that nursing science is female dominated, it can take advantage of what Berman and Bourne recently characterized as the priority for gender diversity in data science to exude its influence (Berman & Bourne, 2015). The influence is likely to be broad and deep, but only two aspects are highlighted here: consideration of individuals in context and adherence to bioethical principles. First, nursing science has a long history of studying individuals in the context of their social (e.g., family, culture) and physical environments. This has implications for data science in terms of the variety of data sources that must be wrangled (i.e., obtained, scrubbed, filtered, and so on). Second, bioethics has been an area of inquiry for nurse scientists with particular attention to ethics associated with research participation. This has resulted in explication of issues as well as development of approaches to ensure the validity of the informed consent process and enhance the participation of those typically underrepresented in research (E. Cohn & Larson, 2007; E. G. Cohn, Jia, Smith, Erwin, & Larson, 2011; Larson et al., 2015; Larson, Cohn, Meyer, & Boden-Albala, 2009). While some big data streams are available without informed consent, others are not and careful distinction must be paid to ensure the protection of research participants. In addition, nurse scientists have developed innovative models of engaging underrepresented populations that can be scaled up to inform data science policy. For example, the WICER/WICER 4 U research team developed an approach that integrates participatory design of information visualizations of patient-reported outcomes and other measures (Arcia et al., 2016; Arcia, Velez, & Bakken, 2015; Unertl et al., 2015) with tailored results reporting to research participants not only to motivate self-management and maximize the benefits of the data, but also as a mechanism for continued engagement in the research process. The software that produces the information visualizations, Electronic Tailored Infographics for Community Engagement, Education, and Empowerment (EnTICE[3]; Velez, Bales, Arcia, & Bakken, 2014), as well as the participatory design processes, is being expanded to integrate new data streams including genomic results (Bakken, Arcia, & Woollen, 2016). Such innovations are relevant to the data science and engagement aspects of the PMI cohort.

CONCLUSION

The increasing availability of big data streams combined with data science methods provides the opportunity for advancement of nursing science. Nursing science has generated significant foundations for applying data science. Moreover, there are now examples of interdisciplinary programs of research led by nurse scientists that integrate data science methods. To take full advantage of the opportunities provided by the drivers for data science, nurse scientists must enhance their data science skills as generalists or specialists, establish centers of excellence and pre- and postdoctoral training programs that integrate data science competencies, engage in interdisciplinary collaborative data science teams, and inform the development and implementation of data science resources and tools that meet the diverse needs of nurse scientists. The synergy between nursing science and data science is essential for advancing nursing science that informs health policy.

REFERENCES

Ahalt, S. C., Bizen, C., Evans, J., Erlich, Y., Ginsburg, G. S., Krishnamurthy, A., . . . Wilhelmsen, K. (2014). *Data to discovery: Genes to health: A white paper from the National Consortium for Data Science: The National Consortium for Data Science*. Chapel, NC: University of North Carolina.

Alfaro, E., Dhruva, A., Langford, D. J., Koetters, T., Merriman, J. D., West, C., . . . Miaskowski, C. (2014). Associations between cytokine gene variations and self-reported sleep disturbance in women following breast cancer surgery. *European Journal of Oncology Nursing, 18*(1), 85–93.

American Nurses Association. (2010). *Nursing's social policy statement: The essence of the profession* (3rd ed.). Silver Spring, MD: Author.

Arcia, A., Suero-Tejeda, N., Bales, M. E., Merrill, J. A., Yoon, S., Woollen, J., & Bakken, S. (2016). Sometimes more is more: Iterative participatory design of infographics for engagement of community members with varying levels of health literacy. *Journal of the American Medical Informatics Association, 23*(1), 174–183.

Arcia, A., Velez, M., & Bakken, S. (2015). Style guide: An interdisciplinary communication tool to support the process of generating tailored infographics from electronic health data using EnTICE3. *eGEMS (Washington, DC), 3*(1), 1120.

Bakken, S., Arcia, A., & Woollen, J. (2016). *Integrating community-engaged and informatics-based approaches for precision medicine results reporting to urban Latinos*. AMIA Joint Summits on Translational Science Proceedings, eCollection 2016. Retrieved from https://knowledge.amia.org

Bakken, S., & Reame, N. (2016). The promise and potential perils of big data for advancing symptom management research in populations at risk for health disparities. *Annual Review of Nursing Research, 34*(1), 247–260.

Berman, F. D., & Bourne, P. E. (2015). Let's make gender diversity in data science a priority right from the start. *PLOS Biology, 13*(7), e1002206.

Bowles, K. H., Chittams, J., Heil, E., Topaz, M., Rickard, K., Bhasker, M., . . . Hanlon, A. L. (2015). Successful electronic implementation of discharge referral decision support has a positive impact on 30- and 60-day readmissions. *Research in Nursing and Health, 38*(2), 102–114.

Brennan, P. F., & Bakken, S. (2015). Nursing needs big data and big data needs nursing. *Journal of Nursing Scholarship, 47*(5), 477–484.

Brennan, P. F., Ponto, K., Casper, G., Tredinnick, R., & Broecker, M. (2015). Virtualizing living and working spaces: Proof of concept for a biomedical space-replication methodology. *Journal of Biomedical Informatics, 57*, 53–61.

Brown, D. S., Donaldson, N., Burnes Bolton, L., & Aydin, C. E. (2010). Nursing-sensitive benchmarks for hospitals to gauge high-reliability performance. *Journal of Healthcare Quality, 32*(6), 9–17.

Cashion, A. K., & Grady, P. A. (2015). The National Institutes of Health/National Institutes of Nursing Research intramural research program and the development of the National Institutes of Health Symptom Science Model. *Nursing Outlook, 63*(4), 484–487.

Centers for Disease Control and Prevention. (2015). Social ecological model. Retrieved from http://www.cdc.gov/ViolencePrevention/overview/social-ecologicalmodel.html

Clancy, T. R. (2004). Navigating in a complex nursing world. *Journal of Nursing Administration, 34*(6), 274–282.

Clancy, T. R., Delaney, C. W., Segre, A., Carley, K., Kuziak, A., & Yu, H. (2007). Predicting the impact of an electronic health record on practice patterns using computational modeling and simulation. *AMIA Annual Symposium Proceedings*, 145–149.

Clancy, T. R., Effken, J. A., & Pesut, D. (2008). Applications of complex systems theory in nursing education, research, and practice. *Nursing Outlook, 56*(5), 248–256.

Cohn, E., & Larson, E. (2007). Improving participant comprehension in the informed consent process. *Journal of Nursing Scholarship, 39*(3), 273–280.

Cohn, E. G., Jia, H., Smith, W. C., Erwin, K., & Larson, E. L. (2011). Measuring the process and quality of informed consent for clinical research: Development and testing. *Oncology Nursing Forum, 38*(4), 417–422.

Collins, F. S., & Varmus, H. (2015). A new initiative on precision medicine. *New England Journal of Medicine, 372*(9), 793–795.

Dang, J. H., Rodriguez, E. M., Luque, J. S., Erwin, D. O., Meade, C. D., & Chen, M. S., Jr. (2014). Engaging diverse populations about biospecimen donation for cancer research. *Journal of Community Genetics, 5*(4), 313–327.

Danko, A., Kennedy, R., Haskell, R., Androwich, I. M., Button, P., Correia, C. M., . . . Russler, D. (2003). Modeling nursing interventions in the act class of HL7 RIM Version 3. *Journal of Biomedical Informatics, 36*(4–5), 294–303.

Dey, S., Cooner, J., Delaney, C. W., Fakhoury, J., Kumar, V., Simon, G., . . . Westra, B. L. (2015). Mining patterns associated with mobility outcomes in home healthcare. *Nursing Research, 64*(4), 235–245.

Dunn, K. S. (2005). Testing a middle-range theoretical model of adaptation to chronic pain. *Nursing Science Quarterly, 18*(2), 146–156.

Dykes, P. C., Carroll, D. L., Hurley, A., Lipsitz, S., Benoit, A., Chang, F., . . . Middleton, B. (2010). Fall prevention in acute care hospitals: A randomized trial. *JAMA, 304*(17), 1912–1918.

Fleurence, R. L., Curtis, L. H., Califf, R. M., Platt, R., Selby, J. V., & Brown, J. S. (2014). Launching PCORnet, a national patient-centered clinical research network. *Journal of the American Medical Informatics Association, 21*(4), 578–582.

Hardiker, N. R. (2003). Logical ontology for mediating between nursing intervention terminology systems. *Methods of Information in Medicine, 42*(3), 265–270.

Hardiker, N. R., & Coenen, A. (2007). Interpretation of an international terminology standard in the development of a logic-based compositional terminology. *International Journal of Medical Informatics, 76*(2), S274–S280.

Harris, M. R., Langford, L. H., Miller, H., Hook, M., Dykes, P. C., & Matney, S. A. (2015). Harmonizing and extending standards from a domain-specific and bottom-up approach: An example from development through use in clinical applications. *Journal of the American Medical Informatics Association, 22*(3), 545–552.

Henry, S. B., Holzemer, W. L., Reilly, C. A., & Campbell, K. E. (1994). Terms used by nurses to describe patient problems: Can SNOMED III represent nursing concepts in the patient record? *Journal of the American Medical Informatics Association, 1*(1), 61–74.

Hyun, S., & Bakken, S. (2006). Toward the creation of an ontology for nursing document sections: Mapping section headings to the LOINC semantic model. *AMIA Annual Symposium Proceedings*, 364–368.

Hyun, S., Johnson, S. B., & Bakken, S. (2009). Exploring the ability of natural language processing to extract data from nursing narratives. *Computers, Informatics, Nursing, 27*(4), 215–223.

Hyun, S., Shapiro, J. S., Melton, G., Schlegel, C., Stetson, P. D., Johnson, S. B., & Bakken, S. (2009). Iterative evaluation of the health level 7-logical observation identifiers names and codes clinical document ontology for representing clinical document names: A case report. *Journal of the American Medical Informatics Association, 16*(3), 395–399.

IBM. (2015). The Four V's of Big Data. Retrieved from http://www.ibmbigdatahub.com/infographic/four-vs-big-data

Jing, X., Kay, S., Marley, T., Hardiker, N. R., & Cimino, J. J. (2012). Incorporating personalized gene sequence variants, molecular genetics knowledge, and health knowledge into an EHR prototype based on the Continuity of Care Record standard. *Journal of Biomedical Informatics, 45*(1), 82–92.

Johnson, S. B., Bakken, S., Dine, D., Hyun, S., Mendonca, E., Morrison, F., . . . Stetson, P. (2008). An electronic health record based on structured narrative. *Journal of the American Medical Informatics Association, 15*(1), 54–64.

Kahn, J. P., Vayena, E., & Mastroianni, A. C. (2014). Opinion: Learning as we go: Lessons from the publication of Facebook's social-computing research. *Proceedings of the National Academy of Sciences USA, 111*(38), 13677–13679.

Keeling, J., Pryde, J., & Merrill, J. (2013). The influence of management and environment on local health department organizational structure and adaptation: A longitudinal case study using network analysis. *Journal of Public Health Management & Practice, 19*(6), 598–605.

Knafl, K., & Grey, M. (2008). Clinical translational science awards: Opportunities and challenges for nurse scientists. *Nursing Outlook, 56*(3), 132–137, e134.

Kohen, R., Tracy, J. H., Haugen, E., Cain, K. C., Jarrett, M. E., & Heitkemper, M. M. (2016). Rare variants of the serotonin transporter are associated with psychiatric comorbidity in irritable bowel syndrome. *Biological Research in Nursing, 18*(4), 394–400.

Koleck, T. A., & Conley, Y. P. (2016). Identification and prioritization of candidate genes for symptom variability in breast cancer survivors based on disease characteristics at the cellular level. *Breast Cancer (Dove Med Press), 8*, 29–37.

Kumar, S., Abowd, G. D., Abraham, W. T., al'Absi, M., Beck, J. G., Chau, D. H., . . . Wetter, D. W. (2015). Center of excellence for mobile sensor data-to-knowledge (MD2K). *Journal of the American Medical Informatics Association, 22*(6), 1137–1142.

Larson, E. L., Cohn, E. G., Meyer, D. D., & Boden-Albala, B. (2009). Consent administrator training to reduce disparities in research participation. *Journal of Nursing Scholarship, 41*(1), 95–103.

Larson, E. L., Lally, R., Foe, G., Joaquin, G., Meyer, D. D., & Cohn, E. G. (2015). Improving the proficiency of research consent administrators. *Clinical and Translational Science, 8*(4), 351–354.

Lee, Y. J., Boden-Albala, B., Jia, H., Wilcox, A., & Bakken, S. (2015). The association between online health information-seeking behaviors and health behaviors among Hispanics in New York City: A community-based cross-sectional study. *Journal of Medical Internet Research, 17*(11), e261.

Liu, L., Popescu, M., Skubic, M., & Rantz, M. (2014). An automatic fall detection framework using data fusion of Doppler radar and motion sensor network. In *Engineering in Medicine and Biology Society (EMBC), 2014 36th Annual International Conference of the IEEE* (pp. 5940–5943). New York, NY: Institute of Electrical and Electronics Engineers.

Marr, B. (2015). Big data: The 5 Vs. Retrieved from http://www.slideshare.net/BernardMarr/140228-big-data-volume-velocity-variety-varacity-value

Mason, H., & Wiggins, C. (2010). A taxonomy of data science. Retrieved from http://www.dataists.com/2010/09/a-taxonomy-of-data-science

Matney, S. A., Dolin, G., Buhl, L., & Sheide, A. (2016). Communicating nursing care using the health level seven consolidated clinical document architecture release 2 care plan. *Computers, Informatics, Nursing, 34*(3), 128–136.

Matney, S. A., Warren, J. J., Evans, J. L., Kim, T. Y., Coenen, A., & Auld, V. A. (2012). Development of the nursing problem list subset of SNOMED CT(R). *Journal of Biomedical Informatics, 45*(4), 683–688.

Meeker, D. (Producer). (2014). Herding ponies: How big data methods facilitate collaborative analytics. Retrieved from http://slidegur.com/doc/145598/daniella-meeker

Merrill, J., Keeling, J., & Carley, K. (2010). A comparative analysis of 11 local health department organizational networks. *Journal of Public Health Management and Practice, 16*(6), 564–576.

Musen, M. A., Bean, C. A., Cheung, K. H., Dumontier, M., Durante, K. A., Gevaert, O., . . . CEDAR Team. (2015). The Center for Expanded Data Annotation and Retrieval. *Journal of the American Medical Informatics Association, 22*(6), 1148–1152.

The National Commission for the Protection of Human Subjects of Biomedical and Behavioral Research. (1979). *The Belmont report: Ethical principles and guidelines for the protection of human subjects of research.* Washington, DC: U.S. Department of Health and Human Services.

National Institute of Nursing Research. (2016a). NINR Strategic plan. Retrieved from www.ninr.nih.gov

National Institute of Nursing Research. (2016b). NINR "Precision health: From 'Omics' to data science" boot camp. Retrieved from http://www.ninr.nih.gov/training/trainingopportunities intramural/bootcamp#.VyfHG4QrLIU

National Institutes of Health. (2015). The NIH Commons. Retrieved from https://datascience .nih.gov/commons

National Institutes of Health. (2016a). BD2K investments in training. Retrieved from https:// datascience.nih.gov/bd2k

National Institutes of Health. (2016b). Data science. Retrieved from https://datascience.nih.gov/ bd2k/about/what

National Institutes of Health. (2016c). Health data initiative. Retrieved from http://www.health data.gov

National Library of Medicine. (2015). Common data element (CDE) resource portal. Retrieved from https://www.nlm.nih.gov/cde

Odlum, M., & Yoon, S. (2015). What can we learn about the Ebola outbreak from tweets? *American Journal of Infection Control, 43*(6), 563–571.

Patient-Center Information Commons: Standardized Unification of Research Elements. (2016). Creating an information commons for biomedical data centered on the patient. Retrieved from http://www.pic-sure.org

Rantz, M. J., Lane, K., Phillips, L. J., Despins, L. A., Galambos, C., Alexander, G. L., . . . Miller, S. J. (2015). Enhanced registered nurse care coordination with sensor technology: Impact on length of stay and cost in aging in place housing. *Nursing Outlook, 63*(6), 650–655.

Rantz, M. J., Skubic, M., Popescu, M., Galambos, C., Koopman, R. J., Alexander, G. L., . . . Miller, S. J. (2015). A new paradigm of technology-enabled "Vital Signs" for early detection of health change for older adults. *Gerontology, 61*(3), 281–290.

Redeker, N. S., Anderson, R., Bakken, S., Corwin, E., Docherty, S., Dorsey, S. G., . . . Grady, P. (2015). Advancing symptom science through use of common data elements. *Journal of Nursing Scholarship, 47*(5), 379–388.

Riegel, B., Jaarsma, T., & Stromberg, A. (2012). A middle-range theory of self-care of chronic illness. *Advances in Nursing Science, 35*(3), 194–204.

Roy, C. (2011). Research based on the Roy adaptation model: Last 25 years. *Nursing Science Quarterly, 24*(4), 312–320.

Sampselle, C. M., Knafl, K. A., Jacob, J. D., & McCloskey, D. J. (2013). Nurse engagement and contributions to the clinical and translational science awards initiative. *Clinical and Translational Science, 6*(3), 191–195.

Shaibi, G. Q., Coletta, D. K., Vital, V., & Mandarino, L. J. (2013). The design and conduct of a community-based registry and biorepository: A focus on cardiometabolic health in Latinos. *Clinical and Translational Science, 6*(6), 429–434.

Unertl, K. M., Schaefbauer, C. L., Campbell, T. R., Senteio, C., Siek, K. A., Bakken, S., & Veinot, T. C. (2015). Integrating community-based participatory research and informatics approaches to improve the engagement and health of underserved populations. *Journal of the American Medical Informatics Association, 23*(1), 60–73.

Vayena, E., Salathe, M., Madoff, L. C., & Brownstein, J. S. (2015). Ethical challenges of big data in public health. *PLOS Computational Biolology, 11*(2), e1003904.

Velez, M., Bales, M. E., Arcia, A., & Bakken, S. (2014). Electronic tailored infographics for community engagement, education, and empowerment (EnTICE3). *AMIA 2014 Joint Summits in Translational Science (abstract), eCollection 2014.* Retrieved from https://knowledge.amia.org

Weber, G. M., Mandl, K. D., & Kohane, I. S. (2014). Finding the missing link for big biomedical data. *JAMA, 311*(24), 2479–2480.

Westra, B. L., Latimer, G. E., Matney, S. A., Park, J. I., Sensmeier, J., Simpson, R. L., . . . Delaney, C. W. (2015). A national action plan for sharable and comparable nursing data to support practice and translational research for transforming health care. *Journal of the American Medical Informatics Association, 22*(3), 600–607.

Wilcox, A., Weng, C., Bigger, J. T., Boden-Albala, B., Bakken, S., Feldman, P., . . . Kaplan, S. (2011). Beyond Framingham: Creating an informatics infrastructure for patient-centered outcomes research in an at-risk population. *AMIA 2011 Joint Summits in Translational Science, eCollection 2011.* Retrieved from https://knowledge.amia.org

Wilcox, A. B., Gallagher, K., & Bakken, S. (2013). Security approaches in using tablet computers for primary data collection in clinical research. *eGEMS (Wash DC), 1*(1), 1008.

Wilkinson, M. D., Dumontier, M., Aalbersberg, I. J., Appleton, G., Axton, M., Baak, A., . . . Mons, B. (2016). The FAIR guiding principles for scientific data management and stewardship. *Science Data, 3,* 160018.

Yoon, S., & Bakken, S. (2010). What can we learn about physical activity from tweets? *Proceedings of the AMIA Symposium, 2010,* 1318.

Yoon, S., Elhadad, N., & Bakken, S. (2013). A practical approach for content mining of tweets. *American Journal of Preventive Medicine, 45*(1), 122–129.

Yoon, S., Hunter, B., & Bakken, S. (under review). Visualization of topics from Twitter and focus groups as the foundation for insights about dementia caregiving. *Proceedings of the AMIA Symposium, 2016.*

Yoon, S., Shaffer, J., Momberg, J., & Bakken, S. (2013). Examining motivation in physical activity Tweets. *Proceedings of the AMIA Symposium, 2013.*

Yoon, S., Wilcox, A., & Bakken, S. (2013). Comparison of a community health behavior survey and a National Health Behavior survey. *eGEMs, 1*(1), 1–5, 9.

7

Self-Management of Illness in Teens

Margaret Grey and Kaitlyn Rechenberg

It is increasingly recognized that self- and family management of chronic conditions is an essential aspect of today's health care (Newman, Steed, & Mulligan, 2009). *Self-management* has been defined in several ways in the literature, but it is usually defined as a dynamic, interactive, and daily process in which individuals engage to manage a chronic illness (Ruggiero et al., 1997). It also is defined as the ability of the individual, in conjunction with family, community, and health care professionals, to manage symptoms, treatments, lifestyle changes, and psychosocial, cultural, and spiritual consequences of health conditions. Corbin and Strauss (1991) were among the first to describe the work related to living with a chronic illness, and they defined the work as illness-related work (e.g., managing symptoms or crisis prevention, often named *illness management*), everyday life work (e.g., managing work or household tasks, often described as *role management*), and biographical work (e.g., managing emotions or identity). In a report from the Institute of Medicine (IOM), *self-management* was defined as including the tasks related to management of medical or behavioral treatments, role management, and emotional management (Adams, Greiner, & Corrigan, 2004).

Self-management by those with chronic conditions and their families is critical to ensuring the best possible outcomes. Thus, interventions that provide patients and their families with information and skills that enhance their ability to participate in their health care (e.g., communicate with health professionals, identify relevant information, manage symptoms, perform health behaviors, adhere to multiple treatment requirements) are increasingly recognized, not only as an essential component of management of chronic conditions, but also as part of secondary prevention and as a way of reducing the burden of chronic conditions on individuals, families, and communities. Accordingly, self- and family management of chronic conditions is receiving increased attention in health care reform. Supporting patient self-management is, for example, a key component of Wagner's Chronic Care Model (Wagner et al., 2001) and the patient-centered medical home (Parekh, Goodman,

Gordon, Koh, & HHS Intra-agency Workgroup on Multiple Chronic Conditions, 2011), and is one of the four goals in the U.S. Department of Health and Human Services framework for addressing complex chronic conditions (U.S. Department of Health & Human Services, 2011). An IOM report pointed to the importance of identifying family-level risk and protective factors that contribute to the health and well-being of family members (IOM & National Research Council, 2011).

Nursing plays a central role in addressing the challenges of chronic condition management, as reflected in the recent recommendations by the IOM and the National Institute of Nursing Research (IOM, 2010; NINR, 2011). The enhancement of individuals' and families' capacities to prevent or manage chronic conditions is a core activity of nursing that is supported by a growing body of knowledge. Enhancing self- and family management to improve quality of life and health outcomes continues to be a scientific priority supported by the NINR (2011). As noted in the new NINR Strategic Plan (2016), "NINR supports research to discover new ways to promote health and prevent disease" and "on new and better ways to manage symptoms of acute and chronic illness." Both of these scientific areas require the understanding of and interventions to improve self-management.

Chronic conditions in childhood and adolescence require not just the development of self-management skills and behaviors for the affected youth, but also partnership with the family and health care providers to ensure better health and quality of life outcomes. In this chapter, we provide a review of prominent clinical trial research in the area of self-management of illness in teens and discuss those that have moved to public policy in detail.

SCOPE OF THE REVIEW

We searched the electronic databases Medline, Embase, PsychINFO, and CINAHL. The initial search terms included "self-management," "self-efficacy," and "chronic disease" (or chronic illness), and these were used consistently in each database when the search term matched a keyword. When "self-management" was not a keyword, the included search term was "self-management-ti.ab." For example, the search strategy for PsychINFO was as follows: (a) exp Self-Management, (b) exp Self-Efficacy, and (c) exp Chronic Illness, with the following limitations: published in English within the past 10 years with participants 18 years old or younger. The entire search yielded 248 articles, 136 of which were eliminated because they either did not include a pediatric population, or because they were not topically appropriate. The final sample of the initial search consisted of 112 articles.

Keywords from articles in the final sample and from articles known to be important in the field were reviewed to ensure that all relevant search terms were included. The reference lists of included articles were also reviewed to assess for outliers. Two additional searches were conducted. Keywords from the second search were "psychoeducation," "self-care," and "chronic disease" (or chronic illness), and from the third search included "technology," "Internet," and "chronic disease" (or chronic illness). When "psychoeducation" was not a keyword, "psychoeducation-ti.ab." was used. The same limitations described in the preceding paragraph were used. After removal of duplicates and review of articles for relevance, 13 articles were retained from the second search and four articles were retained from the third search. Detailed search strings for all databases are available upon request. In addition, we searched for articles authored by people well known to have conducted research with teens with chronic conditions.

The full citations of all identified titles, including bibliographic details, keywords, abstract, and web addresses (when available), were imported into the online bibliographic management program *RefWorks*™ and combined into a database. Articles were included if they were published between 2005 and 2015, evaluated a pediatric population, and included a self-management intervention. Excluded articles were (a) topically not appropriate, (b) written in a language other than English, (c) case studies, and (d) duplicates. The titles and abstracts of all articles were reviewed for relevance. Potentially relevant articles were retained for further review. The articles remaining in the final sample were read and organized into the following categories: (a) interventions, (b) exploratory/descriptive studies, (c) family focused, (d) transitional care, (e) review articles, and (f) other. This process was repeated for each search.

APPROACHES TO IMPROVING SELF-MANAGEMENT IN TEENS

Although self-management is critical across a variety of chronic conditions, and there are commonalities in self-management (Grey, Knafl, Schulman-Green, & Reynolds, 2015), the majority of interventions that have been tested in rigorous studies focus on a single condition. Therefore, we have divided our presentation of the studies according to conditions where there was at least one randomized clinical trial. Study details of the trials included in this review can be found in Table 7.1.

Asthma

Asthma is the most common chronic illness in childhood. Management of asthma and avoiding high-risk exacerbations requires not only adherence to asthma medications but also to regular testing of respiratory capacity to detect early changes. Barriers to self-management in adolescents include being unwilling to give up things providers tell them to, difficulty in remembering to do self-management, and trying to forget that they have asthma (Rhee, Belyea, Ciurzynski, & Brasch, 2009). Thus, as is true with many conditions, youth with asthma require substantial self-management support.

Early approaches to self-management support for adolescents with asthma were educational in nature. In a meta-analysis of randomized controlled trials conducted prior to 2001, such educational interventions were found to be less effective in improving lung function and self-efficacy than more comprehensive behavioral self-management approaches (Guevara, Wolf, Grum, & Clark, 2003). Rhee et al. (2011)

TABLE 7.1　*Descriptions of Trials of Self-Management Interventions in Teens*

Author(s) (Date)	Sample	Intervention	Findings
Asthma			
Rhee, Belyea, Hunt, and Brasch (2011)	112 youth, 13–17 years, attending a day camp	Peer-led asthma self-management program	More positive attitudes, higher quality of life, improved spirometry results
Velsor-Friedrich et al. (2012)	137 African American youth, 15–18 years	Coping skills training with standard asthma education delivered in high schools	Increased asthma quality of life, knowledge, and self-efficacy; decreases in symptom days and asthma-related school absences
Type I Diabetes			
Grey, Boland, Davidson, Li, and Tamborlane (2000)	90 youth, age 12–20	Group-based coping skills training	Improved glycemic control, self-efficacy, and quality of life
Grey et al. (2013)	324 youth, age 11–14, 27% minority	Internet-based coping skills training and advanced diabetes education	Improved glycemic control, quality of life, social acceptance, perceived stress, and reduced family conflict
Whittemore et al. (2015)	124 youth, 25% minority	Internet-based coping skills training and advanced diabetes education	Improved glycemic control and quality of life, lower perceived stress
Laffel, Brackett, Ho, and Anderson (1999)	171 youth, 10–15 years	Care Ambassadors to assist with logistical issues related to keeping appointments	Improved glycemic control, reduced risk of hypoglycemia and hospitalizations
Svoren, Butler, Levine, Anderson, and Laffel (2003)	299 youth, 7–16 years	Care Ambassadors plus eight 30-minute psychoeducational models delivered at clinic visits	Improved clinic visit frequency, reduced rates of hospitalization
Laffel et al. (2003)	105 children and adolescents, 8–17 years	Family-focused teamwork delivered to teens transitioning to adolescence	Improved glycemic control, but not in family conflict or quality of life
Raiff and Dallery (2010)	4 teens, 12–18 years	Contingency management to reward performance of daily self-management tasks	More blood glucose tests performed
Stanger et al. (2013)	17 teens, age 12–17 years, 12 non-Hispanic White, 4 African American, 2 multiracial	Contingency management plus motivational interviewing	More frequent blood glucose monitoring and improved glycemic control
Holmes, Chen, Mackey, Grey, and Streisand (2014)	226 youth, age 11–14 years, 28% minority	Clinic-based teamwork and coping skills training	Both groups showed no deterioration in outcomes over time, but the teamwork group had greater improvements in adherence to self-management and glycemic control

(continued)

TABLE 7.1 *Descriptions of Trials of Self-Management Interventions in Teens (continued)*

Author(s) (Date)	Sample	Intervention	Findings
Obesity			
Melnyk et al. (2007)	23 overweight teens, 63% Black	COPE Healthy Lifestyles TEEN program, educational information, and CBT	Reduction in weight and BMI
Melnyk et al. (2009)	19 Hispanic youth	COPE Healthy Lifestyles TEEN program	Increased healthy lifestyles choices and decreased depressive and anxiety symptoms
Melnyk et al. (2013)	779 (70% Latino), 14–16 years	COPE Healthy Lifestyles TEEN program	Increased physical activity, lower BMI, higher health course grades
Grey, Whittemore, et al. (2009)	198 7th grade students at high risk for type 2 diabetes, 45% Hispanic, 43% African American	Nutrition and physical activity education plus coping skills training and weekly coaching for behavior change	Improvement in weight, lipids, depressive symptoms, and reduction of metabolic risk on oral glucose tolerance tests. No change in BMI
Whittemore, Jeon, and Grey (2013)	384 high school pupils, 70% minority	HEALTH[e]TEEN, an Internet-based program of healthy eating, physical activity, and behavioral support to reduce obesity and overweight	Improvements in health behaviors, but not weight
Family			
Sullivan-Bolyai, Bova, Leung, Trudeau, and Gruppuso (2010)	42 mothers of children with newly diagnosed diabetes	Family social support for parents of children <13 years with newly diagnosed type 1 diabetes	Improved overall family management of diabetes

BMI, body mass index; CBT, cognitive behavioral training; COPE, Creating Opportunities for Personal Empowerment; TEEN, Thinking, Emotions, Exercise, and Nutrition.

conducted a randomized clinical trial of a peer-lead asthma self-management program for adolescents compared to a conventional adult-led asthma program. The peer-led program yielded greater improvements in attitudes, quality of time, and spirometry results compared to the control group. In a more recent randomized clinical trial conducted in low-income urban African American schools, Velsor-Friedrich et al. (2012) found that both a coping skills training (CST) program and a traditional asthma education program led to increases in asthma-related quality of life, knowledge, and self-efficacy as well as decreases in symptom days and asthma-related school absences, but that CST did not improve on the educational program's results.

Type 1 Diabetes

Type 1 diabetes is also one of the most common severe chronic illnesses in children, affecting more than 200,000 youth in the United States (Chiang, Kirkman, Laffel,

Peters, & Type 1 Diabetes Sourcebook authors, 2014). Youth with type 1 diabetes are at a high risk of negative psychosocial and physiological outcomes, particularly during adolescence. There are considerable demands associated with living with the condition. The treatment regimen is complex and demanding, requiring constant monitoring of blood glucose and carbohydrate intake, performing daily insulin therapy, and adjusting insulin dose to match diet and activity (Chiang et al., 2014). Appropriate self-management of these daily tasks helps to reduce short- and long-term diabetes-related complications (Grey, Whittemore, et al., 2009). In teens who are struggling for independence, self-management often suffers. Thus, improvement of self-management in youth has the potential not only to enhance diabetes management, but also to promote psychosocial adjustment.

CST is a method of improving competence and mastery by modifying ineffective coping behaviors into more constructive behaviors (Grey, Whittemore, et al., 2009). CST is based on social cognitive theory, which suggests that individuals can impact many areas of their lives, particularly with regard to coping style and health behaviors (Bandura, 1997). This approach aims to enhance self-efficacy through the development and rehearsal of new behaviors, such as the use of stress reduction techniques (Grey, Boland, Davidson, Li, & Tamborlane, 2000). These authors designed a CST program for youth with type 1 diabetes that aimed to improve sense of competence and mastery by modifying nonconstructive coping styles. The coping skills of social problem solving, stress management, assertiveness, and reducing negative thinking were emphasized. In a randomized controlled trial, Grey, Boland, et al. (2000) provided the training in small groups of two to three participants and compared their outcomes to a group receiving only intensive diabetes management. The trainer leading the CST groups used role playing to model appropriate coping behaviors. Six weekly sessions of approximately 1 hour were conducted, followed by monthly visits over the 12-month follow-up period. As compared to the control group, those who received CST had improved outcomes, including improved glycemic control, self-efficacy, and quality of life.

After determining the efficacy of group-based CST in youth with type 1 diabetes, this intervention was adapted to an Internet-based format (TEENCOPE) to reach teens who could not attend group sessions (Grey, Whittemore, Liberti, et al., 2012; Whittemore, Grey, Lindemann, Ambrosino, & Jaser, 2010). Another rationale for moving to the Internet was to deliver the intervention in a manner that would not interrupt clinic flow. Providing psychoeducational interventions in an online platform allowed for wider distribution of the program, especially as 93% of youth regularly use the Internet nationwide (Pew Research Center, 2015; Whittemore, Grey, et al., 2010). In a multisite randomized control trial, TEENCOPE was compared to an Internet-based diabetes management educational intervention (Managing Diabetes). Grey, Whittemore, Jeon, et al. (2013) reported the 18-month outcomes of this study, after participants were offered the opportunity to cross over to the other intervention at 12 months. There were no significant differences between groups at 18 months, with all participants showing improvements in glycosylated hemoglobin, quality of life, social acceptance, self-efficacy, perceived stress, and family conflict. It was concluded that these Internet interventions improved outcomes in youth with type 1 diabetes, but that both diabetes management education and CST were both necessary.

This research group then developed Teens.Connect, a combined program of TEENCOPE and Managing Diabetes (Whittemore, Liberti, et al., 2015). In a randomized controlled trial, Teens.Connect was compared to a website designed by the American Diabetes Association (ADA) that provided age-appropriate diabetes education. Six-month outcomes indicated that both Teens.Connect and the control program led to improved outcomes in youth with type 1 diabetes. Teens.Connect users, however, reported lower perceived stress than the control group.

Laffel et al. (1999) designed the Care Ambassador intervention to increase ambulatory medical visits for youth with type 1 diabetes. Care Ambassador participants received assistance with appointment scheduling and confirmation, and their families received help with logistical issues related to diabetes care. Compared to standard care, participants in the intervention group had lower glycosylated hemoglobin levels and a reduced risk of severe hypoglycemia and hospitalization at 24 months. Svoren et al. (2003) combined the Care Ambassador intervention with eight 30-minute psychoeducational modules delivered at each clinic visit by the Care Ambassadors. Three groups were compared: the Care Ambassador intervention, the Care Ambassadors plus the psychoeducational modules, and standard care. Both the Care Ambassadors and the Care Ambassadors plus psychoeducation module interventions improved clinic visit frequency compared to standard care. However, Care Ambassadors plus psychoeducation modules reduced rates of hospitalization and hypoglycemia as compared to the Care Ambassador intervention alone and standard care.

A family-focused teamwork intervention was developed by Laffel et al. (2003) with the goal of improving glycemic control, family conflict, and quality of life in youth with type 1 diabetes transitioning to adolescence. The intervention involved structured meetings with patients and parents at quarterly diabetes visits. Importantly, the focus of the discussion was on issues that are of concern to both parents and youth with diabetes about developing self-management and addressing conflict as the youth seek more independence. The research assistant presented brief modules addressing sharing diabetes tasks and resolving conflict, and then provided a forum for patients and parents to discuss the topic. After the intervention, the research assistant helped the family to negotiate a responsibility-sharing plan, in which each individual's responsibility for maintaining various components of the treatment regimen was outlined. Each session of the intervention lasted approximately 15 minutes. In a randomized controlled trial, the teamwork group showed improvements in glycemic control after 1 year, compared to a group receiving standard multidisciplinary diabetes care. However, the teamwork intervention did not lead to significant improvements in family conflict or quality of life.

Contingency management is designed to motivate participants to complete adherence behaviors by providing a reward for performing daily self-management tasks. Raiff and Dallery (2010) studied an Internet-based contingency management intervention to improve blood glucose testing in youth with type 1 diabetes.

Participants uploaded daily videos showing their blood glucose testing to a secure website, for which they received monetary rewards. In a one-group pretest–posttest study, participants completed significantly more blood glucose tests per day during the contingency management intervention. Similarly, Stanger et al. (2013) tested a combined motivational interviewing and contingency management intervention. During the motivational interviewing, therapists reviewed blood glucose management and diabetes-related self-care over 14 weeks. In addition, youth who checked their blood glucose six or more times daily were rewarded $10 weekly after blood glucose meter data were downloaded at the clinic. In a pretest–posttest study, youth monitored their blood glucose significantly more after the intervention and showed significantly improvements in glycemic control.

Obesity

The incidence of overweight and obesity in youth has increased dramatically over the past decade. Approximately 14.9% of youth in the United States are overweight and an additional 16.9% are obese (Fryar, Carroll, & Ogden, 2014; Ogden, Carroll, Kit, & Flegal, 2014). The rise in obesity is partially due to an increase in sedentary activities and changes in food consumption patterns (Melnyk et al., 2007). Overweight and obese youth are at a higher risk of myriad adverse health conditions than their non-overweight peers, including type 2 diabetes, hypertension, dyslipidemia, sleep apnea, increased asthma severity, and a shortened life span (Centers for Disease Control and Prevention [CDC], 2005; Stabouli, Kotsis, Papamichael, Constantopoulos, & Zakopoulos, 2005). Overweight and obese youth are also vulnerable to school and mental health problems, including anxiety and depression (Bell & Morgan, 2000; Melnyk & Moldenhauser, 2006; Sjöberg, Nilsson, & Leppert, 2005). Lifestyle changes required for managing obesity and preventing the development of obesity-related complications requires ongoing support and follow-up (Jefferson et al., 2011).

Cognitive behavioral therapy is based on the notion that the way an individual thinks impacts emotions and behaviors (Beck, Rush, Shaw, & Emery, 1979). This theory implies that a person who has negative thoughts is more likely to have negative emotions and therefore perform negative behaviors. Melnyk et al. (2007) designed the Creating Opportunities for Personal Empowerment (COPE) Healthy Lifestyles Thinking, Emotions, Exercise, and Nutrition (TEEN) program to provide overweight and obese youth with educational information and cognitive behavioral skills to enhance their beliefs about their ability to perform healthy lifestyle behaviors. The COPE TEEN sessions were manualized and delivered to youth by trained interventionists. Youth received homework assignments between sessions. Compared to a control group that received a youth-specific safety education intervention, youth who received the COPE TEEN intervention demonstrated a significantly greater reduction in weight and body mass index (BMI). In follow-up studies, Melnyk et al. (2009, 2013) studied the COPE TEEN program in Latino adolescents and found that the program led to improved physical activity, lower BMI, and higher health course grades than an education-only control group.

Because CST was effective in youth with type 1 diabetes and was associated with less weight gain despite better metabolic control, Grey, Whittemore, et al. (2009) designed a CST-based intervention for multiethnic youth at a high risk for type 2 diabetes. The intervention included a nutrition education component and a physical activity component, CST classes, and 5- to 10-minute weekly health coaching sessions provided by health professionals. In a randomized controlled trial, one group was randomized to a general education intervention that included only nutrition and physical activity education, while the other group received CST and health coaching in addition to general education. At the end of 12 months, both groups showed improvement in weight, lipids, and depressive symptoms, but not BMI. The intervention group showed significantly more improvement in indicators of metabolic risk as measured by oral glucose tolerance tests, however, than the control group.

Health coaching is a patient-centered process that includes goal setting, problem solving, and mobilizing support systems and are based on Bandura's social cognitive theory (Bandura, 1997). These interventions aim to achieve behavior change through the practice and reinforcement of more adaptive behaviors. Health coaching has been shown to be a promising intervention for reducing BMI and increasing healthy behaviors in youth (Grey, Berry, et al., 2004). Jefferson et al. (2011) designed the telephone-delivered health coaching intervention based on CST for youth in the Grey, Whittemore, et al. (2009) study. Telephone-delivered health coaching was provided in the intervention group of Grey et al.'s larger CST intervention for youth at risk for type 2 diabetes. Coaching began after the 6-week classroom component and occurred weekly for 12 months. Health coaches focused on teaching social problem solving, social skills, communication skills, stress reduction techniques, and conflict resolution. The authors described ways that telephone-delivered health coaching can be used to model and reinforce lifestyle changes in order to improve self-efficacy in youth, including improving social problem solving, communication skills, assertiveness, stress management, conflict resolution skills, and self-talk.

This group developed HEALTH[e]TEEN, an interactive education program that provided eight lessons on healthy eating and physical activity as well as behavioral support to try to reduce obesity and overweight in three high schools with high minority attendance and overweight students (Whittemore, Jeon, & Grey, 2013). The program was developed using a participatory approach with feedback from targeted users and were based on the telephone-delivered interventions described earlier. The program included lessons, self-assessments, questions on content, and individualized feedback. Self-management behavioral strategies included self-monitoring, goal setting, interaction with a health coach, and journaling. In a study involving 384 pupils, student participation and satisfaction with the program was high. The program was adopted and implemented in the schools (Whittemore, Jeon, & Grey, 2013).

Family Management of Chronic Conditions

Of the 6.5 million youth in the United States with a chronic health condition, the majority live in families who must manage the daily demands of these chronic conditions as a unit (Perrin, Bloom, & Gortmacher, 2007; Wollenhaupt, Rodgers, & Sawin, 2012). In many cases, caregivers are responsible for adherence to the daily treatment regimen of most chronic conditions until the child or adolescent is able to manage independently, if possible. Family functioning plays a critical role in disease management in youth with chronic conditions. For example, family functioning and parent–child relationship quality has been linked to improved physiological and psychosocial outcomes in youth with type 1 diabetes (Whittemore, Kanner, & Grey, 2004). Knafl and Deatrick (1990) developed the Family Management Style Framework through a series of qualitative studies and integrative reviews to describe the overall family response to chronic conditions in youth. The framework combines the views of individual family members into a description of the overall family response to the chronic condition.

In the framework, Knafl and Deatrick (1990) described three major components that contribute to overall family management: definition of the situation, management behaviors, and perceived consequences. They found that overall family functioning was closely tied to the sum of how individual family members defined and managed these key aspects of the chronic condition. From this conceptual framework, Knafl and Deatrick went on to design the Family Management Measure (FaMM), a method of assessing how families manage caring for a child with a chronic health condition and the extent to which the condition is incorporated into daily family life. An improved understanding of family management style may enhance the ability of providers to develop and customize interventions to improve overall family adaptation to the illness (Knafl et al., 2011).

The FaMM has been employed in a variety of different chronic childhood conditions as a means of testing interventions to improve overall family management. For example, Sullivan-Bolyai et al. (2010) used the FaMM to develop and test their family management intervention in parents of children with type 1 diabetes. They found that their social support intervention for parents of children newly diagnosed with type 1 diabetes improved overall family management of the disease (Sullivan-Bolyai et al., 2010). The FaMM has also been suggested for use in families of children with cancers and children undergoing palliative care in the home environment (Bousso, Misko, Mendes-Castillo, & Rossato, 2012; Nelson, Deatrick, Knafl, Alderfer, & Ogle, 2006).

INTERVENTIONS THAT HAVE MOVED TO PUBLIC POLICY

We defined interventions that have moved to public policy as those that have been adopted into regular clinical practice either in the clinic setting or through legislation and policy. To our knowledge, none of the well-studied interventions have reached legislative mandates at either the local, state, or federal level. Several, however, have been incorporated into clinical practice.

Asthma self-management education is a standard of care. Several education programs have been recommended by the National Heart, Lung, and Blood Institute

(NHLBI). For example, the EPR3 Guidelines were promulgated by NHLBI and they recommend that all adolescents receive education in self-monitoring and use of a written action plan (Srof, Toboas, & Velsor-Friedrich, 2012). The education alone, however, does not consistently result in clinical improvements in adolescents with asthma even if the programs are developmentally appropriate for teens. Rhee and colleagues' work with peer-led programs appear to have potential for implementation, but we did not find evidence of their adoption clinically.

With regard to interventions for type 1 diabetes self-management, Grey et al.'s CST intervention has been adopted clinically in more than 150 diabetes practices. Clinicians have been trained in the approach and adapt the program to meet their clinical needs. Clinicians, especially certified diabetes educators and nurse practitioners, have reported that the approach helps them to identify barriers to self-management and provide important skills to the youth with which they are working.

The potential for dissemination and implementation for the widespread use of Teens.Connect is great, due to its availability on the Internet. Further, in an implementation study, Whittemore, Liberti, et al. (2015) found that providers in two diabetes clinics were supportive of providing prescriptions for the use of the program to youth with type 1 diabetes. They also found that without regular reminders as were provided in the randomized clinical trial, youth were less likely to complete most of the intervention sessions. Currently, they are developing dissemination strategies to engage providers, parents, and youth to go to the program online, as well as automated text reminders to complete the program. Such reminders may be gain-framed or neutral. Nonetheless, these investigators get regular requests from teens and parents to access the program.

Another example of an intervention that has been integrated into clinical practice is the teamwork intervention developed and studied by Laffel et al. (2003). Because the intervention was so successful and was designed to be delivered in the context of care, the teamwork program is now a routine part of the program at the Joslin Center and Baylor University. Another group of investigators combined the teamwork intervention with CST for youth with type 1 diabetes transitioning to adolescence (Holmes et al., 2014). They found that the addition of CST to the teamwork intervention did not enhance outcomes. CST, as well as the teamwork intervention, is suggested as an appropriate intervention in two of the major guidelines for care of youth with type 1 diabetes (Chiang et al., 2014; Delamater et al., 2009).

A number of studies, including those by Grey and colleagues, have informed recommendations by the ADA to screen youth with type 1 diabetes for depressive symptoms at least yearly. These recommendations followed a number of studies showing that the prevalence of high levels of depressive symptoms was nearly twice that of the general adolescent population and was associated with a significant risk for suicidal ideation and/or intent.

Aspects of the type 2 prevention intervention have been adopted by the local schools that participated in those trials. Teachers have incorporated some of the lessons on healthy eating into the school curriculum. HEALTH[e]TEEN has not yet been incorporated into the classrooms in the community.

Much of Melnyk's work has focused on children's mental health and her program, Keep your children/yourself Safe and Secure (KySS; Melnyk et al., 2001), has been adopted by the National Association of Pediatric Nurse Practitioners. The organization regularly sponsors training programs to educate nurses and others on knowledge and skills of addressing mental health concerns in children and adolescents. Further, Melnyk's work in health lifestyles has been adopted by the American Academy of Nursing's Health Behavior Expert Panel. Melnyk herself has used the materials in creating a wellness program at the Ohio State University where she is dean.

Aside from the teamwork intervention, none of the family approaches discussed earlier have yet made their way into routine practice. This gap may be due to the fact that family-based interventions are in their infancy.

CONCLUSION

Sadly, few tested interventions have yet been adopted into policy or practice. This results stands in strong contrast to the work of Lorig et al. (2001), whose programs have been adopted by the National Arthritis Institute and others as the standard of care. A number of health care settings, including Kaiser and others, provide this self-management program, led by lay leaders, to all of their clients.

We can only speculate as to why this gap is present in the care of children and teens. The dearth of high-quality dissemination and implementation trials in this age group may be due to a number of issues. The first is that in many settings (e.g., schools), there is not a critical mass of youth with individual chronic conditions who would benefit from broad inclusion of self-management approaches. This prevalence distribution makes recruitment of participants for the large studies that are necessary to determine effectiveness difficult. While larger numbers of youth with chronic conditions can be found at academic centers, these samples suffer from bias toward more middle- and upper-class families who can afford to travel for care, thus creating a problem with representation. Another key issue is that until recently, dissemination and implementation studies have not been understood by the community and thus may be underfunded. Although it seems that this problem is being addressed, it will take time for the results of such studies to make themselves felt in practice or policy.

We make a number of recommendations, not the least of which is that investigators working in the field of improving self-management in youth need to move beyond the usual randomized clinical trials to pragmatic trials and dissemination and implementation studies. Only by demonstrating what interventions work on what participants will such interventions be ready for wider adoption, not only as part of specialized care for chronic conditions but also as part of school and community-based approaches toward the achievement of population health.

The perception of many clinicians (and potentially policy makers) that most interventions are just too complex and require too much training to provide in routine care leads many to conclude that they are just not feasible to try. As nurse scientists and clinicians, it is critical that we think beyond trials to approaches to implement these efficacious interventions in practice and, if appropriate, policy, and to study what happens. After all, helping people is the point of our work, not just scientific advancement.

Further, it is critically important that scholars working in the area of self-management interventions talk to clinicians as well as those who will benefit from such interventions. This kind of community-engaged or patient-centered approach will allow interventions to be developed that are not only theory-based but reality-based and able to be incorporated into care. The work of Grey and colleagues, Lorig and colleagues, Anderson, and Laffel in their various studies demonstrates the success of this approach.

REFERENCES

Adams, K., Greiner, A. C., & Corrigan, J. M. (2004). *Report of a summit. The 1st annual crossing the quality chasm summit: A focus on communities.* Washington, DC: Government Printing Office.

Bandura, A. (1997). The anatomy of stages of change. *American Journal of Health Promotion, 12*(1), 8–10.

Beck, A. T., Rush, A. J., Shaw, B. F., & Emery, G. (Eds.). (1979). *Cognitive therapy of depression.* New York, NY: Guilford Press.

Bell, S. K., & Morgan, S. B. (2000). Children's attitudes and behavioral intentions toward a peer presented as obese: Does a medical explanation for the obesity make a difference? *Journal of Pediatric Psychology, 25*(3), 137–145.

Bousso, R. S., Misko, M. D., Mendes-Castillo, A. M. C., & Rossato, L. M. (2012). Family management framework and its use with families who have a child undergoing palliative care at home. *Journal of Family Nursing, 18*(1), 91–122.

Centers for Disease Control and Prevention. (2005). Children and teens told by doctors that they were overweight—United States, 1999–2002. *MMWR: Morbidity and Mortality Weekly Report, 54*(34), 848–849.

Chiang, J. L., Kirkman, M. S., Laffel, L. M. B., Peters, A. L., & Type 1 Diabetes Sourcebook authors. (2014). Type 1 diabetes through the lifespan: A position statement of the American Diabetes Association. *Diabetes Care, 37,* 2034–2054.

Corbin, A. M., & Strauss, A. (1991). A nursing model for chronic illness managemetn based on the Trajectory Framework. *Scholarly Inquiry for Nursing Practice, 5,* 155–174.

Delamater, A. M. (2009). Psychological care of children and adolescents with diabetes. *Pediatric Diabetes, 10*(Suppl. 12), 175–184.

Fryar, C. D., Carroll, M. D., & Ogden, C. L. (2014). *Prevalence of overweight and obesity among children and adolescents: United States, 1963–1965 through 2011–2012.* Atlanta, GA: National Center for Health Statistics.

Grey, M., Berry, D., Davidson, M., Galasso, P., Gustafson, E., & Melkus, G. D. (2004). Preliminary testing of a program to prevent type 2 diabetes in high-risk youth. *Journal of School Health, 74,* 10–15.

Grey, M., Boland, E. A., Davidson, M., Li, J., & Tamborlane, W. V. (2000). Coping skills training for youth with diabetes mellitus has long-lasting effects on metabolic control and quality of life. *Journal of Pediatrics, 137*(1), 107–113.

Grey, M., Jaser, S. S., Holl, M. G., Jefferson, V., Dziura, J., & Northrup, V. (2009). A multifaceted school-based intervention to reduce risk for type 2 diabetes in at-risk youth. *Preventive Medicine, 49*(2), 122–128.

Grey, M., Knafl, K., Schulman-Green, D., & Reynolds, N. (2015). A revised self- and family management framework. *Nursing Outlook, 63,* 162–170.

Grey, M., Whittemore, R., Jaser, S., Ambrosino, J., Lindemann, E., Liberti, L., . . . Dziura, J. (2009). Effects of coping skills training in school-aged children with type 1 diabetes. *Research in Nursing and Health, 32,* 405–418.

Grey, M., Whittemore, R., Jeon, S., Murphy, K., Faulkner, M. S., Delamater, A., & TeenCope Study Group. (2013). Internet psycho-education programs improve outcomes in youth with type 1 diabetes. *Diabetes Care, 36*(9), 2475–2482.

Grey, M., Whittemore, R., Liberti, L., Delamater, A., Murphy, K., & Faulkner, M. S. (2012). A comparison of two Internet programs for adolescents with type 1 diabetes: Design and methods. *Contemporary Clinical Trials, 33*(4), 769–776.

Guevara, J. P., Wolf, F. M., Grum, C. M., & Clark, N. M. (2003). Effects of educational interventions for self management of asthma in children and adolescents: Systematic review and meta-analysis. *British Medical Journal, 326,* 1308–1315.

Holmes, C. S., Chen, R., Mackey, E., Grey, M., & Streisand, R. (2014). Randomized clinical trial of clinic-integrated, low intensity treatment to prevent deterioration of disease care in adolescents with type 1 diabetes. *Diabetes Care, 37,* 1535–1543.

Institute of Medicine. (2010). *The future of nursing: Leading change, advancing health.* Washington, DC: Author.

Institute of Medicine & National Research Council. (2011). *Toward an integrated science of research on families.* Washington, DC: Government Printing Office.

Jefferson, V., Jaser, S. S., Lindemann, E., Galasso, P., Beale, A., Holl, M. G., & Grey, M. (2011). Coping skills training in a telephone health coaching program for youth at risk for type 2 diabetes. *Journal of Pediatric Health Care, 25*(3), 153–161.

Knafl, K., & Deatrick, J. A. (1990). Family management style: Concept analysis and development. *Journal of Pediatric Nursing, 5,* 4–14.

Knafl, K., Deatrick, J. A., Gallo, A., Dixon, J., Grey, M., Knafl, G., & O'Malley, J. (2011). Assessment of the psychometric properties of the family management measure. *Journal of Pediatric Psychology, 36,* 494–505.

Laffel, L. M., Brackett, J., Ho, J., & Anderson, B. J. (1999). Changing the process of diabetes care improves metabolic outcomes and reduces hospitalizations. *Quality Management in Healthcare, 7*(3), 53–62.

Laffel, L. M., Vangsness, L., Connell, A., Goebel-Fabbri, A., Butler, D., & Anderson, B. J. (2003). Impact of ambulatory, family-focused teamwork intervention on glycemic control in youth with type 1 diabetes. *Journal of Pediatrics, 142*(4), 409–416.

Lorig, K., Ritter, P., Stewart, A. L., Sobol, D. S., Brown, B. W., & Bandura, A. (2001). Chronic disease self-management: 2-year health status and health care utilization outcomes. *Medical Care, 39,* 1217–1223.

Melnyk, B. M., Jacobson, D., Kelly, S., Belyea, M., Shaibi, G., Small, L., . . . Marsiglia, F. F. (2013). Promoting healthy lifestyles in high school adolescents: A randomized controlled trial. *American Journal of Preventive Medicine, 45,* 407–415.

Melnyk, B. M., Jacobson, D., Kelly, S., O'Haver, J., Small, L., & Mays, M. Z. (2009). Improving mental health, healthy lifestyle choices, and physical health of Hispanic adolescents: A randomized controlled pilot study. *Journal of School Health, 79,* 575–584.

Melnyk, B. M., & Moldenhauser, Z. (2006). *The KySS guide to child and adolescent mental health screening, early intervention and health promotion.* Cherry Hill, NJ: National Association of Pediatric Nurse Practitioners.

Melnyk, B. M., Moldenhauer, Z., Veenema, T., Gullo, S., McCurrtrie, M., O'Leary, E., . . . Tuttle, J. (2001). The KySS Campaign: A national effort to reduce psychosocial morbidities in children and adolescents. *Journal of Pediatric Health Care, 15*(2), 31A–34A.

Melnyk, B. M., Small, L., Morrison-Beedy, D., Strasser, A., Spath, L., Kreipe, R., . . . O'Haver, J. (2007). The COPE healthy lifestyles TEEN program: Feasibility, preliminary efficacy, & lessons learned from an after school group intervention with overweight adolescents. *Journal of Pediatric Health Care, 21*(5), 315–322.

National Institute of Nursing Research. (2011). NINR strategic plan: Bringing science to life. Retrieved from https://www.ninr.nih.gov/sites/www.ninr.nih.gov/files/ninr-strategic-plan -2011.pdf

National Institute of Nursing Research. (2016). NINR strategic plan. Retrieved from http://www .ninr.nih.gov/aboutninr/ninr-mission-and-strategic-plan/strategicplan2016#.V0M_dVJa690

Nelson, A. E., Deatrick, J. A., Knafl, K. A., Alderfer, M. A., & Ogle, S. K. (2006). Consensus state- ments: The family management style framework and its use with families of children with cancer. *Journal of Pediatric Oncology Nursing, 23*(1), 36–38.

Newman, S., Steed, L., & Mulligan, K. (2009). *Chronic physical illness: Self-management and behavioural interventions*. Maidenhead, UK: McGraw-Hill Open University Press.

Ogden, C. L., Carroll, M. D., Kit, B. K., & Flegal, K. M. (2014). Prevalence of childhood and adult obesity in the United States, 2011–2012. *JAMA, 311*, 806–814.

Parekh, A. K., Goodman, R. A., Gordon, C., Koh, H. K., & HHS Intra-agency Workgroup on Mul- tiple Chronic Conditions. (2011). Managing multiple chronic conditions: A strategic frame- work for improving outcomes and quality of life. *Public Health Reports, 126*, 460–471.

Perrin, J. M., Bloom, S. R., & Gortmaker, S. L. (2007). The increase of childhood chronic conditions in the United States. *JAMA, 297*(24), 2755–2759.

Pew Research Center. (2015). Teens, social media, and technology. Retrieved from http://www .pewinternet.org/2015/04/09/teens-social-media-technology-2015

Raiff, B. R., & Dallery, J. (2010). Internet based contingency management to improve adherence with blood glucose testing recommendations for teens with type 1 diabetes. *Journal of Applied Behavior Analysis, 43*(3), 487–491.

Rhee, H., Belyea, M. J., Ciurzynski, S., & Brasch, J. (2009). Barriers to asthma self-management in adolescents: Relationships to psychosocial factors. *Pediatric Pulmonology, 44*, 183–191.

Rhee, H., Belyea, M. J., Hunt, J. F., & Brasch, J. (2011). Effects of a peer-led asthma self-manage- ment program for adolescents. *Archives of Pediatric and Adolescent Medicine, 165*, 513–519.

Ruggiero, L., Glasgow, R., Dryfoos, J. M., Rossi, J. S., Prochaska, J. O., Orleans, C. T., . . . Johnson, S. (1997). Diabetes self-management. Self-reported recommendations and patterns in a large population. *Diabetes Care, 20*, 568–576.

Sjöberg, R. L., Nilsson, K. W., & Leppert, J. (2005). Obesity, shame, and depression in school-aged children: A population-based study. *Pediatrics, 116*(3), e389–e392.

Srof, B., Taboas, P., & Velsor-Friedrich, B. (2012). Adolescent asthma education programs for teens. *Journal of Pediatric Health Care, 26*, 418–426.

Stabouli, S., Kotsis, V., Papamichael, C., Constantopoulos, A., & Zakopoulos, N. (2005). Ado- lescent obesity is associated with high ambulatory blood pressure and increased carotid intimal-medial thickness. *Journal of Pediatrics, 147*(5), 651–656.

Stanger, C., Ryan, S. R., Delhey, L. M., Thrailkill, K., Li, Z., Li, Z., & Budney, A. J. (2013). A multi- component motivational intervention to improve adherence among adolescents with poorly controlled type 1 diabetes: A pilot study. *Journal of Pediatric Psychology, 38*(6), 629–637.

Sullivan-Bolyai, S., Bova, C., Leung, K., Trudeau, A., & Gruppuso, P. A. (2010). Social support to empower parents (STEP): An intervention for parents of children newly diagnosed with type 1 diabetes. *Diabetes Educator, 36*, 88–97.

Svoren, B. M., Butler, D., Levine, B. S., Anderson, B. J., & Laffel, L. M. (2003). Reducing acute adverse outcomes in youths with type 1 diabetes: A randomized, controlled trial. *Pediatrics, 112*(4), 914–922.

U.S. Department of Health & Human Services. (2011). HHS initiative on multiple chronic condi- tions. Retrieved from http://www.hhs.gov/ash/initiatives/mcc

Velsor-Friedrich, B., Militello, L. K., Richards, M. H., Harrison, P. R., Gross, I. M., Romero, E., & Bryant, F. B. (2012). Effects of coping skills training in low-income urban African American adolescents with asthma. *Journal of Asthma, 49*, 372–379.

Wagner, E. H., Austin, B. T., Davis, C. E., Hindmarsh, M., Schaefer, J., & Bonomi, A. (2001). Improv- ing chronic illness care: Translating evidence into action. *Health Affairs, 20*(6), 64–78.

Whittemore, R., Chao, A., Jang, M., Jeon, S., Liptak, T., Popick, R., & Grey, M. (2013). Implementation of a school-based Internet obesity prevention program for adolescents. *Journal of Nutrition Education and Behavior, 45,* 586–594.

Whittemore, R., Grey, M., Lindemann, E., Ambrosino, J., & Jaser, S. (2010). Development of an Internet coping skills training program for teenagers with type 1 diabetes. *Computers, Informatics, Nursing, 28*(2), 103–111.

Whittemore, R., Jeon, S., & Grey, M. (2013). An Internet obesity prevention program for adolescents. *Journal of Adolescent Health, 52,* 439–447.

Whittemore, R., Kanner, S., & Grey, M. (2004). The influence of family on physiological and psychosocial health in youth with type 1 diabetes: A systematic review. In B. Melnyk & E. Fineout-Overholt (Eds.), *Evidence-based practice in nursing and healthcare: A guide to best practice* (pp. CD22-73–CD22-87). Philadelphia, PA: Lippincott Williams & Wilkins.

Whittemore, R., Liberti, L. S., Jeon, S., Chao, A., Minges, K. E., Murphy, K., & Grey, M. (2015). Efficacy and implementation of an Internet psychoeducational program for teens with type 1 diabetes. *Pediatric Diabetes, 17*(8), 567–575.

Wollenhaupt, J., Rodgers, B., & Sawin, K. J. (2012). Family management of a chronic health condition: Perspectives of adolescents. *Journal of Family Nursing, 18*(1), 65–90. doi: 10.1177/1074840711427545

8

Self-Management of Illness in Adults

Barbara Riegel, Victoria Vaughan Dickson, and Christopher S. Lee

Self-management refers to the day-to-day management of chronic conditions by individuals over the course of an illness (Lorig & Holman, 2003). A variety of terms are used to capture this behavior: *self-management, self-care,* and *self-monitoring* are some of the most common terms (Grady & Gough, 2014). In our work, we use *self-care* as an umbrella term to capture both self-management and healthy lifestyle behaviors or maintenance (Figure 8.1). The management element of our work reflects the process described by Grady and colleagues (Grady & Daley, 2014; Grady & Gough, 2014) and is the focus of this chapter. Here we describe the evolution of our research and how that research has influenced policy in the United States and internationally.

EARLY INFLUENCES

Interest in self-care grew out of Riegel's early experiences as a clinical nurse researcher at Sharp HealthCare in San Diego, California, between 1990 and 2002. Upon completion of a doctoral degree at the University of California at Los Angeles, she assumed responsibility for clinical research in the cardiovascular service line. Although now heart failure (HF) is recognized as an exceptionally prevalent and expensive condition (Heidenreich et al., 2013), in the early 1990s hospitals were not yet aware that these patients were being rehospitalized repeatedly. After publication of a monograph from the Cardiology Preeminence Roundtable in 1994 (Cardiology Preeminence Roundtable, 1994) and publication of a seminal study describing a successful multidisciplinary HF disease management study in 1995 (Rich et al., 1995), Riegel pursued funding for a similar multidisciplinary disease management study to be conducted at Sharp HealthCare. After early internal resistance to the idea reflecting the "fill the beds" mindset of the times, Riegel received funding from Merck Foundation to conduct a small trial (Riegel, Carlson, Glaser, & Hoagland, 2000).

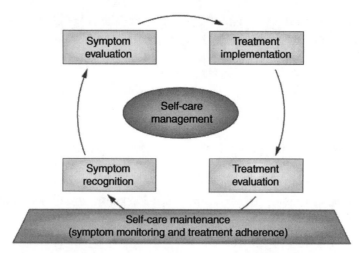

FIGURE 8.1   Model of heart failure self-care. In this model, self-care maintenance is the foundation of effective self-care management. Self-care maintenance and management are connected through the process of symptom monitoring, which is the prerequisite for symptom recognition and subsequent steps in the process of self-care management.

Source: Riegel, Lee, and Dickson (2011).

As Riegel and colleagues designed their multidisciplinary disease management intervention, they pondered the mechanism underlying the intervention. During discussions with nurses, physicians, pharmacists, dieticians, social workers, and physical therapists, it became clear that each element of the intervention approach focused on helping patients with this chronic illness to take better care of themselves (Riegel, Thomason, et al., 1999). Measuring the mechanism of HF self-care in our disease management trial was critical—but at that time there was no instrument measuring HF self-care in the manner in which we defined it. Riegel decided to devise such a measure and in doing so started a long career focused on the development of self-care theory and measurement.

THEORY AND MEASUREMENT DEVELOPMENT

Early efforts in understanding self-care evolved from discussions with clinicians. The nurses described how adults with HF commonly retained 20 to 30 pounds of fluid in their legs before seeking care. Patients who recognized their early signs (e.g., weight gain) and symptoms (e.g., shortness of breath), knew that these changes were abnormal, and did something about it (e.g., call the physician, take an extra diuretic) were most likely to avoid hospitalization. Literature from other patient populations suggested that patients who evaluated the success of behavioral strategies were most likely to become experts in self-care (Paterson & Thorne, 2000a, 2000b). This assessment of the process engaged in by patients resulted in a linear model delineating four stages of management: recognizing a change in signs and symptoms, evaluating the change, implementing a treatment strategy, and evaluating the treatment.

After specifying our vision of the self-management process, in 1995 Riegel engaged an advanced practice nurse to telephone HF patients to assess content validity of the proposed process. She telephoned 25 patients and engaged them in a discussion of their thoughts and decisions surrounding signs and symptoms (Riegel, Carlson, & Glaser, 2000). Those discussions confirmed the four-step process described earlier. Following each semistructured interview, patients were engaged in a discussion to determine if additional stages were involved in self-management. Lack of confidence in the ability to manage symptoms was repeatedly identified as a barrier to treatment success. Confidence did not appear to be a stage of management itself, but rather an important factor influencing self-management ability.

Measurement of these concepts was the ultimate goal, and the original measurement effort produced a 65-item instrument with six subscales measuring the self-management of signs and symptoms of HF (Riegel, Carlson, & Glaser, 2000). The subscales measured the four stages of management described earlier (recognize a change in signs and symptoms, evaluate the change, implement a treatment strategy, and evaluate the treatment) as well as ease in evaluating signs and symptoms and confidence in the ability to self-manage. Early psychometric properties were promising, but six different symptoms were included; few patients have all six symptoms, so a skip-pattern format was used, which was confusing to patients and complicated for scoring.

In 1999, the concept of maintenance was added to the model to reflect patients' efforts to stay healthy and avoid symptoms. Self-care maintenance reflected primarily adherence to treatments and lifestyle recommendations intended to maintain physiologic stability (Figure 8.2). An important element of self-care maintenance

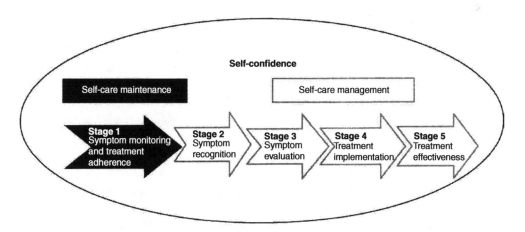

FIGURE 8.2 Visual depiction of the self-care process. Self-care is defined as a process of maintaining health through treatment adherence and symptom monitoring. When signs and symptoms occur, decision making of self-care management is required. Self-care is positively influenced by self-confidence in one's abilities.

Source: Riegel, Carlson, et al. (2004). Used with permission of Elsevier Publishers.

is medication adherence, a behavior we have focused on in recent years (Dickson, Knafl, & Riegel, 2015; Knafl & Riegel, 2014; Riegel & Dickson, 2016; Riegel & Knafl, 2014; Riegel, Lee, et al., 2012; Riegel, Moelter, et al., 2011; Wu et al., 2009). At that point we began referring to the process as self-care with both maintenance and management components. Self-care management did not change from our early work described previously.

In this early work, self-care was defined as a rational process involving purposeful choices and behaviors that reflected knowledge and thought (Riegel, Carlson, & Glaser, 2000). Although we referred to naturalistic decision making, we focused on attention, inference, and judgment—elements of a logical decision-making process. When we published the situation-specific theory of HF self-care in 2008 (Riegel & Dickson, 2008), we de-emphasized logic and emphasized self-care as a naturalistic decision-making process involving the choice of behaviors that maintain physiologic stability (maintenance) and the response to symptoms when they occur (management).

Soon after publishing the 65-item self-management of HF scale, we began work on a shorter version addressing the entire construct of self-care (i.e., maintenance, management) and confidence in the ability to perform self-care. The major change that allowed us to shorten the instrument was a focus on one symptom, shortness of breath, which is experienced by most adults with HF. Our effort to shorten the scale resulted in the Self-Care of Heart Failure Index (SCHFI) with three scales (Riegel, Carlson, et al., 2004). The version of the SCHFI published in 2004 was a 15-item instrument using a 4-point response scale. Scores on each scale were standardized to a 0–100 score. This instrument was updated in 2009 as version 6.2 (Riegel, Lee, Dickson, & Carlson, 2009). Major changes in 2009 were the addition of items to the maintenance and confidence scales. The scoring procedure was refined and the formula for computing standardized scores was improved. A cut point for adequacy of self-care was specified (i.e., ≥ 70 on the standardized score). When internal coherence reliability of the SCHFI scales was assessed with factor score determinacy, maintenance coefficients ranged from .75 to .83, management ranged from .68 to .76, and confidence ranged from .84 to .90 (Barbaranelli, Lee, Vellone, & Riegel, 2014, 2015). Construct and predictive validity have been demonstrated. We have made the SCHFI freely available to anyone who wishes to use it by posting it on our website: www.self-careofheartfailureindex.com. Currently there are 18 foreign-language versions freely available to users, along with local contact users.

After publishing the situation-specific theory of HF self-care in 2008 (Riegel & Dickson, 2008), researchers began e-mailing with requests to use the model for other conditions. Subsequently, Riegel and colleagues published a middle range theory of self-care of chronic illness where self-care was defined as a process of maintaining health through health-promoting practices and managing illness, noting that self-care is performed in both healthy and ill states (Riegel, Jaarsma, & Stromberg, 2012). Again, naturalistic decision making was noted as the process used to make self-care decisions. A key difference in the middle range theory was the addition of *monitoring* as a key conceptual element. The theme of symptom monitoring was picked up again in the revised and updated situation-specific theory of HF self-care where self-care was operationally defined as a process of: (a) maintenance; (b) symptom perception; and (c) management (Figure 8.3; Riegel, Dickson, & Faulkner, 2015). The addition of symptom perception focuses on the observations that persons with HF do not respond rapidly to their early symptoms. We suspect that the difficulty in perceiving symptoms may be related to age-related changes in interoception (Riegel, Dickson, Cameron, et al., 2010). We have now devised an instrument that measures self-care of HF in a manner consistent with the updated theory and one that measures self-care of chronic illness in general; those instruments are currently in psychometric testing.

Since these early efforts, we have continued to study self-care (both maintenance and management) in adults with chronic illness including HF. In what follows, we summarize our research conducted to date and then discuss the influence of this program of research on policy in the United States and internationally.

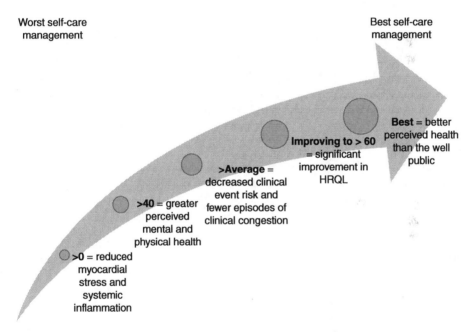

FIGURE 8.3 Illustration of the relationship between self-care management and outcomes.

Note. On a standardized scale ranging from 0 (indicating the worst self-care management) to 100 (indicating the best self-care management), different levels of heart failure self-care management were associated with improvements in health outcomes, and changes in the odds of having higher levels of biomarkers of myocardial stress and systemic inflammation. That is, patients engaged in low levels of self-care management may benefit by having less myocardial distension and inflammation, whereas patients who have levels of self-care management above 40 will likely have improvements in perceived health. Those who are engaged in above-average self-care management cut their chances of being hospitalized or dying in half, and are much less likely to have episodes of preclinical congestion than patients engaged in poor self-care management. Patients engaged in above-average self-care management who have episodes of congestion experience them less frequently and in shorter duration than patients who practice poor self-care management. Those who improve in HF self-care management to above a score of 60 have significant and clinically meaningful improvements in quality of life compared with patients who decrease in their self-care management over time in whom quality of life does not change. Patients engaged in the best self-care management perceive their health as being better than the general well population.

HRQL, health-related quality of life.

SELF-MANAGEMENT IS CHALLENGING

Through the years we have demonstrated repeatedly that HF self-management is difficult for patients to master. Most patients experience multiple symptoms, yet their knowledge of the importance of signs and symptoms is often poor, early recognition is difficult, and misperceptions are common (Carlson, Riegel, & Moser, 2001). When we explored in focus groups how HF influenced patients' lives, how they performed self-care, and how their life situations facilitated or impeded HF self-care, we identified physical limitations, debilitating symptoms, difficulties coping with treatment, lack of knowledge, emotional distress, multiple comorbidities, and personal struggles that impeded self-care. Atypical symptoms such as faintness were rarely attributed to HF (Riegel & Carlson, 2002).

Evolution of Expertise

The development of expert in self-management is important. Using latent class mixture modeling, we identified three distinct profiles of self-management (novice, inconsistent, and expert). As physical symptoms worsened, self-management improved (Lee, Gelow, et al., 2015). These results are consistent with those found repeatedly over the years: Persons with HF rarely perform self-care when they are asymptomatic; as symptoms worsen over time, self-care improves (Riegel, Lee, & Dickson, 2011). We attribute this observation to changes in experience and attitude. Experience with symptoms and responses leads to mastery for some patients (Carlson et al., 2001; Riegel, Lee, et al., 2011). An attitude that is receptive to the need for self-care is also necessary. Persons with negative attitudes rarely master self-management (Dickson, Deatrick, & Riegel, 2008). Fighting against the need to deal with symptoms lowers the odds of developing expert-level management behaviors.

Comorbid Conditions

Many of the themes we identified in the early years have been explored in detail in subsequent years. In a series of descriptive, exploratory, and comparative studies, we have confirmed that multimorbidity greatly impairs the ability of adults with HF to perform self-care (Bidwell et al., 2015; Buck et al., 2015; Dickson, Buck, & Riegel, 2013). Individuals with multiple comorbid conditions report difficulty differentiating HF symptoms from those of other conditions (Dickson, Buck, & Riegel, 2011) and lack confidence in their ability to implement treatment (Dickson et al., 2013). Impaired cognition, found in 25% to 50% of HF patients (Gure et al., 2012), is one particularly challenging condition that interferes with self-care (Bidwell et al., 2015; Dickson et al., 2008; Dickson, Tkacs, & Riegel, 2007; Lee et al., 2013). Yet, confidence in the ability to perform self-care appears to promote successful maintenance and management, even when cognition is impaired (Vellone et al., 2015). This is exciting work because few interventions successfully improve cognition—but perhaps we can address confidence and thereby improve self-care in these patients.

Race, Ethnicity, and Social Norms

Blacks with HF have different and more risk factors than Whites for poor medication adherence (maintenance; Dickson et al., 2015), but racial differences in management have not been found. Rather, cultural beliefs and social norms that vary by ethnic group influence day-to-day decisions about both self-care maintenance and management practices (Dickson, McCarthy, Howe, Schipper, & Katz, 2013). For example, in a mixed-methods study examining the sociocultural influences on self-care in an ethnic minority Black population with HF, we reported that the cultural meaning ascribed to HF, symptoms, and perceived role (Dickson, Kuhn, Worrall-Carter, & Riegel, 2011) in performing self-care influence how patients respond (Dickson et al., 2013). Similarly, although social support is known to promote self-care (Bidwell et al., 2015; Sayers, Riegel, Pawlowski, Coyne, & Samaha, 2008), social norms may interfere with a willingness to access social support, including help with daily self-care practices. Low-income ethnic minority patients reported difficulty with dietary adherence due to a conflict with cultural food preferences, cooking techniques, and family roles (Dickson et al., 2013).

Gender

Gender-specific differences in self-care behaviors are minimal (Bidwell et al., 2015; Lee, Riegel, et al., 2009). However, gender-specific barriers and facilitators greatly influence the choice of self-care behaviors (Riegel, Dickson, Kuhn, Page, & Worrall-Carter, 2010). Specifically, there are distinct gender differences in the decisions made in interpreting and responding to symptoms. Men may be better than women at interpreting their symptoms as being related to HF and in initiating treatment. Gender differences may also simply reflect differences in social support, confidence, and mood (Riegel, Dickson, Kuhn, et al., 2010). Self-care of HF has been studied more extensively in men compared with women; hence, there is more work to be done to gain insight into the role of gender in self-care.

SELF-MANAGEMENT INFLUENCES OUTCOMES

For some time now, we have known that interventions designed to enhance HF self-care maintenance generally reduce rates of HF hospitalization (Ditewig, Blok, Havers, & van Veenendaal, 2010; Jonkman et al., 2016; Jovicic, Holroyd-Leduc, & Straus, 2006; McAlister, Stewart, Ferrua, & McMurray, 2004). In contrast, there is limited evidence of the influence of self-care management on health outcomes of any type. To tackle this critical knowledge gap, we engaged in a collaborative research endeavor to first put forth hypothetical mechanisms by which HF self-care management might influence outcomes and second to generate foundational empirical evidence to support our hypotheses. Based on an extensive synthesis of knowledge on HF self-care and cardiovascular pathogenesis, our overarching hypothesis was that effective HF self-care maintenance and management were cardioprotective and complementary to medical management in improving outcomes (Lee, Tkacs, & Riegel, 2009). Specifically, we proposed that effective HF self-care would (a) facilitate partial blockade and partial deactivation of deleterious neurohormones, (b) limit inflammatory processes, (c) decrease the need for pharmacological agents that may be detrimental, and (d) minimize myocardial hibernation (Lee, Tkacs, & Riegel, 2009). Having disseminated our hypotheses in 2009, we moved on to generating the empirical evidence in support of these hypotheses with an intentional focus on self-care management behaviors, about which we knew the least.

In 2009, we published a secondary analysis of cross-sectional data collected on adults with HF living in Thailand to test our hypothesis that effective self-care was associated with better health status (Lee, Suwanno, & Riegel, 2009). In that paper, we provided the first evidence of a positive and nonlinear influence of self-care management on better health status that interestingly was contingent on self-care confidence. That is, better self-care management was associated with better health status, but only when self-care confidence was high (Lee, Suwanno, & Riegel, 2009). In 2011, we published another secondary analysis of data collected on adults with symptomatic HF to test the hypothesis that better self-care management was associated with better clinical-event-free survival (Lee, Moser, Lennie, & Riegel, 2011). In that analysis, we provided the first evidence that patients who engage in higher levels of self-care management have a significant reduction in 1-year clinical event risk compared with similar patients who engage in poor self-care management. Remarkably, patients who engaged in higher levels of self-care management had a similar event risk compared with patients who were asymptomatic and did not have to engage in self-care management (Lee, Moser, Lennie, & Riegel, 2011). In combination, results from these studies provided the first empirical evidence of the association between self-care management and both patient-oriented and clinical outcomes we had proposed (Lee, Tkacs, & Riegel, 2009). The next step was to test our specific mechanistic hypotheses.

In 2011, we published a secondary analysis of cross-sectional data collected on adults with symptomatic HF to test our hypothesis that effective self-care is associated with less myocardial stress and systemic inflammation (Lee, Moser, Lennie, Tkacs, et al., 2011). We demonstrated that each 1-point increase in self-care management score (range, 15–100) on the SCHFI was associated with a 12.7% reduction in the odds of having levels of the biomarkers amino-terminal pro-B-type natriuretic peptide (Nt-proBNP) and soluble tumor necrosis factor α receptor type 1 (sTNFαR1) at or greater than the sample median. This was the first evidence supporting our proposition that early symptom recognition and management of symptoms may decrease myocardial stress and systemic inflammation (Lee, Tkacs, & Riegel, 2009).

The 2011 study was our first evidence that effective self-care is associated with better pathophysiological outcomes (Lee, Moser, Lennie, Tkacs, et al., 2011). Also in 2011, we published results of another study to test the hypothesis that better HF self-care was associated with less objectively measured clinical congestion (i.e., the accumulation of fluid in the lungs that is a common hallmark of worsening HF; Rathman, Lee, Sarkar, & Small, 2011). In that paper, we provided the first evidence that better HF self-care was associated with less frequent episodes and shorter duration of clinical congestion. It is well known that neurohormonal activation and systemic inflammation contribute significantly to clinical congestion in HF (Packer, 1992; Seta, Shan, Bozkurt, Oral, & Mann, 1996). Hence, evidence of a link between HF self-care and clinical congestion added credibility to our prior finding of a link between better HF self-care and lower biomarkers of myocardial stress and systemic inflammation.

Later we published prospective evidence that HF self-care management is related to health-related quality of life (HRQL; Lee, Mudd, et al., 2015). Using growth mixture modeling, we identified two unique trajectories of change in self-care management: (a) a significant decline in management over time and no change in HRQL, and (b) marked improvements in management and HRQL. Together these studies demonstrated that different levels of HF self-care are associated with better or worse health outcomes (Figure 8.3). Specifically, patients who engage in even low levels of self-care may derive benefit by having less myocardial distension and inflammation. Those who have moderate levels of self-care will likely have improvements in their perceived health. Those who engage in above-average self-care cut their chances of being hospitalized or dying in half, and are much less likely to have episodes of preclinical congestion than patients who are poor in self-care. These patients may still have episodes of congestion, but they experience them less frequently and in shorter duration than patients who practice poor self-care. Patients who improve in their HF self-care management have significant improvements in HRQL compared with patients who decline in HF self-care, in whom HRQL does not change. Patients engaged in the best self-care perceive their health as being better than the general well population.

WAYS TO IMPROVE SELF-CARE

Disease Management

Over the past 20 years Riegel and colleagues have pioneered a variety of HF disease management programs, all of which were designed to improve HF self-care and outcomes, including hospital readmission (Riegel, Carlson, Kopp, et al., 2002; Riegel, Carlson, Glaser, & Hoagland, 2000; Riegel, Carlson, Glaser, & Romero, 2006). Numerous meta-analyses including our work with multidisciplinary and telephonic approaches have demonstrated that disease management is efficacious (Ara, 2004; Gohler et al., 2006; Gonseth, Guallar-Castillon, Banegas, & Rodriguez-Artalejo, 2004; Leppin et al., 2014; McAlister, Lawson, Teo, & Armstrong, 2001;

Ofman et al., 2004; Roccaforte, Demers, Baldassarre, Teo, & Yusuf, 2005; Savard, Thompson, & Clark, 2011; Whellan, Hasselblad, Peterson, O'Connor, & Schulman, 2005). When some of the major investigators in HF disease management pooled results to identify what component of disease management is most important, we found that multidisciplinary teams and in-person interaction were needed to reduce hospital readmissions (Sochalski et al., 2009). However, individual trials have shown inconsistent results, so we recently performed an individual data meta-analysis to determine whether subgroups of patients respond differently to approaches intended to improve self-care. When data from 20 studies representing 5,624 patients were analyzed, self-management interventions reduced risk of time to the combined end point of HF-related hospitalization or all-cause death (hazard ratio [HR], 0.80; 95% CIs [0.71, 0.89]), time to HF-related hospitalization (HR, 0.80; 95% CIs [0.69, 0.92]), and improved 12-month HRQL (standardized mean difference 0.15; 95% CIs [0.00, 0.30]; Jonkman et al., 2016). When we analyzed effective program characteristics, we found that a longer intervention duration improved outcomes.

Self-Care Skills

In our ongoing work (Dickson & Riegel, 2009; Riegel, Dickson, & Topaz, 2013; Riegel, Lee, Albert, et al., 2011) we have shown that effective self-care management requires skill, which evolves over time and with practice as patients gain experience in recognizing and successfully managing symptoms. This work builds on our earlier observation about the importance of experience in mastering self-care (Carlson et al., 2001). In a qualitative descriptive meta-analysis assessing what self-care skills patients with HF perceive that they need and how they develop the skills needed to perform self-care (Dickson & Riegel, 2009), we found that tactical and situational skills are needed to perform adequate self-care. That is, patients reported needing skill in specific self-care behaviors as well as in specific situations (Dickson & Riegel, 2009). Individuals who lack situational skill ("what to do when" faced with special circumstances) were at risk for poor self-care management (Dickson, Deatrick, & Riegel, 2008). We concluded that traditional patient education is poor at developing self-care skill and moved into testing ways to improve skill and commitment to engage in self-care.

In our first skill-building pilot intervention study, we tested an HF symptom monitoring and response intervention called *HF SMART* (Jurgens, Lee, Reitano, & Riegel, 2013). An interactive exercise was used to compare sensations of dyspnea and fatigue at rest and immediately after administration of a 6-minute walk test. Participants were helped to recognize their symptoms and engaged in a discussion of the symptoms experienced and their response to those symptoms. In the intervention group, clinically meaningful improvements were seen in self-care maintenance and confidence but not in management. Although the intervention was theoretically based and innovative, the effect sizes achieved were not sufficiently promising to pursue this approach.

We moved on to testing a skill-building intervention delivered by lay health educators in community-based samples. In our first test of this approach, we succeeded in improving HF self-care, knowledge, and HRQL in an ethnically diverse sample of patients with HF (53% female; 31% Hispanic, 24% Black; mean age 69.9 ± 10 years). Skill building significantly improved self-care maintenance, management, and HF knowledge after three months (Dickson, Melkus, et al., 2014). Through focus group feedback, participants described building both tactical and situational skill through practice with reinforcement by peers and the lay health educator, which increased self-efficacy. In the next study, we focused on Hispanics with HF and piloted the skill-building intervention translated into Spanish and delivered by a bilingual health educator (Dickson, Combellick, et al., 2012). We adapted the self-care management content of our skill-building intervention to simplify the symptom monitoring and management concepts for use in a low-literacy, multilingual HF population (Dickson, Chyun, Caridi, Gregory, & Katz, 2016). This cultural adaptation was guided by feedback from Hispanic adults with HF and community liaisons and focused on skill building with sensitivity to cultural beliefs and preferences. This intervention was successful in improving knowledge and self-care maintenance but not self-care management. Focus group feedback confirmed the importance of the culturally appropriate intervention and the role of family in the process of self-care. Collectively, these results confirm our belief that skill building is essential to self-care. Further work is needed to determine why maintenance improves consistently but not management.

Motivational Interviewing

We have tested the effectiveness of motivational interviewing (MI) in engaging HF patients in self-care (Riegel, Dickson, et al., 2006). In our first study we identified the elements of MI that were most important in influencing patients' intentions to perform self-care. Reflective listening and empathy by the interventionist were essential to helping patients learn how to make self-care decisions. Acknowledging cultural beliefs and addressing barriers and constraints helped patients identify skill deficits and develop an action plan to incorporate self-care into daily life. The intervention was also effective in facilitating the transition from hospital to home, which included activating necessary social supports and services.

In our most recent study we tested MI in a small randomized controlled trial (Masterson Creber et al., 2015). The primary outcome of this trial was HF self-care maintenance, which improved in statistically significant and clinically meaningful ways over a 3-month period compared to usual care (Masterson Creber et al., 2016). In a mixed-methods study of a subset of eight of these study participants, we found quantitative evidence of dramatic improvement in self-care. Qualitative data revealed that most participants described improvements in self-care maintenance, particularly in the areas of dietary adherence and symptom monitoring. When the quantitative and qualitative data were integrated, congruence between the quantitative and qualitative data was 98%. When the qualitative data were analyzed to describe how the intervention was effective and what MI strategies were most successful in this sample, we confirmed that reflective listening and empathy are key. The nurse interventionist used (a) reflection and reframing to support development of self-efficacy, (b) goal setting, and (c) a communication style with empathy, affirmation, and humor. These techniques stimulated openness to goal setting, positive self-talk, perceived ability to overcome barriers, and change talk in study participants. We are now designing an intervention that integrates skills-based education with MI to improve HF self-care.

INFLUENCE ON POLICY

Individuals have been taking care of themselves—performing self-care—long before our organized health care system evolved, but the need for self-care has never been greater. Especially in the United States, we have rising costs and decreasing accessibility of health care (Bali, Troshani, Goldberg, & Wickramasinghe, 2013). At the same time, we have a growing burden of chronic illness. In a recent study of Medicare beneficiaries, 68.4% had two or more chronic conditions and 36.4% had four or more chronic conditions (Lochner & Cox, 2013). A study of a national sample of children showed that more than 50% had at least one chronic condition (Van Cleave, Gortmaker, & Perrin, 2010). Promoting self-care, with a combination of maintenance and management, may be the best solution for the pervasive problem of chronic illness (Kennedy et al., 2007).

INTERNATIONAL POLICY

Our approach to influencing policy has been to think globally, act locally. We have engaged an army of collaborators studying and raising awareness of self-care around the world through wide and free dissemination of the SCHFI via a website (www.self-careofheartfailureindex.com). In this way, we have come to appreciate the pervasiveness of poor self-care worldwide. We pooled data on self-care obtained from 2,082 adults from two developed (United States and Australia) and two developing (Thailand and Mexico) countries; see Riegel, Driscoll, et al. (2009). Self-management was inadequate (<70 on the standardized scale) in most of the samples, but it was worst in the Thai sample, where only 5% of the sample performed adequate self-care. In the combined sample, significant determinants of management were younger age, more comorbid illnesses, and country, but these factors explained only 18% of the variance in management, illustrating the complexity of the issues. In another study, we pooled data on self-care obtained from 5,964 HF patients from the United States, Europe, Australasia, and South America (Jaarsma et al., 2013). Only maintenance behaviors could be compared in this study because not all the data were collected using the SCHFI, but we found, for example, that exercise and weight monitoring were low in all these different countries.

Self-care has been adopted as an emphasis of education and research in Swedish and Italian schools of nursing. We have collaborated with faculty in many of these schools to disseminate the results of our studies and build a cadre of investigators in the field. Through our work with colleagues in Sweden, we developed the middle range theory of self-care of chronic illness (Riegel, Jaarsma, & Stromberg, 2012). This theory has been used to support the development of theoretically grounded self-care research in the areas of diabetes, inflammatory bowel disease, hypertension, end-of-life care, ventricular assist device recipients, and coronary heart disease.

Governmental Policy

Based on the results of this international work, we have advocated for changes in health care systems and national policies to support patients with chronic illness to increase their self-care behavior. One nation that has mandated policies related to self-care is Sweden, which is known for its progressive social policies. In 2009 the National Board of Health and Welfare (Socialstyrelsen), a government agency under the Ministry of Health and Social Affairs, ruled that health care professionals are responsible for assessing patients' abilities and the availability of support before prescribing self-care practices (SOSFS 2009:6). This statute is now being implemented collaboratively between primary, secondary, and community care providers in Sweden. We have written about the importance of the initiative, encouraging other countries to adopt similar measures (Stromberg, Jaarsma, & Riegel, 2012).

Recently we joined forces with the International Self-Care Foundation (ISF); Riegel is a member of their Academic Advisory Board. The ISF was initially established in China in 2011 and separately in 2014 as ISF Global, run out of the United Kingdom. Both organizations are registered as charities, which helps ensure that ISF is independent of vested interests and free to work with any interested party. The mission of ISF is to support the development of evidence-based self-care concepts, practices, and policies and to promote the role of self-care, defined in a manner consistent with our middle range theory of self-care (Riegel, Jaarsma, & Stromberg, 2012) in health. To promote self-care, ISF has named July 24 as International Self-Care Day. The ultimate objective is to have this day accepted as an official United Nations annual commemorative day. Toward that goal, ISF successfully promoted a U.S. Senate resolution to this effect (www.congress.gov/bill/113th-congress/senate-resolution/515) in 2014. ISF is currently working on an "ISF World Healthy City Award," to be presented to cities that have taken significant steps toward creating a living environment conducive to self-care and healthy lifestyles. This award will recognize best practices of policy makers in the urban environment.

Professional Health Care Policy

At a professional level, we have promoted the importance of self-care in clinical guidelines and scientific statements. In 2009 we led a multidisciplinary scientific statement from the American Heart Association, which highlighted concepts and evidence important to understanding and promoting self-care in persons with HF. That statement has been cited 539 times in major interdisciplinary journals such as the *Journal of the American Medical Association* (*JAMA*) published worldwide. We are currently finalizing a new version of this scientific statement advocating self-care of cardiovascular disease, to be published by the American Heart Association in 2017. Our work on self-care has been used in HF clinical guidelines from the Heart Failure Society of America, the American Heart Association, and the European Society of Cardiology guidelines for the diagnosis and treatment of acute and chronic HF.

In 2013, The Joint Commission's Center for Transforming Healthcare incorporated the SCHFI into their Targeted Solutions Tool™ (TST) for use in one of their center projects focused on preventing avoidable decompensation events (and therefore acute care visits) for patients with HF. The TST is a program that guides health care organizations through a step-by-step process to accurately measure their organizations' actual performance, identify their barriers to excellent performance, and direct them to proven solutions that are customized to address each organization's particular barriers. Many national health care systems and organizations that were involved in the Preventing Avoidable Heart Failure Hospitalizations project with the Joint Commission have used the SCHFI, and the Joint Commission promotes the use of the SCHFI to organizations as one approach to assisting with tailoring education and care planning. They have promoted use of the SCHFI in their international efforts as well.

CONCLUSION

This chapter has described the evolution of our work in self-care from a site-specific effort to understand a specific intervention designed for a single group of patients to a worldwide collaborative effort involving patients with a wide variety of illnesses. This brief summary of our research describes advances in theory and measurement over the 25 years that we have been studying the manner in which people with chronic illness care for themselves. Through the process of theoretical development, empirical testing, and significant contributions from many of our colleagues, we have learned immense amounts about self-care. Our work has demonstrated that self-care in general, and management in particular, is extremely challenging for patients. Those who engage in self-care have better outcomes. What we know about self-care is truly the product of global teams with a mission of improving outcomes of persons with chronic illnesses such as HF and their families. Helping patients to become experts in self-care is the focus of our current and future work. As a team, we bring unique skills that we leverage to advance the science of self-care.

With acknowledgment of both maintenance and management, we have introduced a language that helps to integrate the inconsistencies that plague the self-care literature. That is, not all of self-care involves management; sometimes we maintain stability and sometimes we manage illness. Investigators working worldwide in a wide variety of illnesses are now acknowledging this approach as a means to rectify the language disarray in the field. Our policy successes have been robust in some realms, but efforts must be redoubled to continue the push.

REFERENCES

Ara, S. (2004). A literature review of cardiovascular disease management programs in managed care populations. *Journal of Managed Care Pharmacy, 10*(4), 326–344.

Bali, R., Troshani, I., Goldberg, S., & Wickramasinghe, N. (Eds.). (2013). *Pervasive health knowledge management*. New York, NY: Springer. doi:10.1007/978-1-4614-4514-2

Barbaranelli, C., Lee, C. S., Vellone, E., & Riegel, B. (2014). Dimensionality and reliability of the self-care of heart failure index scales: Further evidence from confirmatory factor analysis. *Research in Nursing & Health, 37*(6), 524–537. doi:10.1002/nur.21623

Barbaranelli, C., Lee, C. S., Vellone, E., & Riegel, B. (2015). The problem with Cronbach's alpha: Comment on Sijtsma and van der Ark (2015). *Nursing Research, 64*(2), 140–145. doi:10.1097/NNR.0000000000000079

Bidwell, J. T., Vellone, E., Lyons, K. S., D'Agostino, F., Riegel, B., Juarez-Vela, R., . . . Lee, C. S. (2015). Determinants of heart failure self-care maintenance and management in patients and caregivers: A dyadic analysis. *Research in Nursing & Health, 38*(5), 392–402. doi:10.1002/nur.21675

Buck, H. G., Dickson, V. V., Fida, R., Riegel, B., D'Agostino, F., Alvaro, R., & Vellone, E. (2015). Predictors of hospitalization and quality of life in heart failure: A model of comorbidity, self-efficacy and self-care. *International Journal of Nursing Studies, 52*(11), 1714–1722. doi:10.1016/j.ijnurstu.2015.06.018

Cardiology Preeminence Roundtable. (1994). *Beyond four walls: Cost-effective management of chronic congestive heart failure*. Washington, DC: Advisory Board Company.

Carlson, B., Riegel, B., & Moser, D. K. (2001). Self-care abilities of patients with heart failure. *Heart & Lung: The Journal of Acute and Critical Care, 30*(5), 351–359. doi:10.1067/mhl.2001.118611

Dickson, V. V., Buck, H., & Riegel, B. (2011). A qualitative meta-analysis of heart failure self-care practices among individuals with multiple comorbid conditions. *Journal of Cardiac Failure, 17*(5), 413–419.

Dickson, V. V., Buck, H., & Riegel, B. (2013). Multiple comorbid conditions challenge heart failure self-care by decreasing self-efficacy. *Nursing Research, 62*(1), 2–9. doi:10.1097/NNR.0b013e31827337b3

Dickson, V. V., Chyun, D., Caridi, C., Gregory, J. K., & Katz, S. (2016). Low literacy self-care management patient education for a multi-lingual heart failure population: Results of a pilot study. *Applied Nursing Research, 29*, 122–124. doi:10.1016/j.apnr.2015.06.002

Dickson, V. V., Combellick, J., Malley, M., Sanchez, L., Squires, A., Katz, S., & Riegel, B. (2012). Developing a culturally-relevant self-care intervention for Hispanic adults with heart failure. *Journal of Cardiac Failure, 18*(8 Suppl.), S104–S105.

Dickson, V. V., Deatrick, J., & Riegel, B. (2008). A typology of heart failure self-care management in non-elders. *European Journal of Cardiovascular Nursing, 7*(3), 171–181. doi:10.1016/j.ejcnurse.2007.11.005

Dickson, V. V., Knafl, G. J., & Riegel, B. (2015). Predictors of medication nonadherence differ among black and white patients with heart failure. *Research in Nursing & Health, 38*(4), 289–300. doi:10.1002/nur.21663

Dickson, V. V., Kuhn, L., Worrall-Carter, L., & Riegel, B. (2011). Whose job is it? Examining gender differences in perceptions about the heart failure self-care role. *Journal of Nursing and Healthcare of Chronic Illness, 3*(2), 99–108.

Dickson, V. V., McCarthy, M., Howe, A., Schipper, J., & Katz, S. (2013). Socio-cultural influences on heart failure self-care among an ethnic minority black population. *Journal of Cardiovascular Nursing, 28*(2), 111–118.

Dickson, V. V., Melkus, G. D., Katz, S., Levine-Wong, A., Dillworth, J., Cleland, C. M., & Riegel, B. (2014). Building skill in heart failure self-care among community dwelling older adults: Results of a pilot study. *Patient Education and Counseling, 96*(2), 188–196. doi:10.1016/j.pec.2014.04.018

Dickson, V. V., & Riegel, B. (2009). Are we teaching what patients need to know? Building skills in heart failure self-care. *Heart & Lung: The Journal of Acute and Critical Care, 38*(3), 253–261.

Dickson, V. V., Tkacs, N., & Riegel, B. (2007). Cognitive influences on self-care decision making in persons with heart failure. *American Heart Journal, 154*(3), 424–431. doi:10.1016/j.ahj.2007.04.058

Ditewig, J. B., Blok, H., Havers, J., & van Veenendaal, H. (2010). Effectiveness of self-management interventions on mortality, hospital readmissions, chronic heart failure hospitalization rate and quality of life in patients with chronic heart failure: A systematic review. *Patient Education and Counseling, 78*(3), 297–315. doi:10.1016/j.pec.2010.01.016

Gohler, A., Januzzi, J. L., Worrell, S. S., Osterziel, K. J., Gazelle, G. S., Dietz, R., & Siebert, U. (2006). A systematic meta-analysis of the efficacy and heterogeneity of disease management programs in congestive heart failure. *Journal of Cardiac Failure, 12*(7), 554–567. doi:10.1016/j.cardfail.2006.03.003

Gonseth, J., Guallar-Castillon, P., Banegas, J. R., & Rodriguez-Artalejo, F. (2004). The effectiveness of disease management programmes in reducing hospital re-admission in older patients with heart failure: A systematic review and meta-analysis of published reports. *European Heart Journal, 25*(18), 1570–1595. doi:10.1016/j.ehj.2004.04.022

Grady, P. A., & Daley, K. (2014). The 2013 national nursing research roundtable: Advancing the science of chronic illness self-management. *Nursing Outlook, 62*(3), 201–203. doi:10.1016/j.outlook.2013.12.001

Grady, P. A., & Gough, L. L. (2014). Self-management: A comprehensive approach to management of chronic conditions. *American Journal of Public Health, 104*(8), e25–e31. doi:10.2105/AJPH.2014.302041

Gure, T. R., Blaum, C. S., Giordani, B., Koelling, T. M., Galecki, A., Pressler, S. J., . . . Langa, K. M. (2012). Prevalence of cognitive impairment in older adults with heart failure. *Journal of the American Geriatrics Society, 60*(9), 1724–1729. doi:10.1111/j.1532-5415.2012.04097.x

Heidenreich, P. A., Albert, N. M., Allen, L. A., Bluemke, D. A., Butler, J., Fonarow, G. C., . . . Stroke Council. (2013). Forecasting the impact of heart failure in the United States: A policy statement from the American Heart Association. *Circulation: Heart Failure.* doi:10.1161/HHF.0b013e318291329a

Jaarsma, T., Stromberg, A., Ben Gal, T., Cameron, J., Driscoll, A., Duengen, H. D., . . . Riegel, B. (2013). Comparison of self-care behaviors of heart failure patients in 15 countries worldwide. *Patient Education and Counseling, 92*(1), 114–120. doi:10.1016/j.pec.2013.02.017

Jonkman, N. H., Westland, H., Groenwold, R. H., Agren, S., Atienza, F., Blue, L., . . . Hoes, A. W. (2016). Do self-management interventions work in patients with heart failure? An individual patient data meta-analysis. *Circulation, 133*(12), 1189–1198. doi:10.1161/CIRCULATIONAHA.115.018006

Jovicic, A., Holroyd-Leduc, J. M., & Straus, S. E. (2006). Effects of self-management intervention on health outcomes of patients with heart failure: A systematic review of randomized controlled trials. *BMC Cardiovascular Disorders, 6,* 43.

Jurgens, C. Y., Lee, C. S., Reitano, J. M., & Riegel, B. (2013). Heart failure symptom monitoring and response training. *Heart & Lung: The Journal of Acute and Critical Care, 42*(4), 273–280. doi:10.1016/j.hrtlng.2013.03.005

Kennedy, A., Reeves, D., Bower, P., Lee, V., Middleton, E., Richardson, G., . . . Rogers, A. (2007). The effectiveness and cost effectiveness of a national lay-led self care support programme for patients with long-term conditions: A pragmatic randomised controlled trial. *Journal of Epidemiology & Community Health, 61*(3), 254–261. doi:10.1136/jech.2006.053538

Knafl, G. J., & Riegel, B. (2014). What puts heart failure patients at risk for poor medication adherence? *Patient Preference and Adherence, 8,* 1007–1018. doi:10.2147/PPA.S64593

Lee, C. S., Gelow, J. M., Bidwell, J. T., Mudd, J. O., Green, J. K., Jurgens, C. Y., & Woodruff-Pak, D. S. (2013). Blunted responses to heart failure symptoms in adults with mild cognitive dysfunction. *Journal of Cardiovascular Nursing, 28*(6), 534–540. doi:10.1097/JCN.0b013e31826620fa

Lee, C. S., Gelow, J. M., Mudd, J. O., Green, J. K., Hiatt, S. O., Chien, C., & Riegel, B. (2015). Profiles of self-care management versus consulting behaviors in adults with heart failure. *European Journal of Cardiovascular Nursing, 14*(1), 63–72. doi:10.1177/1474515113519188

Lee, C. S., Moser, D. K., Lennie, T. A., & Riegel, B. (2011). Event-free survival in adults with heart failure who engage in self-care management. *Heart & Lung: The Journal of Acute and Critical Care, 40*(1), 12–20. doi:10.1016/j.hrtlng.2009.12.003

Lee, C. S., Moser, D. K., Lennie, T. A., Tkacs, N. C., Margulies, K. B., & Riegel, B. (2011). Biomarkers of myocardial stress and systemic inflammation in patients who engage in heart failure self-care management. *Journal of Cardiovascular Nursing, 26*(4), 321–328. doi:10.1097/JCN.0b013e31820344be

Lee, C. S., Mudd, J. O., Hiatt, S. O., Gelow, J. M., Chien, C., & Riegel, B. (2015). Trajectories of heart failure self-care management and changes in quality of life. *European Journal of Cardiovascular Nursing, 14*(6), 486–494. doi:10.1177/1474515114541730

Lee, C. S., Riegel, B., Driscoll, A., Suwanno, J., Moser, D. K., Lennie, T. A., . . . Worrall-Carter, L. (2009). Gender differences in heart failure self-care: A multinational cross-sectional study. *International Journal of Nursing Studies, 46*(11), 1485–1495. doi:10.1016/j.ijnurstu.2009.04.004

Lee, C. S., Suwanno, J., & Riegel, B. (2009). The relationship between self-care and health status domains in Thai patients with heart failure. *European Journal of Cardiovascular Nursing, 8*(4), 259–266. doi:10.1016/j.ejcnurse.2009.04.002

Lee, C. S., Tkacs, N. C., & Riegel, B. (2009). The influence of heart failure self-care on health outcomes: Hypothetical cardioprotective mechanisms. *Journal of Cardiovascular Nursing, 24*(3), 179–187; quiz 188–179. doi:10.1097/JCN.0b013e31819b5419

Leppin, A. L., Gionfriddo, M. R., Kessler, M., Brito, J. P., Mair, F. S., Gallacher, K., . . . Montori, V. M. (2014). Preventing 30-day hospital readmissions: A systematic review and meta-analysis of randomized trials. *JAMA Internal Medicine, 174*(7), 1095–1107. doi:10.1001/jamainternmed.2014.1608

Lochner, K. A., & Cox, C. S. (2013). Prevalence of multiple chronic conditions among Medicare beneficiaries, United States, 2010. *Preventing Chronic Disease, 10*, E61. doi:10.5888/pcd10.120137

Lorig, K. R., & Holman, H. (2003). Self-management education: History, definition, outcomes, and mechanisms. *Annals of Behavioral Medicine, 26*(1), 1–7.

Masterson Creber, R., Patey, M., Decesaris, M., Gee, W. H., Dickson, V. V., & Riegel, B. (2015). Motivational interviewing tailored interventions for heart failure (MITI-HF): Study design and methods. *Contemporary Clinical Trials, 41*, 62–68.

Masterson Creber, R., Patey, M., Lee, C. S., Kuan, A., Jurgens, C., & Riegel, B. (2016). Motivational interviewing to improve self-care for patients with chronic heart failure: MITI-HF randomized controlled trial. *Patient Education and Counseling, 99*(2), 256–264. doi:10.1016/j.pec.2015.08.031

McAlister, F. A., Lawson, F. M., Teo, K. K., & Armstrong, P. W. (2001). A systematic review of randomized trials of disease management programs in heart failure. *American Journal of Medicine, 110*(5), 378–384.

McAlister, F. A., Stewart, S., Ferrua, S., & McMurray, J. J. (2004). Multidisciplinary strategies for the management of heart failure patients at high risk for admission: A systematic review of randomized trials. *Journal of the American College of Cardiology, 44*(4), 810–819.

Ofman, J. J., Badamgarav, E., Henning, J. M., Knight, K., Gano, A. D., Jr., Levan, R. K., . . . Weingarten, S. R. (2004). Does disease management improve clinical and economic outcomes in patients with chronic diseases? A systematic review. *American Journal of Medicine, 117*(3), 182–192.

Packer, M. (1992). The neurohormonal hypothesis: A theory to explain the mechanism of disease progression in heart failure. *Journal of the American College of Cardiology, 20*(1), 248–254.

Paterson, B., & Thorne, S. (2000a). Developmental evolution of expertise in diabetes self-management. *Journal of Clinical Nursing, 9*(4), 402–419.

Paterson, B., & Thorne, S. (2000b). Expert decision making in relation to unanticipated blood glucose levels. *Research in Nursing & Health, 23*(2), 147–157.

Rathman, L. D., Lee, C. S., Sarkar, S., & Small, R. S. (2011). A critical link between heart failure self-care and intrathoracic impedance. *Journal of Cardiovascular Nursing, 26*(4), E20–E26. doi:10.1097/JCN.0b013e3181ee28c8

Rich, M. W., Beckham, V., Wittenberg, C., Leven, C. L., Freedland, K. E., & Carney, R. M. (1995). A multidisciplinary intervention to prevent the readmission of elderly patients with congestive heart failure. *New England Journal of Medicine, 333*(18), 1190–1195. doi:10.1056/NEJM199511023331806

Riegel, B., & Carlson, B. (2002). Facilitators and barriers to heart failure self-care. *Patient Education and Counseling, 46*(4), 287–295.

Riegel, B., Carlson, B., & Glaser, D. (2000). Development and testing of a clinical tool measuring self-management of heart failure. *Heart & Lung: The Journal of Acute and Critical Care, 29*(1), 4–15.

Riegel, B., Carlson, B., Glaser, D., & Hoagland, P. (2000). Which patients with heart failure respond best to multidisciplinary disease management? *Journal of Cardiac Failure, 6*(4), 290–299.

Riegel, B., Carlson, B., Glaser, D., & Romero, T. (2006). Randomized controlled trial of telephone case management in Hispanics of Mexican origin with heart failure. *Journal of Cardiac Failure, 12*(3), 211–219.

Riegel, B., Carlson, B., Kopp, Z., LePetri, B., Glaser, D., & Unger, A. (2002). Effect of a standardized nurse case-management telephone intervention on resource use in patients with chronic heart failure. *Archives of Internal Medicine, 162*(6), 705–712.

Riegel, B., Carlson, B., Moser, D. K., Sebern, M., Hicks, F. D., & Roland, V. (2004). Psychometric testing of the self-care of heart failure index. *Journal of Cardiac Failure, 10*(4), 350–360.

Riegel, B., & Dickson, V. V. (2008). A situation-specific theory of heart failure self-care. *Journal of Cardiovascular Nursing, 23*(3), 190–196. doi:10.1097/01.JCN.0000305091.35259.85

Riegel, B., & Dickson, V. V. (2016). A qualitative secondary data analysis of intentional and unintentional medication nonadherence in adults with chronic heart failure. *Heart Lung, 45*(6), 468–474. doi:10.1016/j.hrtlng.2016.08.00

Riegel, B., Dickson, V. V., Cameron, J., Johnson, J. C., Bunker, S., Page, K., & Worrall-Carter, L. (2010). Symptom recognition in elders with heart failure. *Journal of Nursing Scholarship, 42*(1), 92–100. doi:10.1111/j.1547-5069.2010.01333.x

Riegel, B., Dickson, V. V., & Faulkner, K. M. (2015). The situation-specific theory of heart failure self-care: Revised and updated. *Journal of Cardiovascular Nursing*. doi:10.1097/JCN.0000000000000244

Riegel, B., Dickson, V. V., Hoke, L., McMahon, J. P., Reis, B. F., & Sayers, S. (2006). A motivational counseling approach to improving heart failure self-care: Mechanisms of effectiveness. *Journal of Cardiovascular Nursing, 21*(3), 232–241.

Riegel, B., Dickson, V. V., Kuhn, L., Page, K., & Worrall-Carter, L. (2010). Gender-specific barriers and facilitators to heart failure self-care: A mixed methods study. *International Journal of Nursing Studies, 47*(7), 888–895. doi:10.1016/j.ijnurstu.2009.12.011

Riegel, B., Dickson, V. V., & Topaz, M. (2013). Qualitative analysis of naturalistic decision making in adults with chronic heart failure. *Nursing Research, 62*(2), 91–98. doi:10.1097/NNR.0b013e318276250c

Riegel, B., Driscoll, A., Suwanno, J., Moser, D. K., Lennie, T. A., Chung, M. L., . . . Cameron, J. (2009). Heart failure self-care in developed and developing countries. *Journal of Cardiac Failure, 15*(6), 508–516. doi:10.1016/j.cardfail.2009.01.009

Riegel, B., Jaarsma, T., & Stromberg, A. (2012). A middle-range theory of self-care of chronic illness. *Advances in Nursing Science, 35*(3), 194–204. doi:10.1097/ANS.0b013e318261b1ba

Riegel, B., & Knafl, G. J. (2014). Electronically monitored medication adherence predicts hospitalization in heart failure patients. *Patient Preference and Adherence, 8*, 1–13.

Riegel, B., Lee, C., Albert, N., Lennie, T., Chung, M., Song, E., . . . Moser, D. (2011). From novice to expert: Confidence and activity status determine heart failure self-care performance. *Nursing Research, 60*(2), 132–138.

Riegel, B., Lee, C. S., & Dickson, V. V. (2011). Self care in patients with chronic heart failure. *Nature Reviews Cardiology, 8*(11), 644–654. doi:10.1038/nrcardio.2011.95

Riegel, B., Lee, C. S., Dickson, V. V., & Carlson, B. (2009). An update on the self-care of heart failure index. *Journal of Cardiovascular Nursing, 24*(6), 485–497. doi:10.1097/JCN.0b013e3181b4baa0

Riegel, B., Lee, C. S., Ratcliffe, S. J., De Geest, S., Potashnik, S., Patey, M., . . . Weintraub, W. S. (2012). Predictors of objectively measured medication nonadherence in adults with heart failure. *Circulation: Heart Failure, 5*(4), 430–436. doi:10.1161/circheartfailure.111.965152

Riegel, B., Moelter, S. T., Ratcliffe, S. J., Pressler, S. J., De Geest, S., Potashnik, S., . . . Goldberg, L. R. (2011). Excessive daytime sleepiness is associated with poor medication adherence in adults with heart failure. *Journal of Cardiac Failure, 17*(4), 340–348. doi:10.1016/j.cardfail.2010.11.002

Riegel, B., Thomason, T., Carlson, B., Bernasconi, B., Clark, A., Hoagland, P., . . . Watkins, J. (1999). Implementation of a multidisciplinary disease management program for heart failure patients. *Congestive Heart Failure, 5*(4), 164–170.

Roccaforte, R., Demers, C., Baldassarre, F., Teo, K. K., & Yusuf, S. (2005). Effectiveness of comprehensive disease management programmes in improving clinical outcomes in heart failure patients. A meta-analysis. *European Journal of Heart Failure, 7*(7), 1133–1144. doi:10.1016/j.ejheart.2005.08.005

Savard, L. A., Thompson, D. R., & Clark, A. M. (2011). A meta-review of evidence on heart failure disease management programs: The challenges of describing and synthesizing evidence on complex interventions. *Trials, 12,* 194. doi:1745-6215-12-194

Sayers, S. L., Riegel, B., Pawlowski, S., Coyne, J. C., & Samaha, F. F. (2008). Social support and self-care of patients with heart failure. *Annals of Behavioral Medicine, 35*(1), 70–79. doi:10.1007/s12160-007-9003-x

Seta, Y., Shan, K., Bozkurt, B., Oral, H., & Mann, D. L. (1996). Basic mechanisms in heart failure: The cytokine hypothesis. *Journal of Cardiac Failure, 2*(3), 243–249.

Sochalski, J., Jaarsma, T., Krumholz, H. M., Laramee, A., McMurray, J. J., Naylor, M. D., . . . Stewart, S. (2009). What works in chronic care management: The case of heart failure. *Health Affairs, 28*(1), 179–189. doi:10.1377/hlthaff.28.1.179

Stromberg, A., Jaarsma, T., & Riegel, B. (2012). Self-care: Who cares? *European Journal of Cardiovascular Nursing, 11*(2), 133–134. doi:10.1177/1474515111429660

Van Cleave, J., Gortmaker, S. L., & Perrin, J. M. (2010). Dynamics of obesity and chronic health conditions among children and youth. *JAMA, 303*(7), 623–630. doi:10.1001/jama.2010.104

Vellone, E., Fida, R., D'Agostino, F., Mottola, A., Juarez-Vela, R., Alvaro, R., & Riegel, B. (2015). Self-care confidence may be the key: A cross-sectional study on the association between cognition and self-care behaviors in adults with heart failure. *International Journal of Nursing Studies, 52*(11), 1705–1713. doi:10.1016/j.ijnurstu.2015.06.013

Whellan, D. J., Hasselblad, V., Peterson, E., O'Connor, C. M., & Schulman, K. A. (2005). Meta-analysis and review of heart failure disease management randomized controlled clinical trials. *American Heart Journal, 149*(4), 722–729.

Wu, J. R., Moser, D. K., De Jong, M. J., Rayens, M. K., Chung, M. L., Riegel, B., & Lennie, T. A. (2009). Defining an evidence-based cutpoint for medication adherence in heart failure. *American Heart Journal, 157*(2), 285–291. doi:10.1016/j.ahj.2008.10.001

9

Integration of Genomics in Nursing Research: An Example

Karen E. Wickersham and Susan G. Dorsey

The groundbreaking accomplishments of the Human Genome Project (Guttmacher & Collins, 2003) transformed health care research. Innovative studies aimed at understanding the mechanisms underlying acute and chronic conditions have led to the discovery of new therapeutic strategies for many of those conditions (Jenkins, Grady, & Collins, 2005), including cancer, cystic fibrosis, and neuropathic pain. As we transition to an era of precision medicine (Precision Medicine Initiative [PMI] Working Group, 2015), the application of genomic research has implications for the prevention, diagnosis, treatment, and management of acute and chronic conditions, as well as the symptoms associated with these conditions (Jenkins et al., 2005). As the largest and most trusted group of health care workers in the United States and around the world (Calzone et al., 2010), nurses are uniquely positioned to participate in the translation of genomic research from "bench to bedside and back" (Conley & Tinkle, 2007, p. 17). This chapter addresses the integration of genomics in nursing research by:

- Defining the terms *genetics* and *genomics* and providing a brief overview of current technological methods used in genomic research
- Discussing the genomic nursing science blueprint and resulting research questions for nursing inquiry
- Discussing Exemplar 1: Genomic nursing research performed at the National Institute of Nursing Research
- Discussing Exemplar #2: Extramural nursing research examining neuropathic pain related to spinal cord injury
- Summarizing future directions for genomic nursing research

WHAT IS GENETICS/GENOMICS?

Genomic research is one of the many "omics" that are now being investigated in health care research (e.g., transcriptomics, metabolomics, epigenomics and lipidomics, and others; Cheek, Bashore, & Brazeau, 2015). The terms *genetics* and *genomics* are often used interchangeably but, in fact, are different concepts. *Genetics* is the study of single genes and generally refers to heredity and inherited traits. *Genomics* refers to the study of the structure, content, function, and evolution of all nucleotide sequences in the entire genome of a species (Cheek et al., 2015; Johnson, Giarelli, Lewis, & Rice, 2013), and takes into account the influences of the environment, personal lifestyle, and psychosocial and cultural factors (Feero & Collins, 2010).

Current approaches to genomic research (Conley et al., 2013), from a methodological perspective, include sequence-based and array-based platforms (Biesecker, 2012; Rizzo & Buck, 2012). Both of these technology platforms can be used to conduct genomic studies such as genome-wide association studies (GWAS; Marian, 2012), gene expression profiling and transcriptomics analyses (Arao, Matsumoto, Maegawa, & Nishio, 2011), and the examination of differential DNA methylation, which is one important aspect of epigenomic analyses (Emes & Farrell, 2012). While a complete review of all platform technologies and their use is beyond the scope of this chapter, we briefly review the conceptual foundation for the conduct of GWAS, transcriptomics, gene expression analysis, and epigenomics, as well as the relative advantages and disadvantages of each methodological platform.

TYPES OF GENOMIC STUDIES

Genome-Wide Association Studies

GWAS are defined by the National Institutes of Health (NIH) as studies of common genetic variation across the entire human genome, and are designed to identify genetic associations with observable traits (Mitchell, Ferguson, & Ferguson, 2007)—in other words, to observe an association of a phenotype with a particular genotype. The goal of GWAS is to identify single nucleotide polymorphisms (SNPs) in genes that may be associated with disease or symptom susceptibility, or to provide new information about how a particular gene, set of genes, or genes in a canonical signaling pathway might be associated with disease outcomes and/or symptom severity. Several technology platforms, including array-based and sequence-based, can be used to conduct these types of studies. GWAS are performed in unrelated individuals with an attribute of interest (Conley et al., 2013); for example, osteoarthritis pain (Campbell, Trudel, Wong, & Laneuville, 2014; Hsu et al., 2015), which guides the understanding of genetic variation between those with and without disease.

In GWAS, hundreds of thousands of SNPs are examined for an association to a disease in thousands of individuals, ultimately allowing health care professionals to use the information to design effective strategies to screen for or predict disease (Feero & Collins, 2010). The GWAS are not guided by hypotheses. Rather, it is a hypothesis-generating approach that has the potential to identify disease-associated markers in genes that were not previously associated with the particular disease or symptom under study (Wung, Hickey, Taylor, & Gallek, 2013). One major challenge with GWAS as a method is that the GWAS results provide information about the association of functional genetic variants with a phenomenon of interest, but not about causation (Conley et al., 2013). GWAS require large sample sizes, which allows screening for many conditions simultaneously; however, GWAS results are usually limited to the patient sample from which they were developed and do not take into account information about environmental or other nongenetic risk factors (Conley et al., 2013; Pearson & Manolio, 2008). While GWAS results can be used to inform clinical practice and incorporating genomic research findings in clinical practice has been challenging, the results from GWAS can be helpful in initiating conversations with patients about other risk factors for disease (Conley et al., 2013). One example of success in incorporating GWAS findings in clinical practice is the testing of non-small-cell lung cancer (NSCLC) adenocarcinomas for variants in the gene that codes for the epidermal growth factor receptor (EGFR) proteins, which is now considered to be the standard of care (National Comprehensive Cancer Network® [NCCN] guidelines). Searching for these mutations prior to initiating treatment is crucial, because patients with NSCLC adenocarcinoma with sensitizing mutations in *EGFR* generally respond better to EGFR tyrosine kinase inhibitor therapy (Paez et al., 2004; Sequist et al., 2007). However, the mutations themselves are not predictive of patient survival.

Gene Expression Profiling/Transcriptomics

Gene expression profiling, often referred to as *transcriptomics*, investigates the relative expression level of messenger ribonucleic acid (mRNA) in various tissues or circulating plasma. The transcriptome refers to the entire set of mRNAs that are expressed within a single cell or tissue at a specific time or in response to disease or symptom burden (Wang, Gerstein, & Snyder, 2009). As an overall approach, transcriptomics is used to investigate underlying genomic mechanisms in health and disease (Spies et al., 2002). Typically, this involves using either sequence-based or array-based platforms to screen for changes in the expression of hundreds to thousands of genes and transcripts simultaneously (Zhou, Chen, Han, Wang, & Chen, 2014). A *gene* is defined as the locus, or region, of the genome that produces a mature mRNA that is translated into a protein. A transcript refers to the set of alternatively spliced isoforms that are produced by a single gene locus (Gingeras, 2007). Transcriptome analysis is particularly useful to examine the molecular features of a disease or symptom before and after treatment at a specific point in time or to examine expression changes in cases versus controls. Transcriptome data can be used to identify candidate genes or canonical pathways that were altered at the mRNA level that can then be used to predict susceptibility or offer insights into potential new therapeutic targets for further analysis (Harrington, Rosenow, & Retief, 2000; Kurella et al., 2001; Noordewier & Warren, 2001).

Transcriptomic analysis has become especially important in determining the risk of recurrence and survival for women with early-stage breast cancer (Solin et al., 2012). For example, Oncotype DX™ (Genomic Health, Redwood City, California, www. genomichealth.com) is a validated, multigene, expression-based assay that provides information about individualized prognosis, targeted treatment, and surveillance of 21 genes based on the biology of a patient's breast cancer (Albain et al., 2010; Dowsett et al., 2010; Paik et al., 2004, 2006; Solin et al., 2012). The test is meant for use in newly diagnosed women with early-stage (stage I, II, or IIIa), node-negative or node-positive, and estrogen-receptor-positive (ER+), human epidermal growth factor receptor 2 (HER2)-negative breast cancer. Both the American Society of Clinical Oncology® and the NCCN have incorporated Oncotype DX testing into their treatment guidelines for breast cancer (Sparano et al., 2015). Exemplar #2 later in this chapter reviews the use of transcriptomics to identify a potential new therapeutic pathway target to treat chronic neuropathic pain following spinal cord injury (SCI).

Epigenomics

Epigenomics is the study of DNA, using either array-based or sequence-based platforms. But, unlike GWAS, epigenomics produces data related to chemical and structural changes in DNA that impact gene regulation (e.g., changes in methylation) rather than providing nucleotide sequence information (Conley et al., 2013). Disruption of epigenetic networks due to histone modifications, localized changes to chromatin structure, activities of noncoding ribonucleic acids (RNAs), and DNA methylation can result in heritable silencing of genes without changing their coding sequence (Egger, Liang, Aparicio, & Jones, 2004), and can impact injury, illness, pain, and treatment response (Petronis, 2010). For example, because many complex pain conditions such as rheumatoid and osteoarthritis are not associated with heritable factors (Lessans & Dorsey, 2013), epigenomic research has helped to identify potential mechanisms of pain and areas of potential therapeutic response (Lessans & Dorsey, 2013; Mogil, 2012).

METHODS FOR GENETIC AND GENOMIC ANALYSES

Next-Generation Sequencing (NGS)

NGS methods directly examine the DNA or RNA sequence and can be used to conduct high-resolution mapping of 5'—C—phosphate—G—3' (CpG) dinucleotide methylation of DNA to examine epigenomics (Conley et al., 2013; Lan et al., 2011; Metzker, 2010). Genome sequencing uses high-throughput technology to provide information about the order of or methylation status of nucleotide bases in a predetermined length (typically 25–150 base pairs), which is termed a *short read*. Prior genome sequencing technologies accomplished this by examining one molecule at a time using bidirectional Sanger sequencing (Katsanis & Katsanis, 2013); however, advances in technology have made it possible to investigate millions of nucleotides simultaneously (Conley et al., 2013). NGS has become more efficient, with corresponding increases in sequence throughput. Thus, it has also become less expensive over the past 10 years (Figure 9.1; National Human Genome Research Institute [NHGRI], 2015), and it is likely that a sub-$1,000 whole genome sequence will become a reality.

Advantages of NGS include direct capture of sequence data at a digital resolution of individual nucleotides or methylation of CpG sites that can be mapped back to a reference genome; the ability to detect novel SNPs, genes, and transcripts; and the ability to simultaneously interrogate the entire genome, transcriptome, or methylome (Malone & Oliver, 2011). Challenges include the requirement of a multinode computational infrastructure, the need for significant amounts of data storage (files can be terabytes in size), and the need for significant bioinformatics support to implement open-source workflows in R or other programming languages to perform genome alignments and data analysis.

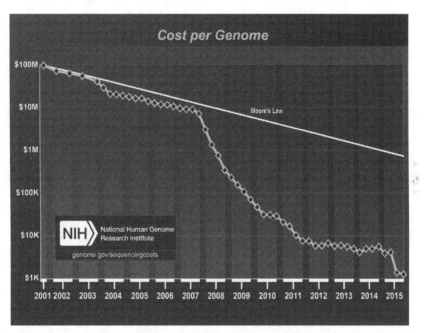

FIGURE 9.1 DNA sequencing costs from the National Human Genome Research Institute (NHGRI). The costs associated with DNA sequencing performed at sequencing centers funded by the NHGRI from 2001 to 2015 (NHGRI, 2015). Costs include labor, administration, management, utilities, reagents, consumables, sequencing instruments and other large equipment, informatics activities directly related to sequence production (e.g., laboratory information management systems and initial data processing), and submission of data to a public database. Data from 2001 to October 2007 represent the costs of generating DNA sequence using Sanger-based chemistries and capillary-based instruments ("first-generation" sequencing platforms). Data beginning in January 2008 represent the costs of generating DNA sequence using "second-generation" (or "next-generation") sequencing platforms.

Source: NHGRI (2015).

Microarray and Other Array-Based Technologies

DNA microarrays can be used to conduct GWAS, transcriptomic, and epigenomic studies. Modern arrays are fabricated on silicon, glass, or plastic substrates and have thousands of probe sets designed to capture small DNA, RNA, or methylated CpG sites (Heller, 2002). In general, labeled complementary (c) RNA or cDNA is hybridized to the arrays and then the fluorescence signal intensity generated by hybridization with individual probe sets is scanned for analysis. Unlike NGS, where each nucleotide is read directly, array-based analysis depends upon transforming the analog fluorescence signal to a value representing relative abundance of gene or transcript expression or calling a SNP for GWAS (DNA). Advantages of microarray technology include relatively short processing time from total RNA or DNA to results that can be analyzed (typically two days), straightforward and mature data analytic workflows that can be implemented in open-source platforms or commercial software packages, the ability to analyze results on most typical desktop computers without the need for advanced computational infrastructure, and relatively small data storage requirements. In our experience, challenges include difficulties inherent in transforming analog to digital signals, off-target hybridization, and limitation of the analysis to the a priori content on the array. So, novel findings are limited.

In sum, we have provided a brief review of current approaches to genomic research that can be used in GWAS, transcriptomic, and epigenomic studies to conduct innovative research aimed at understanding underlying mechanisms of acute and chronic conditions or symptoms and guiding the discovery of new treatments, therapies, or management strategies for those conditions or symptoms. The next section discusses how these approaches may be included in a blueprint for genomic nursing research.

THE BLUEPRINT FOR GENOMIC NURSING SCIENCE

Advances in technologies utilized in conducting genomic research are changing the approach to screening, diagnosis, treatment, prevention, prognosis, and surveillance of chronic illness (Calzone et al., 2012). Because nurses are the largest and most trusted group of health care workers (Calzone et al., 2010; U.S. Department of Health and Human Services, Health Resources and Services Administration [HRSA], Bureau of Health Professions, 2010), they are uniquely poised to implement genomics into clinical nursing and research as a discipline (Calzone et al., 2010). As such, the NIH and HRSA have led several initiatives to prepare nurses to apply genomics in patient care (Jenkins et al., 2005). For example, in 2004, the NHGRI and the National Cancer Institute collaborated to establish the U.S. Genetic/Genomic Nursing Competency Initiative (GGNCI). The GGNCI obtained agreement on essential genomic nursing competencies that apply to all registered nurses regardless of specialty, role, or academic degree (Jenkins & Calzone, 2007). In 2012, the GGNCI published graduate genetic and genomic competencies (Greco, Tinley, & Seibert, 2011). Parallel efforts by the NIH included the Summer Genetics Institute (SGI), which is sponsored by the National Institute of Nursing Research (NINR) and provides participants with a foundation in molecular genetics appropriate for use in research and clinical practice.

In 2012 the NHGRI of the NIH convened a Genomic Nursing State of the Science Advisory Panel to determine gaps in genomic nursing science and to create a blueprint to focus research to address those gaps (Calzone et al., 2013). The primary goals of the advisory panel were to: (a) review and evaluate the available evidence on genetic/genomic competency and nursing practice, and (b) establish a research agenda based on a systematic evaluation of the current state of the science (Calzone et al., 2013). The advisory panel concluded that the two key areas for nursing research would generate evidence about how genomic nursing can contribute to improved client (i.e., person, family, communities, and populations) health outcomes, taking into account the context in which health care is delivered. A description of the blueprint is found in Table 9.1. Four main themes concerning a need for genomic research were identified by the advisory panel: (a) health promotion and disease prevention, including risk assessment, communication, decision support; (b) advancing quality of life for individuals and their families, including symptom management, management of disease states, client self-management; (c) innovation, including technology development, informatics support systems, and environmental influences; and (d) training (e.g., capacity building, education; Calzone et al., 2013). Cross-cutting themes included health disparities, cost, policy, and public education.

As a follow-up to the blueprint, NINR held a Genomic Nursing Science Workshop in August 2013 (NINR, 2013). During this workshop, experts from diverse disciplines identified research questions that were aligned with the NINR's strategic plan and that would guide genomic nursing research in the areas of symptom science, wellness, self-management, end-of life, and palliative care. Specific research questions, which can be located on the NINR website (www.ninr.nih.gov) included:

- What are the biological, physiological, or omic mechanisms underlying symptoms and patient outcomes?
- Based on individual omics, environmental factors, and behavior, what are the most effective and targeted interventions that can be expedited for translation to reduce risk and promote health?
- What are the relative contributions of omic markers and phenomic data in predicting individual responses to therapeutic interventions that improve patient outcomes such as quality of life?
- For high-risk patients who are at the end of life, how can genetic assessment and DNA banking be used to address familial risk?

TABLE 9.1   *Nursing Genomic Science Blueprint Mapping to the NINR Strategic Plan Areas*

NINR Strategic Plan Areas	Specific Nursing Research Categories	Advisory Panel Genomic Nursing Research Topic Areas[a]
Health promotion and disease prevention	Risk assessment	a. Biological plausibility (e.g., pathways, mechanisms, biomarkers, epigenetics, genotoxicity) b. Comprehensive screening opportunities (e.g., family history, identify risk level [population-based average and elevated]) c. Components of risk assessment (e.g., biomarkers, family history) d. Risk-specific health care decision making
	Communication	a. Risk communication (e.g., interpretation, timing, risk reports to the health care provider and client)[b] b. Informed consent c. Direct-to-consumer marketing and testing (e.g., uptake, utilization, dissemination)
	Decision support	a. Informed consent b. Match of values/preferences with decision made c. Risk perception/risk accuracy d. Effect of decision support on decision quality (e.g., knowledge, personal utility)
Advancing the quality of life	Family	a. Family context (e.g., family functioning and structure, family relationships, and communication) b. Ethical issues c. Health care provider communication with families
	Symptom management	a. Biological plausibility (e.g., pathways, mechanisms, biomarkers, epigenetics) b. Clinical utility c. Personal utility d. Pharmacogenomics (e.g., therapy selection, medication titration) e. Decision making f. Evidence-based effectiveness of approaches
	Disease states (encompassing acute, common complex and chronic)	a. Genomic-based interventions that reduce morbidity and mortality b. Gene/environment interactions (e.g., epigenetics, genotoxicity) c. Pharmacogenomics d. Evidence-based effectiveness of treatments/support
	Client self-management	a. Collecting and conveying information that informs self-management (e.g., family history) b. Lifestyle behaviors c. Environmental exposure and protection (e.g., occupational) d. Synergy of client and provider expectations (e.g., client/family-centered care) e. Personal utility
Innovation	Technology development	a. Incorporation of new technologies (e.g., whole genome sequencing) b. Ethics

(continued)

TABLE 9.1 *Nursing Genomic Science Blueprint Mapping to the NINR Strategic Plan Areas* (*continued*)

NINR Strategic Plan Areas	Specific Nursing Research Categories	Advisory Panel Genomic Nursing Research Topic Areas[a]
		c. Policy and guidelines to support applications
		d. Applications (e.g., clinical and analytic validity, clinical utility)
		e. Genomic bioinformatics
		f. Translation, dissemination, implementation
		i. Use of technology in information delivery
		ii. Performance improvement by provider (e.g., point-of-care support)
		iii. Resources that support genomic research (e.g., registries of tools, best practices, nursing outcomes)
	Informatics support systems	a. Data storage and use to facilitate research process and outcomes
		b. Facilitate cross-generational sharing of genomic data (e.g., family history, laboratory analyses)
		c. Managing, analyzing, and interpreting genomic information (e.g., sequencing data)
		d. Point-of-care decision support for client and health care provider
		e. Common terminology and taxonomy
		f. Common formats for data storage/exchange and queries
	Environmental influences (encompassing physical, social environments and policy context)	a. Evidence-based guidelines
		b. Health care reform
		c. Economics (e.g., cost-effectiveness)
		d. Regulatory gaps and/or variability
Training	Capacity building	a. Training future nursing scientists in genomics
		b. Preparing nursing faculty in genomics
		c. Education of current and future workforce in genomics (e.g., research nurse coordinators, advanced practice nurses, other health care professionals)
		d. Preparation of nurse scientists to lead interprofessional teams
		e. Preparation of clinical and administrative leaders to advance appropriate genomic/genetic integration into practice
		f. Innovative uses of biorepositories (e.g., informed consent, result interpretation)
		g. Bioethics
	Education	a. Optimal methods to train the existing nursing workforce in genomics
		b. Optimal methods to train the nursing leadership in genomics to support genomic translation, research, and practice
		c. Optimal methods to integrate nursing genomic competencies in basic prelicensure and postlicensure in academic programs

(continued)

TABLE 9.1   *Nursing Genomic Science Blueprint Mapping to the NINR Strategic Plan Areas (continued)*

NINR Strategic Plan Areas	Specific Nursing Research Categories	Advisory Panel Genomic Nursing Research Topic Areas[a]
Cross-cutting themes		
	Health disparities	a. Racial, ethnic, socioeconomic, and cultural influences on disease occurrence and response to disease and treatment
		b. Genomic health equity (e.g., access)
		c. Diseases that disproportionately affect specific groups (e.g., minorities)
		d. Targeted therapeutics
		e. Overcoming misinformation and genomic "myths"
	Cost	a. Cost-effectiveness
		b. Comparative effectiveness
		c. Value
	Policy	a. Policy as context of science
		b. Research to inform policy
	Public education	a. Health literacy
		b. Genomic literacy

[a]The nursing science blueprint serves as a platform for potential interprofessional collaborations that can include but are not limited to the following: any health care discipline, basic and behavioral scientists, ethicists, business, and/or informatics professionals.

[b]*Clients* refers to persons, families, communities, and/or population.

NINR, National Institute of Nursing Research.

Source: Permission from Calzone et al. (2013). In this table, the authors outline the NINR strategic plan areas, discuss specific nursing research categories, and then map those areas to the advisory panel's genomic nursing research priority topical areas.

- How should omic discoveries be used to create and test technologies (such as clinical tools) that can be used to diagnose clinical problems, predict the clinical course, and promote optimal outcomes?
- In what ways can genomic information be used to promote adherence to and improve self-management of chronic conditions?
- How does the social environment interact with gene expression to influence resilience in coping with life challenges?

In summary, advances in genomic research have affected all aspects of health care, in particular the nursing discipline (Calzone et al., 2010). Integration of genomics into nursing research and practice by developing a body of knowledge about the underlying mechanisms and pathways associated clinical phenotypes, including symptom severity, trajectory, and burden, is needed for nurses to develop, test, and implement interventions tailored to a person and his or her genome. The NIH and other federal agencies have collaborated to develop priorities for nursing research that incorporate the latest genomic technologies. The following sections describe examples of such research.

EXEMPLAR 1: GENOMIC RESEARCH PERFORMED AT THE NATIONAL INSTITUTE OF NURSING RESEARCH

The Division of Intramural Research (DIR) of the NINR, led by Dr. Ann Cashion, conducts basic and clinical research to examine the interactions among molecular mechanisms underlying a single symptom or cluster of symptoms and environmental influences on individual health outcomes (www.ninr.nih.gov). Research conducted by members of the DIR is designed to examine individual genomic variability in symptom phenotypes that are associated with several chronic diseases, including digestive disorders, cancer-related fatigue (CRF), traumatic brain injury, and posttraumatic stress disorders, as well as clinical interventions to alleviate these symptoms. This section discusses genomic research on CRF conducted by investigators of the Symptom Management Branch of the DIR.

For patients with cancer, fatigue is one of the most commonly reported symptoms and often results in decreased functional status and health-related quality of life (Saligan et al., 2015). The etiology of CRF is unclear, but it is thought to be caused by a cascade of events resulting in pro-inflammatory cytokine production, hypothalamic–pituitary–adrenal activation dysfunction, metabolic and/or endocrine dysregulation, disruption to circadian rhythm, and neuromuscular function abnormalities (Saligan et al., 2015). Research efforts conducted by the NINR DIR to understand the underlying biobehavioral mechanisms of CRF include investigations of the role of oxidative stress and inflammation in development of fatigue.

For example, a prospective study (Hsiao, Wang, Kaushal, Chen, & Saligan, 2014) explored the potential relationship between changes in gene expression related to mitochondrial biogenesis/bioenergetics and fatigue in men with prostate cancer (N = 50) receiving external beam radiation therapy (EBRT). Data were collected at baseline prior to initiating EBRT and at the midpoint and end of EBRT. Information about fatigue was measured using the Patient-Reported Outcomes Measurement Information System-Fatigue short form. Whole blood samples were collected at each study time point, and the human mitochondria RT2 Profiler™ PCR Array System was used to identify differential expression of mitochondrial biogenesis/bioenergetics-related genes.

The investigators found a significant correlation between fatigue development and increased levels of erythrocyte oxidative stress, as well as differential expression of genes associated with impairment of mitochondrial biogenesis/bioenergetics: two genes involved in critical mitochondrial complexes, BCS1L (β = 1.30), SLC25A37 (β = −2.44), and two genes on the outer mitochondrial membrane vital for mitochondrial integrity: BCL2L1 (β = −1.68) and FIS1 (β = −2.35). Additional research has focused on the association of upregulation of neuro-inflammatory markers, such as alpha-synuclein, and worsening of fatigue symptoms (Saligan et al., 2013) through transcriptomics analysis from peripheral blood samples. Further investigation of these markers includes in vivo, in vitro, and ex vivo experiments to further understand their role in CRF development.

EXEMPLAR 2: A POTENTIAL NOVEL THERAPEUTIC TARGET TO TREAT SPINAL CORD INJURY–INDUCED NEUROPATHIC PAIN

Here we describe our own research, which investigated whether a truncated isoform of the brain-derived neurotrophic factor (BDNF) receptor is a potential novel therapeutic target to treat SCI-induced neuropathic pain (Wu et al., 2016; Wu, Renn, Faden, & Dorsey, 2013).

SCI results in debilitating motor, sensory, and cognitive deficits and also, in 30% to 80% of patients, neuropathic pain resistant to conventional treatments (e.g., opioids, nonsteroidal anti-inflammatories; Modirian et al., 2010; Rose, Robinson, Ells, & Cole, 1988). On average, 69% of SCI patients experience pain, which starts weeks or months after the original insult, and more than one third report that the pain is severe (Siddall, Yezierski, & Loeser, 2002). The latency between the injury and pain onset suggests that there may be a window to intervene to prevent pain development. However, the development of effective interventions is contingent upon understanding the mechanisms underlying maladaptive central nervous system (CNS) plasticity that takes place during the latent period. One such mechanism is central sensitization, a form of long-term memory that forms in the spinal cord following noxious stimulation, such as SCI (Ji, Kohno, Moore, & Woolf, 2003). Given that BDNF signaling is necessary and sufficient to produce long-term potentiation in the CNS (Lu, Christian, & Lu, 2008) and that it is a potent modulator of pain processing in the CNS (Merighi et al., 2008; Miletic, Hanson, & Miletic, 2004; Pezet & McMahon, 2006), we hypothesized that BDNF signaling via its cell surface receptor, tropomyosin-related kinase B (trkB), might be one mechanism underlying SCI-induced neuropathic pain. We chose to focus on a truncated isoform of the BDNF receptor, trkB.T1, since we have shown that mice lacking the receptor (Dorsey et al., 2006) experience less pain following inflammation of the hindpaw (Renn, Lin, Thomas, & Dorsey, 2009), and others have shown that this receptor is specifically upregulated at the level of the lesion in the spinal cord following injury (King, Bradbury, McMahon, & Priestley, 2000; Liebl, Huang, Young, & Parada, 2001).

First, we showed that following a moderate thoracic contusion injury in mice, trkB.T1 protein expression was elevated at the level of the lesion and also in the spinal dorsal horn, at early and late time points, suggesting an important role for this receptor and the development of motor impairment and pain following SCI. This was specific for the truncated isoform of the BDNF receptor; we found no change in the levels of the full-length receptor, trkB.FL. When we compared the development of neuropathic-pain-like behaviors in mice lacking the truncated receptor, trkB.T1, compared with control mice that had normal levels of the receptor, we found that mice lacking trkB.T1 developed significantly less pain and recovered locomotor function more rapidly. These behavioral findings were associated with a smaller lesion volume in the spinal cord and greater sparing of white matter spinal cord tracts. We were quite interested in understanding why mice lacking this receptor would have less pain and improved locomotor recovery. However, since little is known about the physiological and pathological role of trkB.T1 or its signaling capacity, we had to take a hypothesis-generating approach, using transcriptomics analysis, to determine what genes might lie downstream from the receptor that could explain our findings mechanistically.

For this study, we chose to use microarray technology to interrogate the transcriptome rather than NGS. We chose this technology platform because we were primarily interested in gene level data, versus transcript-level analysis of known and novel genes, and we were in possession of the bioinformatics technologies required to analyze the data efficiently. In addition, when this study was conceived and executed, the bioinformatics pipelines necessary to analyze RNA sequence data were in various stages of maturation and we were concerned with the potential time delays relative to moving the work forward.

We designed the study to examine differential gene expression in the spinal cord, at the level of the lesion, at baseline and then 1, 3, and 7 days after SCI in both normal control mice (trkB.T1 WT) and those lacking trkB.T1 (trkB.T1 KO). While we found that thousands of genes were altered within each genotype, when we analyzed only those gene expression changes that occurred in trkB.T1 KO mice versus controls, we found that relatively few gene changes were different (Figure 9.2A). Moreover, most of the significantly different genes were dysregulated 1 day after SCI; by 3 and 7 days, there were few, if any, changes (Figure 9.2A). We next examined a heat map of the N = 193 genes that were changed in the mice lacking the receptor, and found that many of them were genes that control the cell cycle (Figure 9.2B). We conducted unbiased canonical pathway analysis using Ingenuity Pathway Analysis software (Qiagen, Redwood City, California) and noted that of the top 10 significantly enriched pathways in our dataset, half were directly related to cell cycle regulation (Figure 9.2C). This was further delineated in Figure 9.2D, which shows all of the canonical signaling pathways from our dataset and their proximity or relationship with one another.

We were able to validate the gene expression changes at the protein level, and then demonstrated that intrathecal injection of a cell cycle inhibitor, CR8, in trkB.T1 WT mice significantly reduced neuropathic pain and improved locomotor function. In essence, reducing cell cycle activation in wildtype mice produced a post-SCI pain and function phenotype that was no different from the mice lacking trkB.T1. Giving CR8 to trkB.T1 KO mice had no effect, further confirming our findings that trkB.T1 may regulate cell cycle genes early after SCI to activate astrocytes and microglia as inflammation sets in (Gwak, Kang, Unabia, & Hulsebosch, 2012). We further explored the role for cell cycle activation as a mechanism producing chronic pain after SCI in mice and found that early treatment with cell cycle antagonists significantly limited neuropathic pain and locomotor dysfunction; late treatment with the same drugs reduced pain but had no effect on locomotor recovery (Wu et al., 2016).

Taken together, our results suggest that the BDNF receptor, trkB.T1, may signal to activate cell cycle genes in the spinal cord early after SCI to produce inflammation and subsequent behavioral changes including neuropathic pain and locomotor

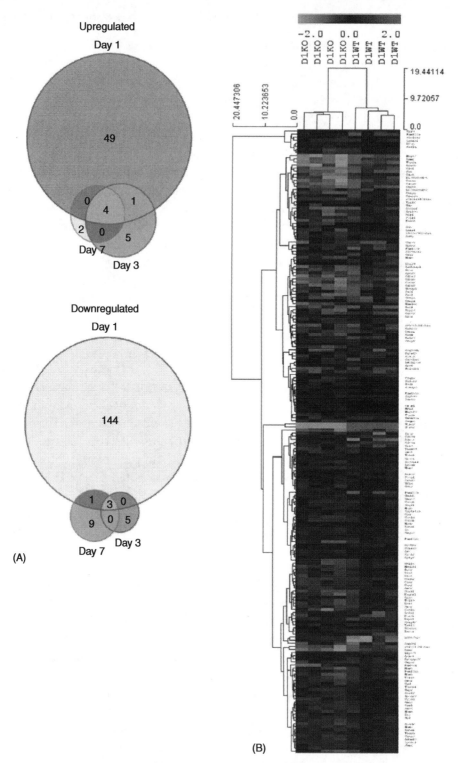

FIGURE 9.2 Cell cycle genes are upregulated in the spinal cord of normal wildtype mice following SCI but not in trkB.T1 KO mice. (A) Differential gene expression analysis in the spinal cord over time shows the number of differentially expressed genes in the trkB.T1 KO mice versus controls. (B) Heat map of genes that cluster by genotype at day one in the KO spinal cord versus controls—the histogram key indicates upregulated genes and downregulated genes. (*continued*)

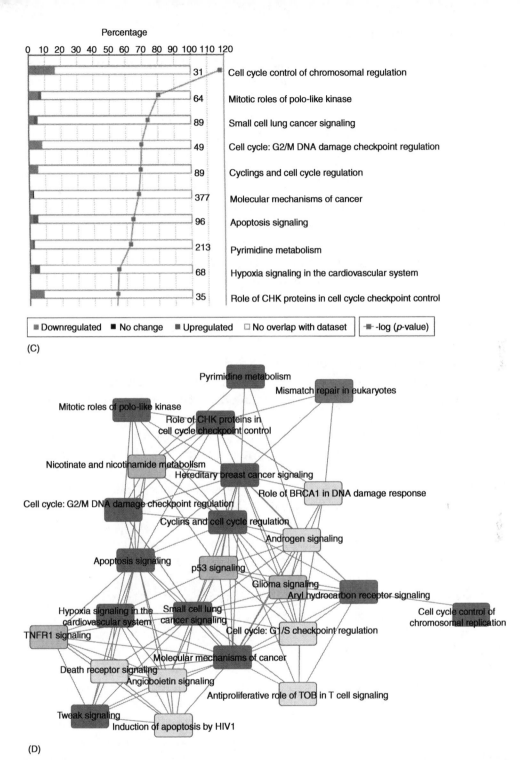

FIGURE 9.2 *(continued)* (C) Unbiased pathway analysis shows that cell cycle genes, and cell cycle pathways, are significantly downregulated in the trkB.T1 KO spinal cord when compared with controls. (D) Overlapping shared gene sets in the database. The darker the gray, the more significant the overlapping pathway is in our gene set using a Fisher's exact test.

CHK, check point; KO, knock out; SCI, spinal cord injury.

Source: Republished with permission from Wu et al. (2013). Permission conveyed through Copyright Clearance Center, Inc.

dysfunction. Blocking cell cycle activation can limit neuropathic pain and locomotor dysfunction if given early, while late treatment with cell cycle antagonists has effects mostly on pain development. They further suggest that the trkB.T1 receptor may be a novel therapeutic target for SCI-induced neuropathic pain treatment, and also shed light on the potential for cell cycle inhibitor use to manage post-SCI pain, acknowledging that further preclinical and clinical studies will be needed.

We highlighted this exemplar to demonstrate how whole transcriptome profiling of gene expression changes can be used to generate new hypotheses regarding the molecular mechanisms underlying the development and severity of symptoms; in this case, chronic neuropathic pain following SCI. Without these studies, we would not have been aware of the potential role for spinal cord cell cycle gene activation in the pain and locomotor phenotype, nor would we have understood the potential role that trkB.T1 has in activating these pathways.

IMPLICATIONS FOR POLICY

In the previous sections, we provided a brief review of current approaches to genomic research, how these approaches may be included in a blueprint for genomic nursing research, and two examples of nursing research that incorporates genomics into research seeking to understand underlying mechanisms of symptoms related to acute and chronic illness and disease. Building a body of evidence for answering these genomic research questions has implications with regard to health policy from several points of view. For example, the Institute of Medicine asserts that there is enough scientific evidence to include genetics, genomics, and pharmacogenomics in an electronic health record (McCormick, 2016). Genomic conditions can be documented using the *International Statistical Classification of Diseases and Related Health Problems 10th Revision (ICD-10)* codes, and the Centers for Medicare and Medicaid now reimburse for nine genetic tests (McCormick, 2016). In addition, the American Nurses Association and other nursing associations have developed guidelines for addressing genomics in nursing practice (McCormick, 2016). Therefore, as nurses, we have a social and professional responsibility to understand and be conversant in laws, guidelines, and policies related to genetic and genomic research (Haig et al., 2016) so that we can guide the use and interpretation of research findings to patients and their families in the best way possible (Badzek, Henaghan, Turner, & Monsen, 2013). The Ethics Committee for the Human Genome Organization recognized this and developed five principles to guide the use of genomics in health care (Kirby, 1997): (a) not to act is to make a decision, (b) use human rights to frame the law, (c) consult the community to obtain input from those who suffer from genetic/genomic conditions, or from those who would benefit from the genomic research, so that researchers and health care professionals can understand the community's concerns and expectations, (d) response to genomics must be based on good science, and (e) to be effective, policies must be global in nature. Unfortunately, access to genomic technologies such as molecular diagnostic technologies in the United States and around the world is unequal (Plun-Favreau et al., 2016). For example, molecular technologies such as the Oncotype DX Breast Cancer Assay discussed earlier in this chapter help oncologists and health care team members make an informed decision about patient treatment and enable integration of precision medicine. Unfortunately, access to these technologies remains unequal across countries and sometimes even within individual countries (Plun-Favreau et al., 2016), including the United States.

In addition, the new PMI (PMI Working Group, 2015) is likely to result in an increase in research focused on genetics, genomics, epigenetics, and other "omics" (Yu et al., 2016), potentially increasing the need for further development of "bio-banks." A *biobank* is a searchable repository of samples and related health data (Rothstein, Knoppers, & Harrell, 2016). Biobanks are beneficial in that they facili-tate analyses of genomic "big data" using large cohorts of participants; however, policies addressing the collection, storage, analysis, curation, and distribution of specimens and data vary from country to country, and within individual countries (Rothstein et al., 2016; Haga & Beskow, 2008). For example, countries with a national biobank, such as the United Kingdom, do not have national legislation specific to the regulation of biobanks. Other countries, such as China, Finland, Thailand, and Estonia, regulate biobanks under the general regulations for the conduct of biomed-ical research. Currently, the United States has no established laws providing over-sight of biobanks, but some provisions have been proposed (Rothstein et al., 2016). Local ethics approval is required for storage and future use of genomic research specimens and data; however, little can be done for a research participant to correct an alleged violation of privacy (U.S. Department of Homeland Security, 2015).

Research continues to focus on elucidating omics biomarkers of symptoms related to chronic illness or self-management of those illnesses. One policy implication for these involves the identification of common data elements (CDEs) that are used in nursing research. For example, the NINR has recently released a set of CDEs for symptom science (Redeker et al., 2015; www.ninr.nih.gov/researchandfunding/cde-main#.V4z6e44mDvA), with recommendations for self-management (Moore et al., 2016) and biomarker CDEs forthcoming. The use of CDEs will facilitate data sharing across sites and investigators and enable big data science.

CONCLUSION

The future includes personalization of information to improve individual health care outcomes through identification of genomic variation, genetic testing, evalu-ation of gene expression changes, gene therapy, changes in the epigenome, or the use of molecular materials to influence gene expression, and other areas of new sci-entific development (Badzek et al., 2013). A significant area for future investments in genomic research will be provided by the Precision Medicine Initiative Cohort Program (PMI-CP) at the NIH, which was announced by President Obama on January 20, 2015, during the State of the Union address. According to the executive summary, questions include examination of the molecular, environmental, and behavioral factors contributing to health and disease so that more efficacious treatment strategies, including identification of novel therapeutic targets, can be realized (www.nih.gov/precision-medicine-initiative-cohort-program). NIH's investment in PMI will focus on: (a) PMI-Oncology, an effort to advance precision oncology and (b) PMI-CP, the creation of a large, voluntary national research cohort. PMI-Oncology will test precision therapies for cancer, including targeted agents and immunotherapies, while also developing a national cancer knowledge system. This work will lay the foundations for precision medicine approaches more broadly, by building a national research cohort of 1 million or more volunteers who are engaged as partners in a longitudinal, long-term effort to identify the molecular, environmental, and behavioral factors that contribute to diverse diseases; to facilitate the development and testing of novel therapies and prevention approaches; and to pioneer mobile Health strategies for improving the efficacy of health care.

In terms of genomic nursing research, there has never been a more opportune time to invest in using genetic and genomic tools to more fully explicate the molecular mechanisms of symptoms associated with chronic disease, including the contribution of individual variation to risk for symptom development, severity, and persistence. Genomic nursing research can also ask questions related to how underlying genetic and genomic differences could account for individual responses to nonpharmacological self-management strategies for symptom management. For example, we know that in humans, exercise and physical activity can alleviate inflammatory, neuropathic, and chronic musculoskeletal pain (Dixit, Maiya, & Shastry, 2014; Hurkmans, van der Giesen, Vliet Vlieland, Schoones, & Van den Ende ECHM, 2009; Wright & Sluka, 2001). In rodents, timed treadmill training and volitional wheel running reverses neuropathic pain produced by nerve injury (Cobianchi, Casal-Diaz, Jaramillo, & Navarro, 2013; Sheahan, Copits, Golden, & Gereau, 2015), and non-weight-bearing exercise (swimming; Shen, Fox, & Cheng, 2013) also reduces neuropathic pain. Other studies, however, have shown that some, but not all, participants experience a benefit from physical activity or exercise (Rooks et al., 2007). An open question remains regarding how these types of self-management strategies work, in whom they work, and what dose is most effective. Much like pharmacogenomic studies of drug responders versus nonresponders, genomic nursing science can use these tools to examine the contribution of individual genetic and genomic variation in response to self-management strategies to reduce or alleviate symptoms associated with chronic disease. These are just several of the areas of genomic science that nursing is uniquely poised to address—it is truly an exciting time to be a nurse scientist!

REFERENCES

Albain, K. S., Barlow, W. E., Shak, S., Hortobagyi, G. N., Livingston, R. B., Yeh, I. T., . . . Hayes, D. F. (2010). Prognostic and predictive value of the 21-gene recurrence score assay in postmenopausal women with node-positive, oestrogen-receptor-positive breast cancer on chemotherapy: A retrospective analysis of a randomised trial. *The Lancet Oncology*, 11(1), 55–65. doi:10.1016/S1470-2045(09)70314-6

Arao, T., Matsumoto, K., Maegawa, M., & Nishio, K. (2011). What can and cannot be done using a microarray analysis? Treatment stratification and clinical applications in oncology. *Biological and Pharmaceutical Bulletin, 34*(12), 1789–1793. Retrieved from http://jlc.jst.go.jp/JST .JSTAGE/bpb/34.1789?from=Google

Badzek, L., Henaghan, M., Turner, M., & Monsen, R. (2013). Ethical, legal, and social issues in the translation of genomics into health care. *Journal of Nursing Scholarship, 45*(1), 15–24. doi:10.1111/jnu.12000

Biesecker, L. G. (2012). Opportunities and challenges for the integration of massively parallel genomic sequencing into clinical practice: Lessons from the ClinSeq project. *Genetics in Medicine: Official Journal of the American College of Medical Genetics, 14*(4), 393–398. doi:10.1038/ gim.2011.78

Calzone, K. A., Cashion, A., Feetham, S., Jenkins, J., Prows, C. A., Williams, J. K., & Wung, S. (2010). Nurses transforming health care using genetics and genomics. *Nursing Outlook, 58*(1), 26–35. doi:10.1016/j.outlook.2009.05.001

Calzone, K. A., Jenkins, J., Bakos, A. D., Cashion, A. K., Donaldson, N., Feero, W. G., . . . Webb, J. A. (2013). A blueprint for genomic nursing science. *Journal of Nursing Scholarship, 45*(1), 96–104. doi:10.1111/jnu.12007

Calzone, K. A., Jenkins, J., Yates, J., Cusack, G., Wallen, G. R., Liewehr, D. J., . . . McBride, C. (2012). Survey of nursing integration of genomics into nursing practice. *Journal of Nursing Scholarship, 44*(4), 428–436. doi:10.1111/j.1547-5069.2012.01475.x

Campbell, T. M., Trudel, G., Wong, K. K., & Laneuville, O. (2014). Genome wide gene expression analysis of the posterior capsule in patients with osteoarthritis and knee flexion contracture. *Journal of Rheumatology, 41*(11), 2232–2239. doi:10.3899/jrheum.140079

Cheek, D. J., Bashore, L., & Brazeau, D. A. (2015). Pharmacogenomics and implications for nursing practice. *Journal of Nursing Scholarship, 47*(6), 496–504. doi:10.1111/jnu.12168

Cobianchi, S., Casals-Diaz, L., Jaramillo, J., & Navarro, X. (2013). Differential effects of activity dependent treatments on axonal regeneration and neuropathic pain after peripheral nerve injury. *Experimental Neurology, 240*, 157–167. doi:10.1016/j.expneurol.2012.11.023

Conley, Y. P., Biesecker, L. G., Gonsalves, S., Merkle, C. J., Kirk, M., & Aouizerat, B. E. (2013). Current and emerging technology approaches in genomics. *Journal of Nursing Scholarship, 45*(1), 5–14. doi:10.1111/jnu.12001

Conley, Y. P., & Tinkle, M. B. (2007). The future of genomic nursing research: Genomics to health. *Journal of Nursing Scholarship, 39*(1), 17–24. doi:10.1111/j.1547-5069.2007.00138.x

Dixit, S., Maiya, A., & Shastry, B. (2014). Effect of aerobic exercise on quality of life in population with diabetic peripheral neuropathy in type 2 diabetes: A single-blind, randomized controlled trial. *Quality of Life Research, 23*(5), 1629–1640.

Dorsey, S. G., Renn, C. L., Carim-Todd, L., Barrick, C. A., Bambrick, L., Krueger, B. K., . . . Tessarollo, L. (2006). In vivo restoration of physiological levels of truncated TrkB.T1 receptor rescues neuronal cell death in a trisomic mouse model. *Neuron, 51*(1), 21–28.

Dowsett, M., Cuzick, J., Wale, C., Forbes, J., Mallon, E. A., Salter, J., . . . Shak, S. (2010). Prediction of risk of distant recurrence using the 21-gene recurrence score in node-negative and node-positive postmenopausal patients with breast cancer treated with anastrozole or tamoxifen: A TransATAC study. *Journal of Clinical Oncology, 28*(11), 1829–1834. doi:10.1200/ JCO.2009.24.4798

Egger, G., Liang, G., Aparicio, A., & Jones, P. A. (2004). Epigenetics in human disease and prospects for epigenetic therapy. *Nature, 429*(6990), 457–463. doi:10.1038/nature02625

Emes, R. D., & Farrell, W. E. (2012). Make way for the "next generation": Application and prospects for genome-wide, epigenome-specific technologies in endocrine research. *Journal of Molecular Endocrinology, 49*(1), 19–27. doi:10.1530/JME-12-0045

Feero, W. G., & Collins, F. S. (2010). Genomic medicine. *New England Journal of Medicine, 362*(21), 2001–2011. doi:10.1056/NEJMra0907175

Gingeras, T. R. (2007). Origin of phenotypes: Genes and transcripts. *Genome Research, 17*, 682–690.

Greco, K. E., Tinley, S., & Seibert, D. (2011). Development of the essential genetic and genomic competencies for nurses with graduate degrees. *Annual Review of Nursing Research, 29,* 173–190.

Guttmacher, A. E., & Collins, F. S. (2003). Welcome to the genomic era. *New England Journal of Medicine, 349*(10), 996–998. doi:10.1056/NEJMe038132

Gwak, Y. S., Kang, J., Unabia, G. C., & Hulsebosch, C. E. (2012). Spatial and temporal activation of spinal glia cells: Role of gliopathy in central neuropathic pain following spinal cord injury in rats. *Experimental Neurology, 234,* 362–372.

Haga, S. B., & Beskow, L. M. (2008). Ethical, legal, and social implications of biobanks for genetics research. *Advances in Genetics, 60,* 505–544.

Haig, S. M., Miller, M. P., Bellinger, R., Draheim, H. M., Mercer, D. M., & Mullins, T. D. (2016). The conservation genetics juggling act: Integrating genetics and ecology, science and policy. *Evolutionary Applications, 9*(1), 181–195. doi:10.1111/eva.12337

Harrington, C. A., Rosenow, C., & Retief, J. (2000). Monitoring gene expression using DNA microarrays. *Current Opinion in Microbiology, 3*(3), 285–291. Retrieved from http://www.ncbi.nlm.nih.gov/pubmed/10851158

Heller, M. J. (2002). DNA microarray technology: Devices, systems and applications. *Annual Review of Biomedical Engineering, 4,* 129–153.

Hsiao, C. P., Wang, D., Kaushal, A., Chen, M. K., & Saligan, L. (2014). Differential expression of genes related to mitochondrial biogenesis and bioenergetics in fatigued prostate cancer men receiving external beam radiation therapy. *Journal of Pain and Symptom Management, 48*(6), 1080–1090. doi:10.1016/j.jpainsymman.2014.03.010

Hsu, Y.-H., Liu, Y., Hannan, M. T., Maixner, W., Smith, S. B., Diatchenko, L., . . . Jordan, J. M. (2015). Genome-wide association meta-analyses to identify common genetic variants associated with hallux valgus in Caucasian and African Americans. *Journal of Medical Genetics, 52*(11), 762–769. doi:10.1136/jmedgenet-2015-103142

Hurkmans, E., van der Giesen, F. J., Vliet Vlieland, T. P., Schoones, J., & Van den Ende ECHM. (2009). Dynamic exercise programs (aerobic capacity and/or muscle strength training) in patients with rheumatoid arthritis. *Cochrane Database of Systematic Review,* (4), CD006853.

Jenkins, J., & Calzone, K. A. (2007). Establishing the essential nursing competencies for genetics and genomics: Genomics to health. *Journal of Nursing Scholarship, 39*(1), 10–16. doi:10.1111/j.1547-5069.2007.00137.x

Jenkins, J., Grady, P. A., & Collins, F. S. (2005). Nurses and the genomic revolution. *Journal of Nursing Scholarship, 37*(2), 98–101. doi:10.1111/j.1547-5069.2005.00020.x

Ji, R. R., Kohno, T., Moore, K. A., & Woolf, C. J. (2003). Central sensitization and LTP: Do pain and memory share similar mechanisms? *Trends in Neurosciences, 26*(12), 696–705.

Johnson, N. L., Giarelli, E., Lewis, C., & Rice, C. E. (2013). Genomics and autism spectrum disorder. *Journal of Nursing Scholarship, 45*(1), 69–78. doi:10.1111/j.1547-5069.2012.01483.x

Katsanis, S. H., & Katsanis, N. (2013). Molecular genetic testing and the future of clinical genomics. *Nature Reviews Genetics, 14*(6), 415–426. doi:10.1038/nrg3493

King, V. R, Bradbury, E. J., McMahon, S. B., & Priestley, J. V. (2000). Changes in truncated trkB and p75 receptor expression in the rat spinal cord following spinal cord hemisection and spinal cord hemisection plus neurotrophin treatment. *Experimental Neurology, 165,* 327–341.

Kirby, M. (1997). Challenges of the genome. *University of New South Wales Law Journal, 20,* 537–549.

Kurella, M., Hsiao, L. L., Yoshida, T., Randall, J. D., Chow, G., Sarang, S. S., . . . Gullans, S. R. (2001). DNA microarray analysis of complex biologic processes. *Journal of the American Society of Nephrology, 12*(5), 1072–1078. Retrieved from http://www.ncbi.nlm.nih.gov/pubmed/11316867

Lan, X., Adams, C., Landers, M., Dudas, M., Krissinger, D., Marnellos, G., . . . Jin, V. X. (2011). High resolution detection and analysis of CpG dinucleotides methylation using MBD-Seq technology. *PLOS ONE, 6*(7), e22226.

Lessans, S., & Dorsey, S. G. (2013). The role for epigenetic modifications in pain and analgesia response. *Nursing Research and Practice, 2013*, 961493. doi:10.1155/2013/961493

Liebl, D. J., Huang, W. Y., Young, W., & Parada, L. F. (2001). Regulation of trk receptors following contusion of the rat spinal cord. *Experimental Neurology, 167*, 15–26.

Lu, Y., Christian, K., & Lu, B. (2008). BDNF: A key regulator for protein-synthesis dependent LTP and long term memory. *Neurobiology of Learning and Memory, 89*, 312–323.

Malone, J. H., & Oliver, B. (2011). Microarrays, deep sequencing and the true measure of the transcriptome. *BMC Biology, 9*, 34.

Marian, A. J. (2012). The enigma of genetics etiology of atherosclerosis in the Post-GWAS era. *Current Atherosclerosis Reports, 14*(4), 295–299. Retrieved from https://doi.org/10.1007/s11883-012-0245-0

McCormick, K. (2016). Understanding new types of evidence ready for translation. *Studies in Health Technology and Informatics, 225*, 686–688.

Merighi, A., Salio, C., Ghirri, A., Lossi, L., Ferrini, F., Betelli, C., & Bardoni, R. (2008). BDNF as a pain modulator. *Progress in Neurobiology, 85*, 297–317.

Metzker, M. L. (2010). Sequencing technologies: The next generation. *Nature Reviews Genetics, 11*, 31–46.

Miletic, G., Hanson, E. N., & Miletic, V. (2004). Brain-derived neurotrophic factor-elicited or sciatic ligation-associated phosphorylation of cyclic AMP response element binding protein in the rat spinal dorsal horn is reduced by block of tyrosine kinase receptors. *Neuroscience Letters, 361*, 269–271.

Mitchell, J., Ferguson, S. M., & Ferguson, S. M. (2007). National Institutes of Health policy for sharing data obtained in NIH supported or conducted genome-wide association studies (GWAS). *Federal Register, 72*(166), 49290–49297.

Modirian, E., Pirouzi, P., Soroush, M., Karbalaei-Esmaeili, S., Shojaei, H., & Zamani, H. (2010). Chronic pain after spinal cord injury: Results of a long-term study. *Pain Medicine, 11*, 1037–1043.

Mogil, J. S. (2012). Pain genetics: Past, present and future. *Trends in Genetics, 28*(6), 258–266. doi:10.1016/j.tig.2012.02.004

Moore, S., Schiffman, R., Waldrop-Valverde, D., Redeker, N., McCloskey, D., Kim, M., . . . Grady, P. (2016). Recommendations of common data elements to advance the science of self-management of chronic conditions. *Journal of Nursing Scholarship, 48*(5), 437–447.

National Human Genome Research Institute. (2015). DNA sequencing costs: Data from the NHGRI genome sequencing program. Retrieved from https://www.genome.gov/sequencingcostsdata

National Institute of Nursing Research. (2013). Advancing genomic nursing science: Workshop summary. Retrieved from https://www.ninr.nih.gov/newsandinformation/genomics-summary

Noordewier, M. O., & Warren, P. V. (2001). Gene expression microarrays and the integration of biological knowledge. *Trends in Biotechnology, 19*(10), 412–415. doi:10.1016/S0167-7799(01)01735-8

Paez, J., Janne, P., Lee, J., Tracy, S., Greulich, H., Gabriel, S., & Meyerson, M. (2004). EGFR mutations in lung cancer: Correlation with clinical response to gefitinib therapy. *Science, 304*, 1497–1500.

Paik, S., Shak, S., Tang, G., Kim, C., Baker, J., Cronin, M., . . . Wolmark, N. (2004). A multigene assay to predict recurrence of tamoxifen-treated, node-negative breast cancer. *New England Journal of Medicine, 351*(27), 2817–2826. doi:10.1056/NEJMoa041588

Paik, S., Tang, G., Shak, S., Kim, C., Baker, J., Kim, W., . . . Wolmark, N. (2006). Gene expression and benefit of chemotherapy in women with node-negative, estrogen receptor-positive breast cancer. *Journal of Clinical Oncology, 24*(23), 3726–3734. doi:10.1200/JCO.2005.04.7985

Pearson, T., & Manolio, T. (2008). How to interpret a genome-wide association study. *JAMA, 299*(11), 1335–1344. doi:10.1001/jama.299.11.1335

Petronis, A. (2010). Epigenetics as a unifying principle in the aetiology of complex traits and diseases. *Nature, 465*(7299), 721–727. doi:10.1038/nature09230

Pezet, S., & McMahon, S. B. (2006). Neurotrophins: Mediators and modulators of pain. *Annual Review of Neuroscience, 29,* 507–538.

Plun-Favreau, J., Immonen-Charalambous, K., Steuten, L., Strootker, A., Rouzier, R., Horgan, D., & Lawler, M. (2016). Enabling equal access to molecular diagnostics: What are the implications for policy and health technology assessment. *Public Health Genomics,* 144–152. doi:10.1159/000446532

Precision Medicine Initiative Working Group. (2015). The Precision Medicine Initiative cohort program: Building a research foundation for 21st century medicine (Precision Medicine Initiative (PMI) Working Group Report to the Advisory Committee to the Director, NIH). Retrieved from http://www.nih.gov/precisionmedicine

Redeker, N., Anderson, R., Bakken, S., Corwin, E., Docherty, S., Dorsey, S., . . . Grady, P. (2015). Advancing symptom science through use of common data elements. *Journal of Nursing Scholarship, 47*(5), 379–388. doi:10.1111/jnu.12155

Renn, C. L., Lin, L., Thomas, S., & Dorsey, S. G. (2009). Full-length tropomyosin-related kinase B expression in the brainstem in response to persistent inflammatory pain. *NeuroReport, 17,* 1175–1179.

Rooks, D. S., Gautam, S., Romeling, M., Cross, M. L., Stratigakis, D., Evans, B., . . . Katz, J. N. (2007). Group exercise, education, and combination self-management in women with fibromyalgia: A randomized trial. *Archives of Internal Medicine, 167*(20), 2192–2200. doi:10.1001/archinte.167.20.2192

Rose, M., Robinson, J. E., Ells, P., & Cole, J. D. (1988). Pain following spinal cord injury: Results from a postal survey. *Pain, 34,* 101–102.

Rothstein, M. A., Knoppers, B. M., & Harrell, H. L. (2016). Comparative approaches to biobanks and privacy. *Journal of Law, Medicine and Ethics, 44*(1), 161–172. doi:10.1177/1073110516644207

Saligan, L. N., Hsiao, C. P., Wang, D., Wang, X. M., John, L. S., Kaushal, A., . . . Dionne, R. A. (2013). Upregulation of alpha-synuclein during localized radiation therapy signals the association of cancer-related fatigue with the activation of inflammatory and neuroprotective pathways. *Brain, Behavior, and Immunity, 27*(1), 63–70. doi:10.1016/j.bbi.2012.09.009

Saligan, L. N., Olson, K., Filler, K., Larkin, D., Cramp, F., Sriram, Y., . . . Mustian, K. (2015). The biology of cancer-related fatigue: A review of the literature. *Supportive Care in Cancer, 23*(8), 2461–2478. doi:10.1007/s00520-015-2763-0

Sequist, L. V., Joshi, V. A., Janne, P. A., Muzikansky, A., Fidias, P., Meyerson, M., . . . Lynch, T. J. (2007). Response to treatment and survival of patients with non-small cell lung cancer undergoing somatic EGFR mutation testing. *The Oncologist, 12,* 90–98. doi:10.1634/theoncologist.12-1-90

Sheahan, T. D., Copits, B. A., Golden, J. P., & Gereau, R. W. (2015). Voluntary exercise training: Analysis of mice in uninjured, inflammatory, and nerve-injured pain states. *PLOS ONE, 10*(7), e0133191. doi:10.1371/journal.pone.0133191

Shen, J., Fox, L. E., & Cheng, J. (2013). Swim therapy reduces mechanical allodynia and thermal hyperalgesia induced by chronic constriction nerve injury in rats. *Pain Medicine, 14*(4), 516–525. doi:10.1111/pme.12057.

Siddall, P., Yezierski, R., & Loeser, J. (2002). In R. Yezierski & K. Burchiel (Eds.), *Spinal cord injury pain: Assessment, mechanisms, management* (Vol. 23, pp. 9–24). Seattle, WA: IASP Press.

Solin, L. J., Gray, R., Goldstein, L. J., Recht, A., Baehner, F. L., Shak, S., . . . Sparano, J. A. (2012). Prognostic value of biologic subtype and the 21-gene recurrence score relative to local recurrence after breast conservation treatment with radiation for early-stage breast carcinoma: Results from the Eastern Cooperative Oncology Group E2197 study. *Breast Cancer Research and Treatment, 134*(2), 683–692. doi:10.1007/s10549-012-2072-y

Sparano, J. A., Gray, R. J., Makower, D. F., Pritchard, K. I., Albain, K. S., Hayes, D. F., . . . Sledge, G. W. (2015). Prospective validation of a 21-gene expression assay in breast cancer. *New England Journal of Medicine, 373*(21), 2005–2014. doi:10.1056/NEJMoa1510764

Spies, M., Dasu, M. R. K., Svrakic, N., Nesic, O., Barrow, R. E., Perez-Polo, J. R., & Herndon, D. N. (2002). Gene expression analysis in burn wounds of rats. *American Journal of Physiology: Regulatory, Integrative and Comparative Physiology, 283*(4), R918–R930. doi:10.1152/ajpregu.00170.2002

U.S. Department of Health and Human Services, Health Resources and Services Administration, Bureau of Health Professions. (2010). The registered nurse population: Findings from the 2008 National Sample Survey of Registered Nurses. Rockville, MD: Author. Retrieved from https://bhw.hrsa.gov/sites/default/files/bhw/nchwa/rnsurveyfinal.pdf

U.S. Department of Homeland Security. (2015). Notice of proposed rulemaking: Federal policy for the protection of human subjects. *Federal Register, 80*(173), 1–131. Retrieved from http://www.hhs.gov/ohrp/humansubjects/regulations/nprm2015summary.html

Wang, Z., Gerstein, M., & Snyder, M. (2009). RNA-seq: A revolutionary tool for transcriptomics. *Nature Reviews Genetics, 10,* 57–63.

Wright, A., & Sluka, K. A. (2001). Nonpharmacological treatments for musculoskeletal pain. *Clinical Journal of Pain, 17*(1), 33–46.

Wu, J., Renn, C. L., Faden, A. I., & Dorsey, S. G. (2013). TrkB.T1 contributes to neuropathic pain after spinal cord injury through regulation of cell cycle pathways. *Journal of Neuroscience: The Official Journal of the Society for Neuroscience, 33*(30), 12447–12463. doi:10.1523/JNEUROSCI.0846-13.2013

Wu, J., Zhao, Z., Zhu, X., Renn, C. L., Dorsey, S. G., & Faden, A. I. (2016). Cell cycle inhibition limits development and maintenance of neuropathic pain following spinal cord injury. *Pain, 157,* 488–503. doi:10.1097/j.pain.0000000000000393

Wung, S. F., Hickey, K. T., Taylor, J. Y., & Gallek, M. J. (2013). Cardiovascular genomics. *Journal of Nursing Scholarship, 45*(1), 60–68. doi:10.1111/jnu.12002

Yu, W., Gwinn, M., Dotson, W. D., Green, R. F., Clyne, M., Wulf, A., . . . Khoury, M. J. (2016). A knowledge base for tracking the impact of genomics on population health. *Genetics in Medicine.* doi:10.1038/gim.2016.63

Zhou, C., Chen, H., Han, L., Wang, A., & Chen, L. A. (2014). Identification of featured biomarkers in different types of lung cancer with DNA microarray. *Molecular Biology Reports, 41*(10), 6357–6363. doi:10.1007/s11033-014-3515-9

Gastrointestinal Symptom Science and Assessment

Margaret M. Heitkemper and Wendy A. Henderson

Symptom science focuses on developing personalized strategies to treat and prevent the adverse symptoms of illness across diverse populations and settings (National Institute of Nursing Research [NINR], 2016). At the same time, symptom science is about understanding mechanisms that account for symptoms so that appropriate therapies can be devised. Nurse scientists are particularly focused on linking patient reports of symptoms with real-time capture of physiological/biological variables that reflect biology and pathophysiology. Equally important is their ability to translate and disseminate the findings into evidence-based practice. In this chapter, we discuss irritable bowel syndrome (IBS) as a prototype of a chronic and life-interfering condition that is associated with intermittent but at times daily symptoms.

IBS is one of the most prevalent gastrointestinal (GI) disorders in the world and its diagnosis is based on patients' symptoms along with exclusion of other diseases. A meta-analysis of 80 studies with more than 260,000 participants reveals that more than 11% of the world's population (Lovell & Ford, 2012) meets the Rome III symptom-based criteria for a diagnosis of IBS. IBS is associated with substantial health care costs, with estimates ranging from $1,562 to $7,537 per year (Nellesen, Yee, Chawla, Lewis, & Carson, 2013). Work productivity of those with IBS is lower than that of other chronically ill populations such as those who have rheumatoid arthritis, migraine headache, and asthma (Taylor, Kosinski, Reilly, & Lindner, 2014). In numerous studies investigators have shown that IBS is associated with reduced quality of life (Monnikes, 2011). IBS is more common in women than men in Western cultures. The most recently revised version of the symptom-based IBS classification is the Rome IV criteria: recurrent abdominal pain on average at least 1 day a week in the past 3 months associated with two or more of the following: related to defecation; associated with a change in a frequency of stool; associated with a change in form (consistency) of stool; and symptoms must have started at least 6 months ago (Palsson et al., 2016). The diagnostic criteria include abdominal pain and alterations (diarrhea, constipation, or mixed diarrhea/constipation) with no discernible pathophysiological cause (e.g., infection, gross inflammation). There is currently no accepted biological marker specific to IBS. Therefore, clinical trials of behavioral therapy and drug therapy rely on self-report of symptoms and symptom intensity.

The biopsychosocial model of IBS first proposed by Drossman (Tanaka, Kanazawa, Fukudo, & Drossman, 2011) is a framework that encompasses the growing list of biological and psychological factors that contribute to the etiology of IBS, some of which are amenable to drug and/or behavioral therapy. In order to better manage symptoms, persons living with IBS need to both self-identify symptom triggers and self-manage to the degree that symptom burden is reduced and quality of life is enhanced. As noted in Figure 10.1, the biopsychosocial model includes pathophysiological factors which, if found to be relevant to symptom experiences, may be important in the design and testing of therapeutic interventions to improve patient-related outcomes.

ALIGNMENT WITH NURSING SCIENCE AND WOMEN'S HEALTH RESEARCH

Prior to the first published criteria for IBS diagnosis known as the Manning criteria in 1989, IBS was generally viewed as a "psychosomatic disorder." The symptoms of abdominal pain and discomfort, diarrhea, and constipation were attributed to personality characteristics such as hysteria and catastrophizing tendencies,

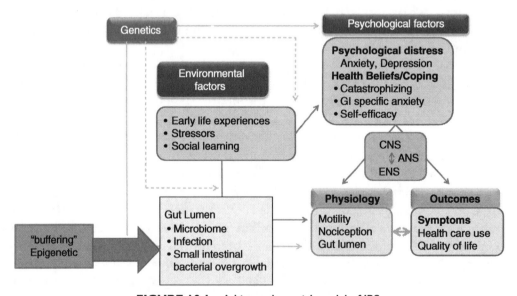

FIGURE 10.1   A biopsychosocial model of IBS.

ANS, autonomic nervous system; CNS, central nervous system; ENS, enteric nervous system; Hx, history; IBS, irritable bowel syndrome.

Source: Adapted from Tanaka, Kanazawa, Fukudo, and Drossman (2011).

depression, and anxiety. Because there was no validated biomarker, the symptoms were often discounted and patients were left seeking medical advice from a series of providers (e.g., gastroenterologists, obstetrics/gynecologists, psychiatrists) with little to guide the management of their symptoms. Such gaps in the literature led to inadequate patient information and in some cases, a bias against those patients, particularly women, reporting symptoms in the absence of overt pathology. At that same time, pharmacologic approaches included agents that were directed at one specific symptom such as constipation, which did little to relieve other intestinal and extra-intestinal symptoms of IBS such as abdominal pain. Relatively recent qualitative studies continue to reveal that patients with IBS often report a sense of frustration, isolation, and dissatisfaction with the medical system and the need for more information (Drossman et al., 2009; Halpert, Rybin, & Doros, 2010).

An early national survey (Heitkemper, Carter, Ameen, Olden, & Cheng, 2002) confirmed the gender gap in the diagnosis and health care–seeking behavior associated with IBS. At that time several researchers noted the overlap of a diagnosis of IBS with other chronic pain disorders such as fibromyalgia, headache with aura, interstitial cystitis, temporomandibular joint disorder, and pelvic pain, all of which were more likely to be diagnosed in women. Abdominal surgical procedures such as cholecystectomy and hysterectomy rates were higher in women with IBS relative to other patient groups. Likewise, other comorbid conditions such as insomnia, fatigue, and psychological distress (anxiety, depression) were more frequently reported by women with IBS relative to men with IBS and non-IBS female patients. Building on this published work, our team of nurse scientists, a psychologist, a gastroenterologist, and a psychiatrist began a series of descriptive studies in which women with a medical diagnosis of IBS were studied using both prospective and retrospective measures of symptoms and health-related quality of life.

These initial studies focused solely on women participants for two primary reasons. First, more women seek health care services for symptoms and they are most likely to be diagnosed with IBS relative to men. Second, in the early 1990s there was an impetus across NIH to include more women in clinical trials, as well as to study conditions that predominantly affect women, so as to reduce gaps in our understanding of sex and gender differences (Kirschstein, 1991). Although fewer in number, men are diagnosed with IBS, most frequently IBS-diarrhea. Women with IBS tend to have more reports of constipation.

Our work in the field of functional gastrointestinal disorders (FGDs) began with the question: Why do women report more GI symptoms? Our hypothesis was that women who experienced/reported more stress (e.g., life events, daily stress) resulting in physiological activation of the hypothalamic–pituitary–adrenal axis and the autonomic nervous system (ANS) would experience more GI symptoms. In our initial model, both of these physiological stress response systems work downstream to influence the GI tract either through increases or decreases in smooth muscle contractions and/or intestinal secretion.

The first project, titled *A Nursing Study of Gut Function in Menstruating Women*, was funded by the Division of Nursing in 1984. The basic premise of this proposal, as well as of subsequent descriptive, mechanistic studies, was that stress and GI symptoms are linked. We postulated that understanding this relationship was important to informing the design of behavioral interventions to reduce GI symptom distress. In this initial study, the focus was on women with and without dysmenorrhea (menstrual cramping pain) as a model for determining first if menstrual cycle phase differences in GI symptoms existed and if symptoms were related to ovarian hormone levels. Both well-validated retrospective (e.g., Symptom Checklist-90, Menstrual Distress Questionnaire) and prospective (i.e., Women's Health Diary [WHD]) for three menstrual cycles) tools were used to characterize the types and severity of symptoms, including GI, menstrual cramping pain, and mood states. The WHD was developed by Woods for the longitudinal Seattle Midlife Women's Study (Mitchell & Woods, 1996) and includes 26 symptoms with items related to sleep, fatigue, pain, and mood. Measures of gastric motility and serum levels of estrogen and progesterone were made in the two groups of women. Urine luteinizing hormone (LH) surge testing at ovulation was used to confirm menstrual cycle phase.

The results of this initial study demonstrated that many women both with and without dysmenorrhea report GI symptoms including diarrhea, constipation, stomach pain, and nausea. For both nondysmenorrheic and dysmenorrheic women, these symptoms are amplified during the late luteal and early menses phases of the menstrual cycle. However, the menses-related symptom amplification was greater in those with dysmenorrhea. We also found that menstrual cycle phase influences stool number/consistency (e.g., looser stools at menses), which is likely due to natural cyclic changes in the ovarian hormones estrogen and progesterone. As hypothesized, there were group differences, with the dysmenorrheic group reporting more moderate to severe pain and bowel symptoms than nondysmenorrheic women. Thus, menstrual cycle phase is a confounder when attempting to make comparisons of symptom frequency/intensity between IBS and non-IBS premenopausal women, as well as men-versus-women comparisons. In addition, menstrual cycle phase is an important consideration when conducting physiological testing in premenopausal women.

Additional secondary data analyses of this and later descriptive studies were used to describe the influence of oral contraceptives and perimenopausal status on GI, mood, and somatic symptoms in healthy control and women with IBS (Heitkemper, Cain, Jarrett, et al., 2003). For example, women in the perimenopausal period report an increase in the number of GI, somatic, and psychological distress symptoms. Given the fluctuations in ovarian hormones as well as life stressors during this stage, the cause of the increase in symptoms is likely multifactorial. Women with IBS who also report a history of dysmenorrhea and perimenstrual dysphoria disorder report greater symptoms and cyclic variation than women with IBS alone. This effect is not modified by the use of oral contraceptives (Heitkemper, Cain, Jarrett, et al., 2003). An outcome of the aforementioned early descriptive work is the necessity of gathering a comprehensive medical history that includes gynecologic evaluation when studying women with IBS.

Concurrent with the prior clinical studies were ongoing animal experiments to study the effects of estrogen (estradiol; E_2) and progesterone on GI smooth muscle and intestinal transit under both resting (basal condition) and stress-related peptide (thyrotropin releasing hormone [TRH]) stimulation. Significant findings reported (Heitkemper & Bond, 1995) included that ovariectomized and E_2-treated rats exhibited a blunted response to central (i.e., intracerebroventricular) administration of TRH when compared to sham-ovariectomized females and untreated male rats. Whether this is a direct effect of E_2 on the smooth muscle because estrogen receptors are present in the gut or due to E_2 modulation of vagal input subsequent to TRH administration is unknown.

The notion that gonadal hormone levels can modulate the response to stress-related hormone administered centrally raises the question of whether sex-related differences in stress responsivity are solely present in adult animals when higher levels of gonadal hormones are present. However, recently investigators demonstrated sex differences in visceral pain sensitivity related to altered stress paradigms administered early in neonatal development in a rat model (Prusator & Greenwood-Van Meerveld, 2016). Together these experiments, along with other animal data, support the hypothesis that ovarian hormones may contribute to the documented phenotypic differences in men and women with IBS.

Irritable Bowel Syndrome

In 1990, we began our first study specifically focused on women with IBS. The comparison groups included: women with medically diagnosed IBS; IBS-non-patients (IBS-NP), women who report current symptoms compatible with IBS (i.e., they met Rome I criteria but denied health care–seeking for their GI symptoms); and healthy control women. Data were collected on: (a) daily reports of GI symptoms and stool patterns, (b) daily and reported life time stress, psychological distress, (c) physiological arousal, and (d) diet. The IBS-NP group was chosen as the comparison group because while a significant portion of the U.S. adult population reports daily or monthly symptoms consistent with a diagnosis of IBS, many do not seek health care. Whether this is due to differences in symptom intensity/frequency, the presence of psychological distress, or the degree to which symptoms interfere with daily activity and work or quality of life was not known. An interdisciplinary team including experts in gastroenterology, psychiatry, psychology, bioengineering, and nutrition were brought together to design and conduct the study.

Some of the key findings from these early studies are that daily self-reported stress levels are higher in the IBS compared to the control women and that daily stress predicts next-day GI symptoms, especially pain (Jarrett et al., 1998; Levy, Cain, Jarrett, & Heitkemper, 1997). This confirms what many individuals say anecdotally when asked what they believe triggers their symptoms. Also, in this study it was found that more women in the IBS group (66%) as compared with controls (34%) have a history of symptoms compatible with a *Diagnostic and Statistical Manual of Mental Disorders*, third edition (*DSM-IIIR*; DSM criteria available at that time) diagnosis (e.g., depression, anxiety disorder) and higher scores on a retrospective psychological distress tool (Heitkemper, Jarrett, Cain, et al., 1995). Indeed, the major difference between those seeking health care services and those not was found in the psychological distress variables, with the IBS group reporting more distress than non-health-care seekers. Ideally, a longitudinal study may reveal whether the non-health-care seekers with time ultimately sought health care services for their IBS. Additional variables such as lack of social supports in the environment or individual characteristics such as low resilience may also contribute to health care–seeking behavior. However, these factors are often not included in clinical (primary and tertiary care) and community studies of IBS.

In a separate follow-up study, we examined the role of psychological distress, both current and lifetime, with respect to GI symptoms. A history of psychological distress was measured with the Composite International Diagnostic Interview (CIDI) that determines if their symptoms meet the *Diagnostic and Statistical Manual of Mental Disorders*, fourth edition (*DSM-IV*; version at the time of the study) criteria for a mood or anxiety disorder. Women with severe IBS symptoms were more likely to report a history of posttraumatic stress disorder (PTSD, 30%), social phobia public (SPP, 35%), and somatization (12%) relative to women with mild to moderate IBS symptoms (PTSD, 0%; SPP, 7%; somatization, 0%). Early adverse events including abuse in childhood, especially sexual abuse, are more commonly reported in women with IBS when compared to non-IBS groups. We assessed childhood trauma, including physical and emotional neglect and abuse, with the Childhood Trauma Questionnaire (Heitkamper et al., 2001). More women with severe IBS were likely to report a history of emotional and physical abuse, physical neglect, and sexual abuse as children compared to healthy controls and IBS individuals with mild to moderate symptoms (Heitkemper, Cain, Burr, Jun, & Jarrett, 2011). These findings were among the early studies showing the relationship of early childhood adverse events and symptom severity in IBS. Again, such results are important when considering multicomponent interventions for IBS. These data also reflect the need for a multidisciplinary approach (diet, exercise, stress reduction) to the management of IBS, rather than a focus solely on bowel pattern. In addition, it is clear that early negative childhood experiences may shape the trajectory of future pain-related conditions such as IBS. Hence, there is a need to study sociocultural and environmental factors that predispose to adult health problems. Understanding these as well as times of transitions (e.g., puberty) may be key to management of adult IBS.

The importance of stress exposure and environment and the development of IBS in adulthood is perhaps best exemplified in recent studies of U.S. military personnel. In a review of 314 new-onset cases of IBS from a cohort of more than 41,000 active duty participants, Riddle et al. (2016) described that both increased life stressors and reports of anxiety and depression increased the risk of developing IBS. They found that risk was greatest in those with these features combined with a history of infectious gastroenteritis (Riddle et al., 2016). In another study of 337 women veterans seen in primary care for PTSD, depression, and IBS (prevalence 33%), White et al. found that while depression and PTSD were more common in the women with IBS, this did not fully explain the association between trauma and increased risk of IBS (White et al., 2010). Given the prevalence of IBS in active duty service people and veterans, understanding the linkages among stress, environment (infectious exposure), and gender is an important direction for future work.

ALIGNMENT WITH SYMPTOM SCIENCE

Symptom science focuses on developing personalized strategies to treat and prevent the adverse symptoms of illness across diverse populations and settings. At the same time, symptom science is about understanding mechanisms that account for symptoms so that appropriate therapies may be devised. For example, urine and salivary proteomic measures can serve as potential biomarkers reflective of tissue damage produced by inflammation resulting in pain, nausea, and fatigue. While omics approaches provide information on potential pathophysiological mechanisms at play, they can also serve as outcome measures (e.g., diet changes and microbiome) depending on study design. As such, biological measures provide the opportunity to explicate mechanisms linking comorbid symptoms, such as disturbed sleep, with abdominal pain, and the opportunity to predict and/or monitor responses to nonpharmacological therapies. Explorations of biological alterations may help explain why individuals with the same clinical diagnosis (e.g., IBS) have different symptoms, symptom severity, symptom triggers, or degree of life interference due to symptoms.

One challenge in IBS symptom science research is the wide array of measures and approaches used to capture common symptoms such as poor sleep and pain. To address the general issue of measurement, the NINR center directors led an initiative to address common data elements (CDEs) for symptom science research (Corwin et al., 2014; Redeker et al., 2015). This work built on prior and ongoing NIH initiatives including PROMIS and NeuroQoL. The University of Washington School of Nursing incorporated symptom CDEs for our pilot projects funded through the Center for Research on Management of Sleep Disturbances (P30 NR 011400, 2009–2014) and our Center for Innovation in Sleep Self-Management (P30 NR016585, 2016–2021), as well as several R series grants. For example, we use PROMIS-sleep–pain interference, and Global Health tools in all studies of adults with a disorder or disease for which these symptoms are either examined as descriptors or as outcome measures. Recently, the GI Health PROMIS measures (Spiegel et al., 2014) became available and will be incorporated into future studies of FGDs. At a recent National Institute of Diabetes and Digestive and Kidney Diseases (NIDDK)-sponsored conference on FGD research, a common theme expressed by scientists was the need for a data repository that would link centers of excellence focused on FGDs. This could be much like the NIDDK Multidisciplinary Approach to the Study of Chronic Pelvic Pain (MAPP) project that focuses on urological chronic pelvic pain (www. mappnetwork.org).

As noted earlier, in many studies, daily symptom recordings provide not only a snapshot of a day's experience, but also patterns within weeks, months, or years. Though not perfect, daily recordings attend to one of the important limitations of one-time retrospective measures: response bias, which is the tendency for participants to report their "worst" symptom intensity. Initially, paper-and-pencil diary versions were employed, whereas more recently, electronic diaries have been introduced to capture symptom experiences. Colleagues from medicine, engineering, and computer sciences assisted to test and employ an eDiary symptom log to capture real-time data elements and at the same time allow for symptom pattern recognition, with the goal of using this as a self-management tool. The use of these technologies both for data collection and as tools to enhance self-management enables collaborative industry–academic partnerships.

Pain

Abdominal pain is the most disruptive and distressing symptom reported by individuals with IBS. GI pain is unlike somatic pain in that it is often diffuse and challenging to discover its site of origin. Henderson and colleagues, in 2009, identified the need to develop a more sophisticated tool to help patients and providers to communicate regarding the location of GI symptoms. Together with an interdisciplinary team, they developed an electronic assessment tool, the Gastrointestinal Pain Pointer (GIPP). The GIPP employs a graphical interface, shown in Figure 10.2, where patients identify personal characteristics including gender, body type (normal or overweight) and record the location and intensity of their pain. The graphical interface also includes a list of descriptors from which to select the one that matches best the pain experience, including intensity, location, and qualitative components. At the same time, the provider records the patient's heart rate and blood pressure. In a sample of 93 IBS and non-IBS participants, they found the GIPP to be a practical method of assessing GI symptoms such as bloating and simultaneously entering the data into an electronic medical record (Henderson et al., 2015). The tool is a novel measure of GI symptom intensity that enhances clinicians' ability to better quantify, in real time, patient-related GI outcomes for both clinical care and research (Henderson et al., 2015).

Diet is another area of importance when considering factors that contribute to GI symptoms. As such, dietary assessments are increasingly viewed as important to the management of persons with chronic GI symptoms. Many persons with IBS can self-identify a food trigger that elicits or exacerbates their symptoms. Investigators have identified fermentable oligosaccharides, disaccharides, monosaccharides, and polyols (FODMAPs) as triggers for symptoms such as abdominal pain and discomfort, intestinal gas/bloating, and diarrhea for many persons with IBS (Nanayakkara, Skidmore, O'Brien, Wilkinson, & Gearry, 2016).

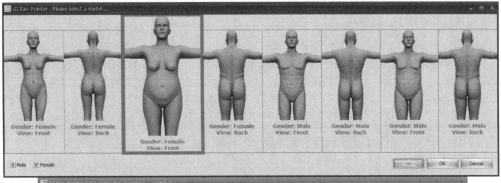

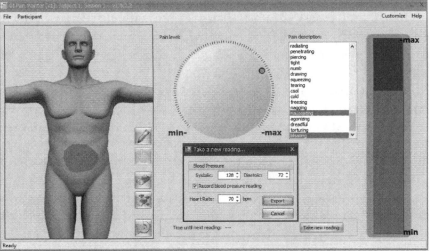

FIGURE 10.2 The Gastrointestinal Pain Pointer.

FODMAPs are short-chain carbohydrates (oligosaccharides, monosaccharides) and generate alcohols that are poorly absorbed in the small intestine. The elimination or restriction of FODMAPs from the diet is difficult to achieve and the long-term impact of such restrictions is unknown. More research in this area is clearly warranted.

The assessment of dietary intake associated with GI symptoms, as well as other chronic, episodic illnesses, is challenging. Recall tools such as the Food Frequency Questionnaire are dependent upon memory and do not provide real-time information about specific food triggers. Working with medical and computer science colleagues, a novel prospective computer-based application (app) for logging GI symptoms over a 2-week period was tested. The investigators found that 73% of IBS participants were able to identify a meal nutrient trigger of their GI symptoms. In another survey, gastroenterology patients were willing to use health-related apps (Zia, Le, Munson, Heitkemper, & Demiris, 2015).

As the necessity of rigorous approaches to symptom assessment moves to the forefront, it is also important to incorporate analytic strategies to consider the reality that a single symptom rarely exists in isolation from other comorbid symptoms. For example, abdominal pain, sleep disturbance, and fatigue are highly correlated and comorbid in individuals with IBS. Building on the work of Miaskowski et al. (Miaskowski et al., 2006; Miaskowski & Aouizerat, 2007), an approach of examining symptom clusters not only as an outcome or a means of identifying subgroups with a heterogeneous condition such as IBS is needed.

OVERLAPPING CONDITIONS: EMPHASIS ON SLEEP

Studies by us and others indicate that patients with IBS report other non-GI symptoms, of which insomnia, frequent awakenings, and fatigue are among the most common. A limited number of studies with small samples using polysom-nography (PSG) measures suggest that objective sleep may be different in IBS patients as compared to nonsymptomatic individuals (Tu, Heitkemper, Jarrett, & Buchanan, 2016). In addition, neuroendocrine factors, ANS imbalances, and psychological distress are known to influence the quality of sleep and are associated with GI symptom distress in women with IBS (Jarrett et al., 1998; Levy et al., 1997). Investigators suggest, based on limited PSG data, that there is a sleep disturbance associated with IBS and that this may lead to the exacerbation of symptoms in a significant subgroup of women. Many studies are not conclusive regarding objective sleep disturbances and IBS, due to methodological weaknesses including the use of a one-night sleep monitoring protocol; failure to attend to important cofactors such as age, gender (including ovarian hormone status or menstrual cycle phase), and psychological comorbidities (e.g., depression); and small sample size (Tu et al., 2016). A "first-night" effect is clearly evident when PSG sleep studies are performed with women with IBS. The phenomenon of sleep misperception (i.e., marked differences between self-report and objective indicators in the sleep laboratory) may be present.

Although our original IBS studies did not specifically include sleep variables, the WHD included three self-report variables: *difficulty in getting to sleep, awakening during the night,* and *early morning awakening.* Women with IBS self-report problems with sleep and these reports are related to report of GI symptoms and psychological distress in almost half of the women with IBS (Jarrett, Heitkemper, Cain, Burr, & Hertig, 2000). Based on these initial observations, we began to incorporate experts in nursing science and sleep physiology onto our research team. With their collaboration we designed two laboratory sleep studies. In these studies, we also stratified the IBS sample by symptom intensity (using items from Bowel Disease Questionnaire, e.g., abdominal pain, diarrhea, constipation) and found that women with the IBS-severe had more sleep complaints than those with IBS-mild–moderate symptoms.

The protocols for the sleep studies involved the recruitment of women with and without IBS between the ages of 20 and 45. Objective indices of sleep were obtained during a standard 3-night PSG study in a school of nursing sleep laboratory, as well as 7-day actigraphy recording. The first night in the sleep laboratory was considered "adaptation," while the second was considered "baseline." The third night involved the insertion of an intravenous line and serial blood drawings for the measurement of catecholamines, adrenocorticotropic hormone, and cortisol. In the second sleep study, a stressor (public speaking) was added to the study protocol. We also measured heart rate with a Holter monitor for the assessment of heart rate variability. Both PSG and actigraphy-determined sleep efficiency the night before are also related to pain and discomfort the next day (Buchanan et al., 2014; Burr, Jarrett, Cain, Jun, & Heitkemper, 2009; Heitkemper, Cain, Deechakawan, et al. 2012; Jarrett et al., 2009). Women with severe IBS-diarrhea consistently showed elevations in markers of vagal tone during the night, while those with IBS-constipation demonstrated reduced vagal tone. Evidence of neuroendocrine dysregulation, in particular elevations in serum cortisol, on the third night was also found. Together, these findings support the notion that there are physiological markers that distinguish IBS from healthy controls and that even within IBS there are differences in these markers based on bowel pattern predominance and symptom severity. Whether these physiological observations contribute to the clinical phenotype of IBS or are the outcome of a chronic condition remains to be determined. It is likely that there is a subgroup of women with IBS who experience disturbed sleep (e.g., prolonged sleep onset latency) and for whom strategies such as sleep hygiene and/or cognitive behavioral therapy-insomnia (CBT-I) may be beneficial for IBS symptom management. Clinically, evidence supports the inclusion of subjective sleep assessment in the comprehensive assessment of persons with IBS.

The observation that poor sleep predicts increased GI symptoms the next day has particular relevance for those who do shiftwork. Researchers conducting studies of nurses in both an American and a Korean medical center found the prevalence of IBS as well GI symptoms to be higher in those doing shiftwork. In the U.S. report, Nojkov, Rubenstein, Chey, and Hoogerwerf (2010) hypothesized that the circadian rhythm disruptions contribute to the pathogenesis of IBS (Nojkov et al., 2010). The development of chronic-pain-related conditions such as IBS is a relevant inclusion in the national dialogue about the impact of sleep disturbances on chronic comorbid symptoms.

SYMPTOM SCIENCE AND INTERVENTION RESEARCH

With our interdisciplinary team of investigators and clinicians, an advanced practice registered nurse (APRN)-delivered comprehensive self-management (CSM) program was designed and tested (Heitkemper, Jarrett, Levy, et al., 2004; Jarrett et al., 2009, 2016; Zia, Barney, Cain, Jarrett, & Heitkemper, 2016). Males and females were recruited to these studies; however, as men seek health care services in fewer numbers, our samples were composed of approximately 20% men. The major findings of these studies are that regardless of approach (in-person or telephone CSM delivery) used, the CSM intervention is effective for up to 12 months in reducing symptoms (as defined by a composite GI symptom score that included pain measures and diarrhea/constipation) and improving quality of life. These effects were found regardless of predominant bowel type in approximately 55% to 60% of those who participated. Qualitative interviews with the participants at the end of the study showed that at the 12-month follow-up, participants continued to employ the strategies such as avoiding diet triggers and performing relaxation response that they learned during the intervention (Zia et al., 2016).

Baseline data from these intervention trials were used for additional secondary analyses. The results of these secondary data analyses have relevance to future behavioral intervention trials and clinical practice. The first is that alcohol and dietary intake patterns are related to GI symptoms, and thus the focus on how best to tailor diet (i.e., exclusion versus restrictive) is an important and timely discussion (Reding, Cain, Jarrett, Eugenio, & Heitkemper, 2013). Second, the CSM intervention also improves sexual quality of life in women (Eugenio, Jun, Cain, Jarrett, & Heitkemper, 2012). This is an important finding in that women with IBS often report reduced satisfaction with sexual activity. Third, although not a primary outcome of the trials, the CSM intervention resulted in reduced self-reported daily stress at 3, 6, and 12 months postrandomization.

Despite these overall group differences, not all patients improved following the CSM program. One goal of the last intervention trial was not only to determine benefit but also to determine if baseline physiological factors (e.g., biomarkers) could predict who is most likely to benefit. Understanding who is most likely to benefit would also enlighten us as to the pathophysiology or etiology of functional GI disorders to identify early on who is most likely to benefit. We have found that IBS patients with higher vagal tone and lower sympathovagal balance at baseline experienced greater symptom reduction following the CSM intervention (Jarrett et al., 2016). It is interesting to note that lower vagal activity and reduced heart rate variability have been linked to a number of risk factors for cognitive impairment and lower cognitive flexibility (Kim et al., 2006; Ylitalo, Airaksinen, Sellin, & Huikuri, 1999). Specifically, in IBS, increased catecholamines may contribute to disease pathophysiology through their roles in pain perception and stress reactivity, particularly as part of the ANS branch of the stress response. There are data to indicate that patients with IBS have imbalances in the ANS, with some but not all patients exhibiting increases in sympathovagal balance as reflected in reduced vagal activity and increased circulating levels of norepinephrine. Whether this sympathetic dominance is a reflection of a genetic predisposition for the degradation of catecholamines or the result of chronic stress and/or environmental exposure is not known (Liu et al., 2014).

Omics and Symptom Assessment in IBS

In 2001, Levy and colleagues conducted an analysis based on more than 10,000 respondents representing 6,060 twin pairs (Levy et al., 2001). The concordance for IBS was significantly greater in monozygotic than in dizygotic twins, leading researchers to consider the potential role that genetics plays in IBS development. In 2014, a large, multinational genome-wide association study was published demonstrating that the genes that encode for *KDELR2* (endoplasmic reticulum protein retention receptor) and *GRID2IP* (glutamate receptor, ionotropic, delta 2 [Grid2] interacting protein) were associated with a risk for IBS (Ek et al., 2015). Building on what is known about the interaction of psychological distress with symptoms, our collaborative laboratories have pursued a targeted genetic approach.

Genomics

Prior to these genetic studies, clinical investigators reported that patients with IBS-diarrhea had higher levels of the urinary metabolite of serotonin (Bearcroft, Perrett, & Farthing, 1998). Following this, Caspi et al., in a Turkish study, reported that individuals who had a genetic polymorphism in the gene that regulates the production of the serotonin reuptake transporter (5-HTTLPR) protein were more vulnerable to life stress (Caspi et al., 2003). Subsequent to this, a number of investigators sought to examine whether the *SERT* gene polymorphisms and later the presence of rare alleles in the gene were associated with IBS (Zhang et al., 2014). Early reports with relatively small samples indicated that *SERT* polymorphisms were not associated with a diagnosis of IBS, but some differences in psychological variables were noted. Kohen examined *SERT* variants in both IBS and healthy control women by use of a combined dataset from the CSM intervention trials with related descriptive/mechanistic studies. While no IBS versus control differences were found in the distribution of alleles, a greater number of women with IBS had rare variants as compared to controls. A larger sample is needed to understand the clinical impact of these rare variants with respect to phenotype and response to treatment.

One of the genes with potential contribution to abdominal pain but also the responsiveness to the CSM intervention is Catechol-O-methyltransferase (*COMT*). This gene codes for an enzyme that is involved in the degradation of the neurotransmitters norepinephrine and dopamine. It was known that COMT plays important roles in neurocognitive processes like pain and emotional processing. The Val158Met polymorphism (rs4680) of the *COMT* gene leads to a substitution of valine (Val) by methionine (Met). The Met allele has less enzymatic activity than the Val allele (Lachman et al., 1996). There is an association between the Met/Met carrier status and cognitive performance and psychiatric conditions as well as pain processing and sensitivity (Gatt, Burton, Williams, & Schofield, 2015; Scheggia, Sannino, Scattoni, & Papaleo, 2012; Tammimaki & Mannisto, 2012).

The literature on *COMT* and IBS is inconsistent with one study in Chinese patients (Wang, Wu, Qiao, & Zhang, 2014) finding a higher preponderance of the Val/Met and a Swedish study (Karling et al., 2011) finding that the Val/Val was more common in IBS. Of interest to our team was the study by Hall and colleagues, who studied 104 U.S. patients with IBS and found that Met/Met homozygotes had the strongest response to a placebo intervention (i.e., the greatest symptom reduction), thus pointing to a possible role of *COMT* Val158Met in moderating the cognitively focused intervention response (Hall et al., 2012).

To determine if *COMT* genotype is associated with response to a behavioral intervention, we used data from two previously reported randomized clinical trials of CSM versus usual care (Jarrett et al., 2009, 2016). In keeping with prior observations of population-specific genotype effects, the analysis was restricted to self-identified European American participants only. Based on the prior literature, daily reports of abdominal pain, depression, anxiety, and feeling stressed were used as the primary outcome measures for analyses. Baseline abdominal pain among IBS patients did not differ by *COMT* genotype. However, study participants who carried at least one Val allele (i.e., either the Val/Met or Val/Val genotype) derived greater benefit, in terms of psychological distress relief, from the CSM program compared to participants with the Met/Met genotype. This finding is consistent with what had been described in other non-IBS populations, particularly those with psychiatric conditions, with respect to *COMT* genotype and response to behavioral therapies. The *COMT* genotype by CSM interactions on psychological distress may reflect the way in which *COMT* genotype shapes signal transmission through dopamine D1 and D2 receptors (Witte & Floel, 2012). *COMT* polymorphisms may confer or participate in cognitive flexibility, which is proposed to be a key factor of response to CBT, due to greater activation of dopamine D2 type receptors (Carroll et al., 2015; Witte & Floel, 2012). Whether this greater cognitive flexibility conveyed by the Val allele is associated with an improved learning capacity required to incorporate CSM strategies of self-management remains to be determined (Carroll et al., 2015). If so, this may have relevance in terms of self-management for other patient groups.

In another study of both men and women with chronic abdominal pain who had either high or low levels of perceived stress, the expression of genes involved in metabolic stress was examined. Henderson et al. found that Interleukin-1 alpha gene (IL1A) was upregulated in females with high stress versus females with low stress. Similarly, IL1A was upregulated in participants with high stress and chronic abdominal pain versus those with low stress and chronic abdominal pain. These findings suggested that the mechanism behind stress-related changes in GI symptoms is pro-inflammatory in nature (Peace et al., 2012). Further, these investigators found that CCL-16 gene expression was upregulated by 7.46-fold in IBS patients when compared with controls. More specifically, CCL-16 was overexpressed by more than 130-fold in IBS-constipation patients when compared with both controls and IBS-diarrhea patients. For some IBS patients, subclinical inflammation, epithelial dysfunction, and dysregulation of inflammatory cells (Del Valle-Pinero et al., 2011) may be important pathophysiological factors.

It is likely that there are multiple genes and/or epigenetic influences related to lifetime exposures, resilience, and personal resources, which influence patient outcomes. Our combined findings contribute to a growing literature exploring the role of genetic factors in individualized self-management and symptom outcomes. Inclusion of omics (e.g., genetics) in future clinical trials may help identify for whom interventions work and under what conditions (Grey, Schulman-Green, Knafl, & Reynolds, 2015; Henly, 2016).

Proteomics and Metabolomics

A biomarker discovery approach that may hold promise for nurse scientists is the examination of the proteome (Voss et al., 2011). *Proteomics* refers to the global analysis of cellular proteins with mass spectrometry (MS)-based techniques, image analysis, reverse-phase protein array, amino acid sequencing, and/or bioinformatics to identify and quantify proteins. Proteomics is focused on cellular or secreted proteins in terms of both their structure and the functional interaction among proteins. Advances in high-throughput proteomics exponentially increased the potential for new clinical biomarkers, particularly using noninvasive sources such as urine and saliva. To date, the majority of studies are focused on cancer detection and tissue injury. However, these approaches are being employed in symptom science research (Voss et al., 2011). Initially, a shotgun proteomics using urine or other body fluids was used to compare patient and healthy control group differences. This broad hypothesis-generating approach allows an initial identification of proteins for further validation studies.

Another biomarker approach that utilizes MS technology is metabolomics. Metabolomics is a multitargeted analysis of low molecular mass (<1000D) of endogenous and exogenous metabolites and their pathways. This approach allows for the systematic study of the unique chemical fingerprints (amino acids, glucose) that are the result of cellular processes. Metabolites are both the intermediates and the products of metabolism. Complementing genomics and proteomics, metabolomics offers investigators the advantage of linking environmental (diet, stress) factors to cellular responses. Metabolites are found in all body fluids. The Human Metabolome Database (www.hmdb.ca) contains a list of those metabolites that are the result of cellular activities. Metabolomic approaches are increasingly used in the study of diabetes, dyslipidemia, cancer, chronic neurological disorders, pharmaceutics, and nutrition. The utility of metabolomics in symptom science is a new area of inquiry. Given the relationship of diet and stress to IBS symptoms, it is conceivable that metabolomics fingerprints may help distinguish those most likely to benefit from dietary restrictions or cognitively focused therapies.

Microbiome

There is growing appreciation of how the environment within us—that is, our microbiome—can affect health. Our physiological health is influenced by the large number of microbes that exist on or in the skin, mouth, respiratory tract, vagina, and urinary and GI tracts (Van Ness, 2016). There is recent evidence of nutritional and gender effects associated with the microbiome in early life (Cong et al., 2016). Of particular relevance to the development of IBS is the interaction of diet, intestinal bacteria, and the host response. When alterations within the microbiome occur due to disease or lifestyle changes, the balance of microbes is disrupted (dysbiosis), leading to local inflammation, immune response, and metabolic changes. Depending on genetic risk, as well as contextual factors, such responses may ultimately result in chronic inflammation. The Human Microbiome Project (HMP) has contributed to an explosive amount of interest in the gut microbiome and its role in chronic illnesses, including lung disease, diabetes, and psychiatric conditions (Taylor, Wesselingh, & Rogers, 2016).

Our team works collaboratively with pediatric gastroenterologists to test the impact of fiber therapy on stool microbiome and symptoms in children with chronic abdominal pain (Shulman et al., 2016). We observed no differences in stool microbiome composition between children treated for 6 weeks with psyllium compared to placebo, despite reductions in the number of pain episodes. It may be that more sustained efforts are needed to see substantial differences in gut microbial communities.

In an exploratory study, differences in the oral microbiome of IBS patients and healthy controls were examined, to see whether the oral microbiome related to GI symptom severity. The oral microbiome of 38 participants was characterized using PhyloChip microarrays. The severity of GI symptoms was assessed by orally administering a GI test solution. Participants self-reported their induced GI symptoms. Abdominal pain severity was highest in IBS patients and was significantly correlated to the abundance of 60 operational taxonomic units (OTUs), four genera, five families, and four orders of bacteria ($r^2 > 0.4$, $p < .001$). Of note is that the patients with IBS who were also overweight reported the greatest symptom severity and exhibited differences in microbiome diversity characteristics. Abdominal pain severity was highly correlated to the abundance of many taxa, suggesting the potential utility of the oral microbiome in GI symptom phenotyping (Fourie et al., 2016).

Omics Toolbox for Symptom Assessments

Taken together, these new "omic" measures may be viewed as part of the "toolbox" for nurse scientists pursuing the biobehavioral basis for symptoms in a condition such as IBS. These tools, as well as the integration of data elements (i.e., systems biology), allow us to uncover the heterogeneity of each individual and open up future possibilities of designing therapies that are personalized or tailored. Nurse scientists, through their multilevel focus on the individual, family, and community, can interweave the sociocultural, behavioral, and biological influences on ability and disability. The toolbox as used by current and future nurse scientists has the potential to utilize the power of omics to address significant health care problems within the context of the person's life.

Despite the impressive growth in technologies, there are challenges in the interpretation, utilization, and translation of omic findings to practice. A number of potential pitfalls associated with varying analytic approaches in testing contribute to false positives, false negatives, and conflicting results (Rehm, Hynes, & Funke, 2016). How and when these approaches are used to enhance patient self-management remains to be determined and is therefore an area much in need of research.

HEALTH POLICY IMPLICATIONS

In the 2015 State of the Union address, President Obama introduced the launching of the Precision Medicine (a.ka. health) Initiative. It is a bold plan to improve health and treat disease (www.whitehouse.gov/precision-medicine). He stated:

> The future of precision medicine will enable health care providers to tailor treatment and prevention strategies to people's unique characteristics, including their genome sequence, microbiome composition, health history, lifestyle, and diet. To get there, we need to incorporate many different types of data, from metabolomics (the chemicals in the body at a certain point in time), the microbiome (the collection of microorganisms in or on the body), and self-report symptom and behavioral data collected by both the health care providers and the patients themselves.

The intent was to move the focus from the "average" patient or "one-size-fits-all" diagnosis and treatments, to individualized health care by including an individual's molecular makeup in concert with environment and lifestyle factors. Such an approach capitalizes on recent advances in technologies that allows scientists and clinicians to characterize individuals and families in terms of health risk and treatment responses.

Symptom science is a necessary and integral component of the personalized precision health care science agenda. It is difficult to imagine a disease or condition that does not result in symptoms. It is these symptoms that often lead to health care–seeking behavior and the use of medications and technology. Thus, understanding the basis of symptoms, both biological and behavioral, is important for early detection as well as monitoring the progression of many diseases and conditions. For example, fatigue is a common and debilitating symptom in heart failure and cancer, and without symptom management may result in the inability to comply with medical management. Fatigue in caregivers often limits their ability to safely care for family members. Understanding the pathophysiological underpinnings may result in the testing and validating of evidence-based approaches to enhance self-care through fatigue reduction.

So, what barriers to the incorporation of symptom science into the national research agenda exist? There are several, including limited federal and foundation funding, beyond the NINR, to invest in future scientists with the capacity to link self-reported symptoms with biological measures; too few national centers of excellence in symptom science that have the infrastructure to develop and maintain a central data repository for new secondary data analytic approaches; and an inadequate focus on diversity/culture and resilience and how these factors contribute to the expression of symptoms, successful utilization of self-management strategies, and health care–seeking behaviors. It is important to continue to include symptom scientists on national and international review committees; increase the incorporation of technology for symptom assessment as well as measures that capture CDEs; enhance training opportunities for early stage and midcareer scientists; and endorse and provide greater support for the NINR, which has clearly established itself as the "home" of symptom science. The scrutiny and publication of negative findings should be encouraged and greater emphasis placed on reproducibility of findings.

Another barrier that exists is the gap between mechanistic symptom science research that incorporates omics measures into evidence-based practice. Ideally, we carefully phenotype individuals based on symptoms or symptom clusters and then disseminate and utilize the findings in community, ambulatory, and bedside care settings and patient/family education. In part, this gap could be addressed by greater collaboration among interdisciplinary practitioners and nursing scientists. Building on efforts in medicine where joint MD/PhD programs exist, development of DNP/PhD programs could open up opportunities for the next generation of nursing faculty scientists.

CONCLUSION

Nursing science studies of patients with chronic GI symptoms are important because health care providers working with IBS patients are challenged by the facts that the underlying pathophysiology remains poorly defined and treatments are not universally effective. New drug therapies are emerging; however, the long-term benefit (including the impact of chronic use) remains to be studied. Our work to date has been helpful in establishing that menstrual cycle phase, stress, psychological distress, and ANS function are related to IBS symptom frequency/intensity. We have also demonstrated that poor sleep contributes to GI symptoms the next day. Understanding stress-induced alterations in sleep and ANS function may provide important clues as to additional self-management strategies to test.

The breadth of this work, including the recruitment and retention strategies, the assay methodologies for omics measures employed, and the integration of mobile health data collection, could not have been possible without the inclusion of interdisciplinary team members. The team was guided by the following shared hypotheses: (a) there are subgroups of patients with IBS who could be characterized by phenotypic characteristics beyond the Rome bowel and pain symptom criteria; (b) there should be standardized assessment strategies that consider the scope of symptoms experienced by this patient population; (c) there is a likelihood that there are yet undiscovered noninvasive biomarkers, which could be developed and applied to clinical practice; and (d) the quality of life of the majority of patients could best be achieved through evidence-based self-management approaches.

Given nursing's tradition of utilizing biobehavioral information in concert with patient and family assessments, the development of nurse scientists with complementary skills in the interpretation and clinical integration (i.e., translation) of data derived from new technologies is imperative. A larger cadre of nurse scientists who develop and utilize such methods to capture and monitor symptoms and omics data to optimize treatment outcomes through individualized "precision" health is needed (Henly, 2016).

REFERENCES

Bearcroft, C. P., Perrett, D., & Farthing, M. J. (1998). Postprandial plasma 5-hydroxytryptamine in diarrhoea predominant irritable bowel syndrome: A pilot study. *Gut, 42*(1), 42–46.

Buchanan, D. T., Cain, K., Heitkemper, M., Burr, R., Vitiello, M. V., Zia, J., & Jarrett, M. (2014). Sleep measures predict next-day symptoms in women with irritable bowel syndrome. *Journal of Clinical Sleep Medicine, 10*(9), 1003–1009. doi:10.5664/jcsm.4038

Burr, R. L., Jarrett, M. E., Cain, K. C., Jun, S. E., & Heitkemper, M. M. (2009). Catecholamine and cortisol levels during sleep in women with irritable bowel syndrome. *Neurogastroenterology & Motility, 21*(11), 1148–e1197. doi:10.1111/j.1365-2982.2009.01351.x

Carroll, K. M., Herman, A., DeVito, E. E., Frankforter, T. L., Potenza, M. N., & Sofuoglu, M. (2015). Catechol-O-methyltransferase gene Val158met polymorphism as a potential predictor of response to computer-assisted delivery of cognitive-behavioral therapy among cocaine-dependent individuals: Preliminary findings from a randomized controlled trial. *American Journal on Addictions, 24*(5), 443–451. doi:10.1111/ajad.12238

Caspi, A., Sugden, K., Moffitt, T. E., Taylor, A., Craig, I. W., Harrington, H., . . . Poulton, R. (2003). Influence of life stress on depression: Moderation by a polymorphism in the 5-HTT gene. *Science, 301*(5631), 386–389. doi:10.1126/science.1083968

Cong, X., Xu, W., Janton, S., Henderson, W. A., Matson, A., McGrath, J. M., . . . Graf, J. (2016). Gut microbiome developmental patterns in early life of preterm infants: Impacts of feeding and gender. *PLOS ONE, 11*(4), e0152751. doi:10.1371/journal.pone.0152751

Corwin, E. J., Berg, J. A., Armstrong, T. S., DeVito Dabbs, A., Lee, K. A., Meek, P., & Redeker, N. (2014). Envisioning the future in symptom science. *Nursing Outlook, 62*(5), 346–351. doi:10.1016/j.outlook.2014.06.006

Del Valle-Pinero, A. Y., Martino, A. C., Taylor, T. J., Majors, B. L., Patel, N. S., Heitkemper, M. M., & Henderson, W. A. (2011). Pro-inflammatory chemokine C-C motif ligand 16 (CCL-16) dysregulation in irritable bowel syndrome (IBS): A pilot study. *Neurogastroenterology & Motility, 23*(12), 1092–1097. doi:10.1111/j.1365-2982.2011.01792.x

Drossman, D. A., Chang, L., Schneck, S., Blackman, C., Norton, W. F., & Norton, N. J. (2009). A focus group assessment of patient perspectives on irritable bowel syndrome and illness severity. *Digestive Diseases and Sciences, 54*(7), 1532–1541. doi:10.1007/s10620-009-0792-6

Ek, W. E., Reznichenko, A., Ripke, S., Niesler, B., Zucchelli, M., Rivera, N. V., . . . D'Amato, M. (2015). Exploring the genetics of irritable bowel syndrome: A GWA study in the general population and replication in multinational case-control cohorts. *Gut, 64*(11), 1774–1782. doi:10.1136/gutjnl-2014-307997

Eugenio, M. A., Jun, S. E., Cain, K. C., Jarrett, M. E., Heitkemper, M. M. (2012). Comprehensive self-management improves sexual quality of life in IBS? *Digestive Diseases & Sciences, 57*,1636–1646.

Fourie, N. H., Wang, D., Abey, S. K., Sherwin, L. B., Joseph, P. V., Rahim-Williams, B., . . . Henderson, W. A. (2016). The microbiome of the oral mucosa in irritable bowel syndrome. *Gut Microbes,* 1–16. doi:10.1080/19490976.2016.1162363

Gatt, J. M., Burton, K. L., Williams, L. M., & Schofield, P. R. (2015). Specific and common genes implicated across major mental disorders: A review of meta-analysis studies. *Journal of Psychiatric Research, 60*, 1–13. doi:10.1016/j.jpsychires.2014.09.014

Grey, M., Schulman-Green, D., Knafl, K., & Reynolds, N. R. (2015). A revised self- and family management framework. *Nursing Outlook, 63*(2), 162–170. doi:10.1016/j.outlook.2014.10.003

Hall, K. T., Lembo, A. J., Kirsch, I., Ziogas, D. C., Douaiher, J., Jensen, K. B., . . . Kaptchuk, T. J. (2012). Catechol-O-methyltransferase val158met polymorphism predicts placebo effect in irritable bowel syndrome. *PLOS ONE, 7*(10), e48135. doi:10.1371/journal.pone.0048135

Halpert, A., Rybin, D., & Doros, G. (2010). Expressive writing is a promising therapeutic modality for the management of IBS: A pilot study. *American Journal of Gastroenterology, 105*(11), 2440–2448. doi:10.1038/ajg.2010.246

Heitkemper, M. M., & Bond, E. F. (1995). Gastric motility in rats with varying ovarian hormone status. *Western Journal of Nursing Research, 17*(1), 9–19; discussion 101–111.

Heitkemper, M. M., Cain, K. C., Burr, R. L., Jun, S. E., & Jarrett, M. E. (2011). Is childhood abuse or neglect associated with symptom reports and physiological measures in women with irritable bowel syndrome? *Biological Research for Nursing, 13*(4), 399–408. doi:10.1177/1099800410393274

Heitkemper, M. M., Cain, K. C., Deechakawan, W., Poppe, A., Jun, S. E., Burr, R. L., & Jarrett, M. E. (2012). Anticipation of public speaking and sleep and the hypothalamic-pituitary-adrenal axis in women with irritable bowel syndrome. *Neurogastroenterology & Motility, 24*(7), 626–631, e270–621. doi:10.1111/j.1365-2982.2012.01915.x

Heitkemper, M. M., Cain, K. C., Jarrett, M. E., Burr, R. L., Hertig, V., & Bond, E. F. (2003). Symptoms across the menstrual cycle in women with irritable bowel syndrome. *American Journal of Gastroenterology, 98*(2), 420–430. doi:10.1111/j.1572-0241.2003.07233.x

Heitkemper, M. M., Carter, E., Ameen, V., Olden, K., & Cheng, L. (2002). Women with irritable bowel syndrome: Differences in patients' and physicians' perceptions. *Gastroenterology Nursing, 25*(5), 192–200.

Heitkemper, M. M., Jarrett, M., Cain, K. C., Shaver, J., Walker, E., & Lewis, L. (1995). Daily gastrointestinal symptoms in women with and without a diagnosis of IBS. *Digestive Diseases and Sciences, 40*(7), 1511–1519.

Heitkemper, M. M., Jarrett, M. E., Levy, R. L., Cain, K. C., Burr, R. L., Feld, A., . . . Weisman, P. (2004). Self-management for women with irritable bowel syndrome. *Clinical Practice Gastroenterology & Hepatology, 2*(7), 585–596.

Heitkemper, M. M., Jarrett, M., Taylor, P., Walker, E., Landenburger, K., & Bond, E. F. (2001). Effect of sexual and physical abuse on symptom experiences in women with irritable bowel syndrome. *Nursing Research, 50*(1), 15–23.

Henderson, W. A., Rahim-Williams, B., Kim, K. H., Sherwin, L. B., Abey, S. K., Martino, A. C., . . . Zuccolotto, A. P. (2015). The gastrointestinal pain pointer: A valid and innovative method to assess gastrointestinal symptoms. *Gastroenterology Nursing.* doi:10.1097/sga.0000000000000210

Henly, S. J. (2016). Individualizing nursing care in the omics era. *Nursing Research, 65*(2), 89–90. doi:10.1097/nnr.0000000000000156

Jarrett, M. E., Cain, K. C., Barney, P. G., Burr, R. L., Naliboff, B. D., Shulman, R., . . . Heitkemper, M. M. (2016). Balance of autonomic nervous system predicts who benefits from a self-management intervention program for irritable bowel syndrome. *Journal of Neurogastroenterology and Motility, 22*(1), 102–111. doi:10.5056/jnm15067

Jarrett, M. E., Cain, K. C., Burr, R. L., Hertig, V. L., Rosen, S. N., & Heitkemper, M. M. (2009). Comprehensive self-management for irritable bowel syndrome: Randomized trial of in-person vs. combined in-person and telephone sessions. *American Journal of Gastroenterology, 104*(12), 3004–3014. doi:10.1038/ajg.2009.479

Jarrett, M.E., Heitkemper, M., Cain, K. C., Burr, R. L., & Hertig, V. (2000). Sleep disturbance influences gastrointestinal symptoms in women with irritable bowel syndrome. *Digestive Diseases and Sciences, 45*(5), 952–959.

Jarrett, M. E., Heitkemper, M., Cain, K. C., Tuftin, M., Walker, E. A., Bond, E. F., & Levy, R. L. (1998). The relationship between psychological distress and gastrointestinal symptoms in women with irritable bowel syndrome. *Nursing Research, 47*(3), 154–161.

Karling, P., Danielsson, A., Wikgren, M., Soderstrom, I., Del-Favero, J., Adolfsson, R., & Norrback, K. F. (2011). The relationship between the val158met catechol-O-methyltransferase (COMT) polymorphism and irritable bowel syndrome. *PLOS ONE, 6*(3), e18035. doi:10.1371/journal.pone.0018035

Kim, D. H., Lipsitz, L. A., Ferrucci, L., Varadhan, R., Guralnik, J. M., Carlson, M. C., . . . Chaves, P. H. (2006). Association between reduced heart rate variability and cognitive impairment in older disabled women in the community: Women's health and aging study I. *Journal of the American Geriatrics Society, 54*(11), 1751–1757. doi:10.1111/j.1532-5415.2006.00940.x

Kirschstein, R. L. (1991). Research on women's health. *American Journal of Public Health, 81*(3), 291–293.

Lachman, H. M., Papolos, D. F., Saito, T., Yu, Y. M., Szumlanski, C. L., & Weinshilboum, R. M. (1996). Human catechol-O-methyltransferase pharmacogenetics: Description of a functional polymorphism and its potential application to neuropsychiatric disorders. *Pharmacogenetics, 6*(3), 243–250.

Levy, R. L., Cain, K. C., Jarrett, M., & Heitkemper, M. M. (1997). The relationship between daily life stress and gastrointestinal symptoms in women with irritable bowel syndrome. *Journal Behavioral Medicine, 20*(2), 177–193.

Levy, R. L., Jones, K. R., Whitehead, W. E., Feld, S. I., Talley, N. J., & Corey, L. A. (2001). Irritable bowel syndrome in twins: Heredity and social learning both contribute to etiology. *Gastroenterology, 121*(4), 799–804.

Liu, L., Liu, B. N., Chen, S., Wang, M., Liu, Y., Zhang, Y. L., & Yao, S. K. (2014). Visceral and somatic hypersensitivity, autonomic cardiovascular dysfunction and low-grade inflammation in a subset of irritable bowel syndrome patients. *Journal of Zhejiang University SCIENCE B, 15*(10), 907–914. doi:10.1631/jzus.B1400143

Lovell, R. M., & Ford, A. C. (2012). Global prevalence of and risk factors for irritable bowel syndrome: A meta-analysis. *Clinical Gastroenterology and Hepatology, 10*(7), 712–721.e4. doi:10.1016/j.cgh.2012.02.029

Miaskowski, C., & Aouizerat, B. E. (2007). Is there a biological basis for the clustering of symptoms? *Seminars Oncology Nursing, 23*(2), 99–105. doi:10.1016/j.soncn.2007.01.008

Miaskowski, C., Cooper, B. A., Paul, S. M., Dodd, M., Lee, K., Aouizerat, B. E., . . . Bank, A. (2006). Subgroups of patients with cancer with different symptom experiences and quality-of-life outcomes: A cluster analysis. *Oncology Nursing Forum, 33*(5), E79–E89. doi:10.1188/06.onf.e79-e89

Mitchell, E. S., & Woods, N. F. (1996). Symptom experiences of midlife women: Observations from the Seattle midlife women's health study. *Maturitas, 25*(1), 1–10.

Monnikes, H. (2011). Quality of life in patients with irritable bowel syndrome. *Journal of Clinical Gastroenterology, 45*, S98–S101. doi:10.1097/MCG.0b013e31821fbf44

Nanayakkara, W. S., Skidmore, P. M., O'Brien, L., Wilkinson, T. J., & Gearry, R. B. (2016). Efficacy of the low FODMAP diet for treating irritable bowel syndrome: The evidence to date. *Clinical and Experimental Gastroenterology, 9*, 131–142. doi:10.2147/ceg.s86798

National Institute of Nursing Research. (2016, May 6). Spotlight on symptom management research. Retrieved from http://www.ninr.nih.gov/researchandfunding/symptommanagement#.V6x-N2dTGM8

Nellesen, D., Yee, K., Chawla, A., Lewis, B. E., & Carson, R. T. (2013). A systematic review of the economic and humanistic burden of illness in irritable bowel syndrome and chronic constipation. *Journal of Managed Care Pharmacy, 19*(9), 755–764. doi:10.18553/jmcp.2013.19.9.755

Nojkov, B., Rubenstein, J. H., Chey, W. D., & Hoogerwerf, W. A. (2010). The impact of rotating shift work on the prevalence of irritable bowel syndrome in nurses. *American Journal of Gastroenterology, 105*(4), 842–847. doi:10.1038/ajg.2010.48

Palsson, O. S., Whitehead, W. E., van Tilburg, M. A., Chang, L., Chey, W., Crowell, M. D., . . . Yang, Y. (2016). Rome IV diagnostic questionnaires and tables for investigators and clinicians. *Gastroenterology, S0016–S5085*(16), 00180–00183. doi:10.1053/j.gastro.2016.02.014

Peace, R. M., Majors, B. L., Patel, N. S., Wang, D., Valle-Pinero, A. Y., Martino, A. C., & Henderson, W. A. (2012). Stress and gene expression of individuals with chronic abdominal pain. *Biological Research for Nursing, 14*(4), 405–411. doi:10.1177/1099800412458350

Prusator, D. K., & Greenwood-Van Meerveld, B. (2016). Sex-related differences in pain behaviors following three early life stress paradigms. *Biology of Sex Differences, 7,* 29. doi:10.1186/s13293-016-0082-x

Redeker, N. S., Anderson, R., Bakken, S., Corwin, E., Docherty, S., Dorsey, S. G., . . . Grady, P. (2015). Advancing symptom science through use of common data elements. *Journal of Nursing Scholarship, 47*(5), 379–388. doi:10.1111/jnu.12155

Reding, K. W., Cain, K. C., Jarrett, M. E., Eugenio, M. D., & Heitkemper, M. M. (2013). Relationship between patterns of alcohol consumption and gastrointestinal symptoms among patients with irritable bowel syndrome. *American Journal of Gastroenterology, 108*(2), 270–276. doi:10.1038/ajg.2012.414

Rehm, H. L., Hynes, E., & Funke, B. H. (2016). The changing landscape of molecular diagnostic testing: Implications for academic medical centers. *Journal of Personalized Medicine, 6*(1). doi:10.3390/jpm6010008

Riddle, M. S., Welsh, M., Porter, C. K., Nieh, C., Boyko, E. J., Gackstetter, G., & Hooper, T. I. (2016). The epidemiology of irritable bowel syndrome in the US military: Findings from the millennium cohort study. *American Journal of Gastroenterology, 111*(1), 93–104. doi:10.1038/ajg.2015.386

Scheggia, D., Sannino, S., Scattoni, M. L., & Papaleo, F. (2012). COMT as a drug target for cognitive functions and dysfunctions. *CNS & Neurological Disorders—Drug Targets, 11*(3), 209–221.

Shulman, R. J., Hollister, E. B., Cain, K., Czyzewski, D. I., Self, M. M., Weidler, E. M., . . . Heitkemper, M. (2016). Psyllium fiber reduces abdominal pain in children with irritable bowel syndrome in a randomized, double-blind trial. *Clinical Gastroenterology and Hepatology, S1542–S3565*(16), 30021–30020. doi:10.1016/j.cgh.2016.03.045

Spiegel, B. M., Hays, R. D., Bolus, R., Melmed, G. Y., Chang, L., Whitman, C., . . . Khanna, D. (2014). Development of the NIH patient-reported outcomes measurement information system (PROMIS) gastrointestinal symptom scales. *American Journal of Gastroenterology, 109*(11), 1804–1814. doi:10.1038/ajg.2014.237

Tammimaki, A., & Mannisto, P. T. (2012). Catechol-O-methyltransferase gene polymorphism and chronic human pain: A systematic review and meta-analysis. *Pharmacogenetics and Genomics, 22*(9), 673–691. doi:10.1097/FPC.0b013e3283560c46

Tanaka, Y., Kanazawa, M., Fukudo, S., & Drossman, D. A. (2011). Biopsychosocial model of irritable bowel syndrome. *Journal of Neurogastroenterology and Motility, 17*(2), 131–139. doi:10.5056/jnm.2011.17.2.131

Taylor, D. C., Kosinski, M., Reilly, K., & Lindner, L. (2014). Comparison of the burden of IBS with constipation on health-related quality of life (HRQOL), work productivity, and health care utilization to asthma, migraine, and rheumatoid arthritis in the US, UK, and France. *Value in Health, 17*(7), A371–A372. doi:10.1016/j.jval.2014.08.849

Taylor, S. L., Wesselingh, S., & Rogers, G. B. (2016). Host-microbiome interactions in acute and chronic respiratory infections. *Cellular Microbiology, 18*(5), 652–662. doi:10.1111/cmi.12589

Tu, Q., Heitkemper, M. M., Jarrett, M. E., & Buchanan, D. T. (2016). Sleep disturbances in irritable bowel syndrome: A systematic review. *Neurogastroenterology & Motility.* doi:10.1111/nmo.12946. [Epub ahead of print].

Van Ness, B. (2016). Applications and limitations in translating genomics to clinical practice. *Translational Research, 168,* 1–5. doi:10.1016/j.trsl.2015.04.012

Voss, J., Goo, Y. A., Cain, K., Woods, N., Jarrett, M., Smith, L., . . . Heitkemper, M. (2011). Searching for the noninvasive biomarker holy grail: Are urine proteomics the answer? *Biological Research for Nursing, 13*(3), 235–242. doi:10.1177/1099800411402056

Wang, Y., Wu, Z., Qiao, H., & Zhang, Y. (2014). A genetic association study of single nucleotide polymorphisms in GNbeta3 and COMT in elderly patients with irritable bowel syndrome. *Medical Science Monitor, 20,* 1246–1254. doi:10.12659/msm.890315

White, D. L., Savas, L. S., Daci, K., Elserag, R., Graham, D. P., Fitzgerald, S. J., . . . El-Serag, H. B. (2010). Trauma history and risk of the irritable bowel syndrome in women veterans. *Alimentary Pharmacology & Therapeutics, 32*(4), 551–561. doi:10.1111/j.1365-2036.2010.04387.x

Witte, A. V., & Floel, A. (2012). Effects of COMT polymorphisms on brain function and behavior in health and disease. *Brain Research Bulletin, 88*(5), 418–428. doi:10.1016/j.brainresbull.2011.11.012

Ylitalo, A., Airaksinen, K. E., Sellin, L., & Huikuri, H. V. (1999). Effects of combination antihypertensive therapy on baroreflex sensitivity and heart rate variability in systemic hypertension. *American Journal of Cardiology, 83*(6), 885–889.

Zhang, Z. F., Duan, Z. J., Wang, L. X., Yang, D., Zhao, G., & Zhang, L. (2014). The serotonin transporter gene polymorphism (5-HTTLPR) and irritable bowel syndrome: A meta-analysis of 25 studies. *BMC Gastroenterology, 14,* 23. doi:10.1186/1471-230x-14-23

Zia, J. K., Barney, P., Cain, K. C., Jarrett, M. E., & Heitkemper, M. M. (2016). A comprehensive self-management irritable bowel syndrome program produces sustainable changes in behavior after 1 year. *Clinical Gastroenterology and Hepatology, 14*(2), 212–219.e211–212. doi:10.1016/j.cgh.2015.09.027

Zia, J. K., Le, T., Munson, S., Heitkemper, M. M., & Demiris, G. (2015). Download alert: Understanding gastroenterology patients' perspectives on health-related smartphone apps. *Clinical and Translational Gastroenterology, 6,* e96. doi:10.1038/ctg.2015.25

11

Caring for Caregivers in an Aging Society: Contributions of Nursing Research to Practice and Policy

Laura N. Gitlin

"The visiting nurse is coming today. Just what the doctor ordered (after I told him this is what we need!)."

"Mom is weaker and having trouble supporting herself in a standing position. Weakening seems to be happening faster than we knew. Never a dull moment. I love our visiting nurse."

"Hospice nurse is coming. Mom was having trouble breathing. She seems to have quieted down after a 2nd small dose of morphine. The gasping was scary."

These excerpts of e-mail communications, from a daughter caring for her mother with dementia to a family member, provide a small window into some of the daily care challenges families confront and the important roles of nurses. Family members, broadly defined as friends, fictive kin, or neighbors, have been, are now, and will continue to be in the future the primary providers of care to older adults with unmet needs or physical or cognitive limitations (Bookman & Kimbrel, 2011; Pruchno & Gitlin, 2012).

Family involvement in the care of older adults is a global phenomenon occurring across all socioeconomic levels, within all racial and ethnic groups, and in low-, middle-, and high-income countries. In the United States alone, estimates of the number of families providing some form of care to an older adult range from a high of 65.7 million (28.5% of the U.S. adult population), most of whom are providing care to adults 50 years of age or older (National Alliance for Caregiving and AARP, 2009), to a low of 3.5 million informal caregivers providing unpaid care to people 65 years or older, as identified in the National Long-Term Care survey (National Institute of Aging and Duke University, 2004). According to the National Study of Caregiving (NSOC), a population-based companion survey to the National Health and Aging Trends Study (NHATS), approximately 17.7 million individuals were caregivers of older adults ($\geq$ 65) in 2011 due to poor health or functioning, with close to half (8.5 million) providing help with two or more self-care needs to older adults (Spillman, Wolff, Freedman, & Kasper, 2014).

Although prevalence estimates may vary based on definitions of caregiving and survey methodologies (Giovannetti & Wolff, 2010), there is strong consensus that the number of older adults in need of caregiving, and consequently the need for and number of families providing care, will only increase as the population ages (Stone, 2015). How nursing supports the efforts of family caregivers in diverse health care settings has been and will continue to be an important focal area of concern in research, practice, and policy. The purpose of this chapter is to provide foundational knowledge about family caregiving from which to understand its implications for nursing. First, key societal drivers that place families front and center in the care of older adults and the range of responsibilities families commonly assumed are described. Then, care interventions to support family caregivers and the principles they are based upon are discussed. Finally, the key competencies for nurses in interacting and engaging with and supporting family caregivers are identified, along with policy implications.

SOCIETAL TRENDS PLACE FAMILIES IN THE FOREFRONT OF HEALTH CARE

Several key pressing societal trends have placed families in the forefront of providing, coordinating, or overseeing long-term care and services for older adults; this is why nursing needs to carefully attend to and support family caregivers, now and into the future. Of most significance is the unprecedented and dramatic demographic shift toward an aging society that is under way in the United States and globally (Ortman, Velkoff, & Hogan, 2014). Whereas today 8.5% (617 million) of the world's population is 65 years or older, this number will leap to almost 17% (1.6 billion) by 2050 (He, Goodkind, & Kowal, 2015). This demographic phenomenon is rapidly sweeping high-, middle-, and low-income countries alike (Beard et al., 2015). As living longer is typically accompanied by age-related deficits, chronic disease, disability, and frailty, most older adults can expect to need some form of assistance during some part of their later life, placing increasing responsibilities upon families to provide this support (B. Coleman & Pandya, 2002; E. A. Coleman, Boult, & American Geriatrics Society Health Care Systems Committee, 2003; National Alliance for Caregiving & AARP, 2009).

Secondly, improvements in medical advances, coupled with shorter hospital and rehabilitation stays accompanied by the expansion of home care technologies, have moved health care from medical centers to homes or residences of older adults. For example, care delivered in the home by nurses versus the hospital results in shorter recovery time, fewer complications, and reduced rehospitalizations even for frail older adults (Leff et al., 1999; Leff & Burton, 1996). Furthermore, emerging medical models such as hospital at home, hospice home care, collaborative primary care models, and care transition models—which all involve nurses at the helm directing, managing, or coordinating care—all assume that a family member will serve as the primary caregiver who will be present and responsible for carrying out care responsibilities at home.

Third, unfortunately, health care organizations and systems of care, particularly in the United States, continue to be based upon an acute care medical model. This, combined with the lack of an integrated, coordinated system of long-term care for older adults, continues to systematically preclude recognition of and an adequate response to the complex, unique, and elongated needs posed by chronic conditions and multimorbidities that present as people age (Aronson, 2015). Common conditions such as heart failure, diabetes, vision impairments, cancer, HIV, and multimorbidities, for which nurses are again in the forefront of managing and overseeing patient self-management, are not responsive to quick fixes, a magic pill or silver bullet, or singular treatments; rather, they require ongoing care, attention to their functional consequences on daily activities of living, and an understanding and evaluation of the social and environmental living space and how it supports, or not, everyday healthy living.

A fourth key and striking trend is the changing structure of families, along with the shrinking pool of family members who are or will be available and able to provide care to older adults. This trend is due to the confluence of several factors: low birth rates (e.g., families are having fewer to no children or having children later in life); geographic mobility and dispersion of families (e.g., fewer families live in geographic proximity to an aging relative); and more women than previously in the workforce (National Academy of Medicine, 2016; Stone, 2015).

These dominant societal features are punctuated as well by an increasingly diverse aging population. Consequently, family members reflect assorted cultures, values, beliefs, practices, preferences, living conditions, literacy levels, and so forth (Gaugler & Kane, 2015). Thus, there is no doubt that nurses now and into the future will need to interact with, include, and elicit the support of highly dissimilar family members throughout or at some point in the course of their own professional lives. These trends also portend that a new science of nursing caregiving is necessary. As families are and will continue to be integral to the fabric of long-term care for older adults, some of the key areas of nursing science with practice implications concern the following: developing, evaluating, and implementing ways to effectively and efficiently identify and engage diverse older adults and families in care decision making; examining the complex psychological, physiological, health, financial, and social effects of caregiving for different conditions and disease trajectories of older adults; and deriving and implementing evidence-based clinical tools for evaluating the capacity of families to engage in expected care tasks and strategies for training and supporting them.

WHO IS A FAMILY CAREGIVER?

Who is a family caregiver is not a straightforward or easy question to answer. The answer often depends upon how caregiving is defined, which has resulted in different prevalence rates and perspectives of roles, responsibilities, and outcomes. As the term "caregiver" is a social construct, families providing care may or may not self-identify as such. Some families reject or do not relate to the term "caregiver," as they consider their role to be a "natural" part of their relationship with their spouse, parent, sibling, friend, or another relative, despite the fact that they are providing assistance commensurate with traditional definitions of a caregiving role. This poses tricky methodological challenges concerning how to effectively identify a family member who is providing care for research or clinical purposes, and how to document caregiving needs in electronic medical records or elsewhere for tracking and identifying appropriate services and support.

Research studies of family caregivers tend to include and evaluate those who self-identify as a "caregiver" and who are able to volunteer their time for study participation, thus potentially limiting our understandings of caregiving to this self-selective group. Individuals who self-identify as a family caregiver may differ in important ways from those involved in the same level and type of care but who do not self-identify as such. For example, study volunteer caregivers, when compared to those who qualified as a "caregiver" in a random-digit-dial survey of families but who did not volunteer, reported higher levels of education and income, were more likely to be married and living with the older adult, more likely to be caring for an older adult diagnosed with dementia or having greater cognitive difficulties, have significantly higher levels of caregiver burden and increased depressive symptomatology, and report more negative and fewer positive relationships with their older adult (Pruchno et al., 2008).

Complicating the landscape as well is the fact that nurses and other health care providers, in addition to researchers, label families differently depending upon the role a family caregiver is perceived to have in a medical encounter. For example, families attending physician appointments with an older relative may be referred to as a "medical visit companion" or "companion" (Wolff & Roter, 2008; Wolff, Boyd, Gitlin, Bruce, & Roter, 2012); families involved in helping older adults transition from hospital to home may be referred to as "informal caregivers" (Burton, Zdaniuk, Schulz, Jackson, & Hirsch, 2003; E. A. Coleman, Parry, Chalmers, & Min, 2006; Vickrey et al., 2006); families who provide medical information for older relatives with cognitive impairments in particular and for diagnostic purposes are often called "proxy" or "key" informants; families involved in end-of-life care or individuals who are incapacitated are called "proxy decision makers" (Winter & Parks, 2008). Nomenclature has research, practice, and policy implications. How we recognize and label family members providing care to older adults in research, practice, or policy affects the way in which they are identified, treated, and integrated into care planning and decision making, as well as their access to supportive interventions including education, counseling, and skills training when needed.

So, who are family members that assume caregiving? Previously, family caregivers were distinguished from formal caregivers with the distinction of providing "unpaid" assistance for a relative; however, this definition is no longer viable because of the relatively recent federal and state programs offering financial offsets or stipends to families (e.g., Money Follows the Person), the rise of familial arrangements in which one member is paid by others to assume caregiving responsibilities, and the recognition of the economic value and toll of family caregiving. Some surveys or research studies narrowly define caregivers as family members providing a particular high level of care provision (e.g., certain number of hours per week or assistance with one or more basic self-care activities). But these boundaries do not reflect the full range of care needs of older adults and consequently the wide array of tasks that family caregivers commonly assume (discussed later; Reinhard, Levine, & Samis, 2012).

Broadly speaking, *family caregiver* refers to a relative, spouse, friend, neighbor, or fictive kin, who provides "extraordinary" physical and mental health support to an older adult who has a vulnerability due to a health condition(s) or disability of some sort requiring assistance, including end-of-life care. As caring is of course core to the essence and definition of being a family, the term "extraordinary" differentiates "caregiving" from normative cultural expectations and everyday practices in which families "care" for each other.

Using this broad definition, we find that most family caregivers are still women in their forties (Schulz & Tompkins, 2010; Wolff, Spillman, Freedman, & Kasper, 2016). As coined by Dr. Brody (2003), this "woman in the middle" typically juggles both childcare and eldercare, as well as possibly the care for more than one impaired parent or relative, in addition to employment and increasing responsibilities and pressures at work (Gaugler & Kane, 2015).

Although this reflects the average profile, there are noteworthy exceptions and a changing demography. First, more men are assuming care responsibilities than previously; this is particularly the case in dementia care, in which over 40% of caregivers are male (Alzheimer's Association, 2016). Second, there is a growing group of long-distance caregivers, although the precise number is not clear (Gitlin & Schulz, 2012). Third, caregiving is not a sole-source job; rather, it is typically a family matter with specific responsibilities often dispersed or delegated to different members. However, there is little understanding of how one person in a family network becomes a primary caregiver, nor how delegation and care decision making occurs among multiple family players.

Characteristics of caregivers also vary by level and type of care provided. Wolff et al. (2016) report that family caregivers providing "substantial help" (defined as assistance with care coordination and medication management) are more likely to be older, and less likely to report having excellent health.

Finally, it cannot be overstated that a defining characteristic of family caregivers as a whole today is their extreme diversity, including but not limited to their race and ethnicity, geographic location, cultural beliefs and values, literacy, care practices, and preferences.

The implications for nursing are manifold. First, in clinical practice, when interacting with a family caregiver, consideration must be given to life trajectory or the point in a person's life in which he or she is needed to provide care. The caregiver role may intersect with other life expectations such as raising children, caring for other family members, work and/or leadership responsibilities, and attending to personal needs for self-fulfillment, health, and well-being.

Second, future nursing research will have to examine who within families assumes the role of caregiver, how life-span dynamics and the health of the caregiver shape this decision and care decision making in general, strategies for maintaining or restoring the health of family caregivers, and how the health condition of the older adult affects the health and well-being of family caregivers. This will require a population perspective, longitudinal designs, and incisive attention to diversity.

WHAT DO FAMILIES DO?

As families form the backbone of health care systems worldwide, and particularly in the United States in which there is not a coherent system of long-term care (Institute of Medicine, Committee on the Future Health Care Workforce for Older Americans & Board on Health Care Services, 2008), understanding the range of tasks and responsibilities families assume is important. Family care responsibilities are highly varied depending upon (of course) the health, living conditions, and needs of the older adult, as well as the abilities, resources, and geographic proximity of the family caregiver. Family caregiver involvement can be broadly categorized as being either episodic, transitional, long-term, or a combination thereof and involving emotional, financial, coordination, and/or instrumental support (Gitlin & Wolff, 2011). Episodic assistance may include, but is not limited to, transporting and/or accompanying older adults to physician appointments, shopping, housekeeping, financial managing, checking in or monitoring housing conditions for safety, or refilling and monitoring medications periodically (Wolff et al., 2012; Wolff & Spillman, 2014). Transitional care responsibilities may involve helping older adults move safely from one care setting to another (hospital to rehabilitation to home, or home to adult day services), and participating in medication reconciliation and compliance (Gitlin & Wolff, 2011). Finally, long-term care typically includes hands-on assistance in instrumental and basic self-care interspersed with episodic and transitional care responsibilities (Schulz & Tompkins, 2010). Even with hospitalization or nursing home or assisted living facility placement, family care responsibilities continue with new tasks, including ensuring that quality of care is provided, coordinating input and decision making across settings and health providers, providing social and emotional support, and attending to instrumental and possibly self-care activities of living (Gitlin & Schulz, 2012).

How families come to assume caregiving may vary depending upon their own resources and abilities as well as the condition and needs of the older adult. As to the latter, for chronic conditions such as diabetes, heart disease, or dementia, family care responsibilities may start slowly, involving periodic or episodic assistance such as providing reminders about medication taking or doctor's appointments to accompanying older adults to medical visits or assisting with shopping and/or finances. Then, with disease progression, more time in caregiving may be needed and involve hands-on assistance, moving from assistance with instrumental activities of living (shopping, medication management, household repairs) to providing supervision and then hands-on care with activities of daily living (e.g., bathing, dressing, toileting, eating). There is an incremental increase in care responsibilities and time spent, as well as the emotional, physical, and financial tolls that may be experienced (Gitlin & Schulz, 2012). Alternately, care responsibilities may be assumed abruptly, such as in the case of an older adult with a sudden stroke or acute acerbation of heart disease for which there are physical, cognitive, or other sequelae that trigger the need for more assistance. Here there may be a sharp bifurcation: one day a family member is not a caregiver, and the next, he or she is.

Over the course of caregiving for an older relative, whether care provision is sudden or incremental, a family caregiver may at some point provide care coordination, care transitions, hands-on assistance with instrumental and basic self-care, health-related services such as medication management and administration, wound care, financial support or management, and/or on-site or long-distance monitoring, as well as emotional and social support (Aneshensel, Pearlin, Mullan, Zarit, & Whitlatch, 1995; Schulz & Tomkins, 2010).

A distinguishing feature of caregiving today compared to previous decades is the complexity of care tasks families are expected to assume. These may include changing and cleaning feeding tubes; administering injections; engaging in wound care; attending to psychiatric conditions such as apathy, depression, hallucinations, or other behavioral disturbances; and/or overseeing or carrying out complex medication regimens. These tasks are typically carried out with little to no training, recourse, or ongoing counsel or support (Reinhard et al., 2012).

WHAT ARE THE CONSEQUENCES OF PROVIDING CARE TO OLDER ADULTS?

Both positive and negative consequences of providing care to older adults have been reported in the research literature. An emerging body of research shows that family caregivers may actually be healthier and live longer than non-caregivers (Brown & Brown, 2014). Similarly, other studies have documented positive outcomes such as an enhanced sense of mastery, improved relationships, or feeling that one is fulfilling an important obligation and giving back (Roth, Dilworth-Anderson, Huang, Gross, & Gitlin, 2016). However, it remains difficult to tease out if family caregivers are healthier prior to assuming the caregiver role, or if it is the act of caring itself that improves health and possibly longevity; it may be, for example, that only the strongest and most robust members of families become caregivers.

Families also may assume care tasks at great cost to themselves (Adelman, Tmanova, Delgado, Dion, & Lachs, 2014). These consequences are amply documented and may include, but are not limited to, financial strain, distress, depressive symptoms, missed doctor's appointments, poor health, loss of work, and/or social isolation (National Academy of Medicine, 2016). A wide array of factors shape the experience of caregiving, whether it be positive, negative, or both, including the condition of the older adult, type of assistance needed, familial resources, gender, age, education, finances, relationship, and so forth. Dementia caregiving, however, remains the most challenging, with this group of caregivers having higher rates of depressive symptoms, stress and burden, and poor health compared to caregivers of older adults with other conditions (Ory & Hoffman, 1999; Schulz, O'Brien, Bookwala, & Fleissner, 1995).

Presenting clinical features also shape the caregiving experience and outcomes. For example, families caring for persons with dementia and managing behavioral symptoms (rejection of care, agitation, aggression) have higher rates of depression compared to those caring for persons without these symptoms. Also, as physical function declines, stress and burden increase along with time allocated to caregiving for dementia caregivers (Jutkowitz et al., in press; Okura & Langa, 2011).

The economic toll of caregiving on families should not be underestimated, although the impact of this stressor on health and well-being is unclear. Although it is difficult to identify the precise economic contributions of family caregiving, it is estimated at $470 billion per year in the United States (Reinhard, Feinberg, Choula, & Houser, 2015). This is more than total Medicaid spending in 2013, including both federal and state contributions for health care and long term, which was estimated to be $449 billion, and greater than the total out-of-pocket spending on health care in 2013 estimated at $339 billion. Out-of-pocket health care expenses seem to vary by the condition of the older adult, with dementia caregiving presenting as one of the most costly to families (Alzheimer's Association, 2016; Delavande, Hurd, Martorell, & Langa, 2013; Jutkowitz et al., in press). Out-of-pocket costs also vary by symptomatology, with functional limitations versus cognitive decline or behavioral symptoms resulting in higher personal costs (Jutkowitz et al., in press).

Despite the magnitude of caregiving, whether episodic, transitional, long-term, or a combination thereof, families often provide care and make care decisions without the benefit of effective training, support, or requisite knowledge and skills. Although most families accept caregiving responsibilities unconditionally, society at large, health care organizations, and providers also presume that families will de facto provide and ensure safe and effective care for an older adult regardless of ability, resources, employment, or other responsibilities. This societal push places families in a tenuous position; it enforces that care responsibilities will be assumed by a family member without determining whether that individual has the necessary resources and capacity. This is disturbing, as many care tasks that families are expected to take on can be complex, such as medication reconciliation and administration, wound care, toileting, dressing, and transferring. Nor are the health, resources, employment status, and needs of family caregivers themselves assessed, recognized, accommodated, or addressed (Family Caregiver Alliance, 2006). Families also may be vilified by health professionals; they can be perceived as not doing enough, as not providing good care, or as "pushy" or interlopers when advocating for their relatives. The lack of attention to and support of and sometimes disdain for caregivers may not only cause undue familial distress, but also compromise quality of care and outcomes for older adults as well (Marx et al.,

2014; Stensletten, Bruvik, Espehaug, & Drageset, 2014; Wolff, Clayman, Rabins, Cooke, & Roter, 2015).

Obtaining the right balance between familial and societal responsibilities has significant policy implications. Moreover, how nurses interact with and impact this complex web of health system failures in long-term care, and attend to the needs of both family caregivers and older adult "patients," remains uncharted territory (Wolff, 2012).

CARING FOR THE CAREGIVER

The past 30-plus years have yielded a significant body of research on family caregiving, focusing on who they are, what they do, consequences (both positive and negative), unmet needs, and supportive interventions (Callahan, Kales, Gitlin, & Lyketsos, 2013). This substantial evolution of research and knowledge generation from descriptive to exploratory and correlational to a focus on intervening to enhance caregiver outcomes is impressive, although more research is certainly needed, particularly as it concerns understanding the changing dynamics and demographics of caregiving, its physiological effects, and best practices for engaging families and intervening to support them. The role of technology and web-based methods for supporting nurse–caregiver interactions in particular is promising, yet undeveloped (Kales et al., 2016; Solli, Hvalvik, Bjørk, & Hellesø, 2015), and more research is needed to develop and test clinical tools to systematically and effectively involve family caregivers to participate in medical encounters (Family Caregiver Alliance, 2006; Wolff et al., 2014).

Of particular importance is the varied array of interventions that have been developed and tested with families and which have immediate, practical application. Taken as a whole, a wide range of interventions have been tested, including education, counseling, care management, and skill building. Collectively, studies report an array of important positive benefits for family caregivers, such as reducing stress, burden, and depression; improving knowledge and skills; and enhancing self-efficacy and mastery (Adelman et al., 2014). Additionally, many interventions targeting family caregivers also result in benefits to older adult recipients—that is, intervening with families can also improve the quality of care and outcomes for older adults as well (Brodaty & Arasaratnam, 2012).

While most intervention research has been conducted with dementia caregivers (Gitlin & Hodgson, 2015), the few focusing on other conditions such as cancer (Northouse, Katapodi, Song, Zhang, & Mood, 2010) are equally promising, although much more intervention research for specific conditions (e.g., stroke, heart failure, multimorbidities) is warranted.

Nursing-based interventions in particular are critical for addressing the wide range of needs of families and for a variety of care settings. Figure 11.1 provides a social ecological conceptualization for understanding nursing-based interventions that can be used to guide future development of interventions, evaluate implementation potential of current interventions, and change practices and policies.

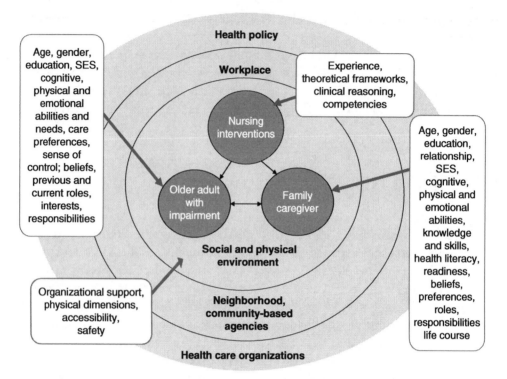

FIGURE 11.1 *Social ecological model of family caregiving and nursing interventions.*

SES, socioeconomic status.

The framework suggests that nursing interventions are embedded within multilayered systems and interacting components or levels of influence that also change over time. These factors and layers of influence include nurse interventionists and what they bring to the care situation, such as their previous experiences and know-how, their competencies working with families, and their clinical reasoning and theoretical frameworks guiding their interactions; older adults with impairment and their demographic, physical, and psychological health profile, as well as cultural beliefs and practices; the family caregiver(s) and their resources, abilities, knowledge/skills, and demographic profile, along with where they are in their own life course; the social and physical environment or setting in which an intervention takes place and the barriers and supports it offers; the community, neighborhood, health care organization, and workplace and their barriers and support for interventions, as well as the health policy and organizational environment, such as reimbursement, staffing, and administrative policies that may directly and indirectly impact the dynamics of delivery and outcomes of an intervention (adopted from Gitlin & Czaja, 2016).

The Care of Persons With Dementia in Their Environments (COPE) intervention for dementia caregivers can be used as an exemplar to understand the significance of this conceptualization (Gitlin, Winter, Dennis, Hodgson, & Hauck, 2010). COPE sought to support capabilities of persons with dementia by reducing environmental stressors, and enhancing family caregiver skills and improving caregiver well-being.

In this multicomponent intervention, families receive up to 10 sessions over 4 months by occupational therapists (OT); and 1 face-to-face session and 1 telephone session by an advanced practice nurse. OTs initially interview caregivers to identify patient routines, previous and current roles, habits and interests, and caregiver concerns. OTs also conduct cognitive and functional testing to identify patients' strengths and deficits in attention, initiation/perseveration, construction, conceptualization, and memory. OTs then train caregivers to modify home environments, daily activities, and communications to support patient capabilities, use problem solving to identify solutions for caregiver-identified concerns, and stress reduction techniques to address their own upset and distress. For each targeted concern, a written action plan is provided, describing treatment goal(s), patient strengths, and specific strategies. In a home visit, the nurse provides caregivers with health-related information (pain detection, hydration, advance directives), obtains patient blood/urine samples, and examines patients for signs of dehydration. Laboratory evaluations include complete blood count (CBC), blood chemistry (Chem 7, thyroid testing of serum samples), and culture and sensitivity of urine samples. Patient medications are reviewed for appropriateness, polypharmacy, and dosing using published guidelines. Caregivers are informed of results by telephone and mailed copies to share with the patients' physicians.

Results from the nurse component alone of the intervention revealed that more than a third of dementia patients had an undetected but treatable medical condition that may have been contributing to their poor functioning and behavioral symptoms (Hodgson, Gitlin, Winter, & Czekanski, 2011). COPE is currently being replicated in the state of Connecticut in home-based community and Medicaid Waiver programs (Fortinsky et al., 2016). Similar to the main trial, of the first 36 persons with dementia evaluated by the nurse interventionist, 36% had a medical or medication issue (Fortinsky et al., 2016).

This intervention illustrates the important role of nursing interventions. Applying the conceptual framework, it shows that this particular intervention attends to both older adults with dementia and caregivers. Thus, the nurse interventionist has to adjust his or her clinical style, approach, and interactions to successfully build rapport along a number of factors listed in Figure 11.1, including the caregiver's level of readiness, or receptivity to learn new strategies for caregiving (Gitlin & Rose, 2016). The intervention occurs in the home, so issues related to accessibility, obtaining blood and urine samples in potentially contaminated environments, and constrained spaces have to be considered. The intervention also involves collaboration with another health professional, OTs, requiring skill and competencies in traversing different languages, conceptual frames of references, and treatment goals (Hodgson & Gitlin, in press). As the workplace was in neighborhoods, access, safety, parking, weather conditions, and time of day were all considerations. Finally, reimbursement or financial support for the nurses' time to travel to homes, provide the needed education, and engage in a clinical evaluation of the person with dementia are all affected by current health policies and the organization of health care such as home care. These factors have significant implications for the spread, uptake, and adoption of the COPE intervention (Gitlin & Czaja, 2016). Knowledge of the characteristics of each of these factors and levels can inform the construction of an impactful intervention.

Using this conceptual framework, several guiding principles for nursing intervention research can be derived. First, interventions must be understood as occurring within a context that includes multiple levels—the individual, the caregiver, the setting in which the intervention will be delivered (e.g., home, clinic, workplace, hospital), formal and informal networks and social support systems, the community, and the policy environment. Health and behavior and hence intervention delivery characteristics may be shaped by factors at each of the levels.

Second, interventions are more likely to be successful and sustainable if factors in each level and the interactions among them are considered. Interventions cannot be designed in isolation or in a vacuum and solely focus on individual-level determinants of health and behaviors. Rather, interventions must consider the independent and joint influences of determinants at all of the specified levels. Levels will be proximal and distal to the immediate outcomes sought (e.g., improving knowledge and skills among diverse family caregivers).

Third, the levels and the interactions among them are dynamic, and determinants may change with time. Therefore, for interventions to be sustainable, their characteristics must be adaptable to potential changes and dynamic relationships over time.

Figure 11.1 also implies that new competencies for nurses may be needed. This includes viewing the family unit as the "patient" or "client" versus the older adult alone; the need to integrate quality indicators such as quality of care and quality of life into national performance measurements along with changes in reimbursement mechanisms to accommodate time spent with the family caregiver; the need for nurses to understand their role on an interprofessional team, the complexities of caregiving, and how to communicate information to families in a supportive and nonjudgmental way. Also, implicit is the need for the use of multidimensional assessments in order to match resources to family needs and the care of older adults and from which to identify strengths of a family caregiver and from which to derive culturally appropriate instructional approaches and care strategies. Finally, the inclusion of family caregivers as part of the unit of care has significant implications for training; new training curriculum in nursing programs is needed to instruct in evidence-informed practices for effectively involving families in care decision making, as well as how to manage family conflict and the involvement of more than one family caregiver or when family members have differing perspectives, treatment goals, and involvement (Gitlin & Hodgson, 2016; Kelly, Reinhard, & Brooks-Danso, 2008).

Regardless of condition of the older adult and/or type of assistance needed, nurses have a critical role in intervening to support family caregivers in any context of care. Table 11.1 outlines some of the key areas of knowledge and skills that families need and which nurses can provide.

TABLE 11.1 *Knowledge and Skills That Family Caregivers May Need and That Nurses Are Instrumental in Providing*

- Disease-specific knowledge
- Managing medications
- Hands-on assistance (transfers, dressing, bathing)
- Avoiding physical strain/injury
- Preventing and managing behavioral symptoms (e.g., rejection of care, agitation, aggression)
- Fall recovery techniques
- Wound care
- Administration of infusions, injections, monitoring blood pressure
- Communicating effectively to health professionals
- Problem solving
- Advocating on behalf of older adult
- Conflict management among family members and care providers
- Reconciling competing health provider information and directions
- Care coordination
- Taking care of self (proper nutrition, exercise, sleep hygiene)

CONCLUSION

This chapter provides a snapshot of the landscape of family caregiving and the implications for nursing research, care, and policy. It highlights key points about family caregiving, including societal trends, prevalence, and relevance of family involvement in providing care to older adults, as well as the burgeoning research on care interventions. As family caregiving represents complex physical, emotional, financial, and social processes, which have physiological and health consequences, nursing science is critical to bridge knowledge gaps, particularly as it concerns who becomes a caregiver, consequences of caregiving, and ways to effectively engage and support family caregivers (Grady & Gough, 2015).

There is no doubt that now and into the future, nurses will need to purposively and effectively involve family caregivers in the care of their older adult patients, particularly individuals with chronic conditions, and/or physical and/or cognitive changes or limitations. Treating the family as a "unit" of care reflects a different paradigm from the acute care singular patient model by which health care is currently organized. Adequately addressing this new paradigm will require new research methodologies to capture the complexities of multiple relationships, the intersection of different life trajectories (carer and care receiver and nurse) and impact on care decision making and outcomes; new competencies in nursing practice that address engaging diverse families in patient care; and new policies that support changes in health care organization, care practices, and funding, as well as training of nurses to work on interprofessional teams involving family caregivers as integral members.

REFERENCES

Adelman, R. D., Tmanova, L. L., Delgado, D., Dion, S., & Lachs, M. S. (2014). Caregiver burden: A clinical review. *JAMA, 311*(10), 1052–1060. doi:10.1001/jama.2014.304

Alzheimer's Association. (2016). 2016 Alzheimer's disease facts and figures. Retrieved from http://www.alz.org/documents_custom/2016-facts-and-figures.pdf

Aneshensel, C. S., Pearlin, L. I., Mullan, J. T., Zarit, S. H., & Whitlatch, C. J. (1995). *Profiles in caregiving: The unexpected career*. San Diego, CA: Academic Press.

Aronson, L. (2015). Necessary steps: How health care fails older patients, and how it can be done better. *Health Affairs, 34*(3), 528–532.

Beard, J. R., Officer, A., de Carvalho, I. A., Sadana, R., Pot, A. M., Michel, J.-P., . . . Chatterji, S. (2015). The world report on ageing and health: A policy framework for healthy ageing. *Lancet (London, England), 387*(10033), 2145–2154. doi:10.1016/S0140-6736(15)00516-4

Bookman, A., & Kimbrel, D. (2011). Families and elder care in the twenty-first century. *Future of Children, 21*(2), 117–140.

Brodaty, H., & Arasaratnam, C. (2012). Meta-analysis of nonpharmacological interventions for neuropsychiatric symptoms of dementia. *American Journal of Psychiatry, 169*(9), 946–953. doi.org/10.1176/appi.focus.11.1.79

Brody, E. M. (2003). *Women in the middle: Their parent-care years (Springer Series on Life Styles and Issues in Aging,* 2nd ed.). New York, NY: Springer Publishing.

Brown, R. M., & Brown, S. L. (2014). Informal caregiving: A reappraisal of effects on caregivers. *Social Issues and Policy Review, 8*(1), 74–102.

Burton, L. C., Zdaniuk, B., Schulz, R., Jackson, S., & Hirsch, C. (2003). Transitions in spousal caregiving. *The Gerontologist, 43*(2), 230–241.

Callahan, C. M., Kales, H. C., Gitlin, L. N., & Lyketsos, C. G. (2013). The historical development and state of the art approach to design and delivery of dementia care services. In *Designing and delivering dementia services* (pp. 17–30). West Sussex, UK: John Wiley & Sons. doi:10.1002/9781118378663.ch2

Coleman, B., & Pandya, S. M. (2002). *Family caregiving and long-term care* [Fact sheet]. Retreived from http://assets.aarp.org/rgcenter/il/fs91_ltc.pdf

Coleman, E. A., Boult, C., & American Geriatrics Society Health Care Systems Committee. (2003). Improving the quality of transitional care for persons with complex care needs. *Journal of the American Geriatrics Society, 51*(4), 556–557.

Coleman, E. A., Parry, C., Chalmers, S., & Min, S. J. (2006). The care transitions intervention: Results of a randomized controlled trial. *Archives of Internal Medicine, 166*(17), 1822–1828. doi:10.1001/archinte.166.17.1822

Delavande, A., Hurd, M. D., Martorell, P., & Langa, K. M. (2013). Dementia and out-of-pocket spending on health care services. *Alzheimer's and Dementia, 9*(1), 19–29. doi:10.1016/j.jalz .2011.11.003

Family Caregiver Alliance. (2006). *Caregiver assessment: Principles, guidelines and strategies for change* (Report from a National Consensus Development Conference, vol. 1). San Francisco, CA: Author.

Fortinsky, R. H., Gitlin, L. N., Pizzi, L. T., Piersol, C. V., Grady, J., Robison, J. T., & Molony, S. (2016). Translation of the care of persons with dementia in their environments (COPE). Intervention in a publicly-funded home care context: Rationale and research design. *Contemporary Clinical Trials, 49*, 155–165. doi:10.1016/j.cct.2016.07.006

Gaugler, J., & Kane, R. (2015). *Family caregiving in the new normal*. Boston, MA: Elsevier.

Giovannetti, E. R., & Wolff, J. L. (2010). Cross-survey differences in national estimates of numbers of caregivers of disabled older adults. *Milbank Quarterly, 88*(3), 310–349.

Gitlin, L. N., & Czaja, S. J. (2016). *Behavioral intervention research: Designing, evaluating and implementing*. New York, NY: Springer Publishing.

Gitlin, L. N., & Hodgson, N. A. (2015). Caregivers as therapeutic agents in dementia care: The evidence-base for interventions supporting their role. In J. Gaugler & R. Kane (Eds.), *Family caregiving in the new normal* (pp. 305–353). Boston, MA: Elsevier.

Gitlin, L. N., & Hodgson, N. A. (2016). Who should assess the needs of and care for a dementia patient's caregiver? *AMA Journal of Ethics, 18*(12), 1171–1181.

Gitlin, L. N., & Rose, K. (2016). Impact of caregiver readiness on outcomes of an intervention to address behavioral symptoms in persons with dementia. *International Journal of Geriatric Psychology, 31*(9), 1056–1063. doi:10.1002/gps.4422

Gitlin, L. N., & Schulz, R. (2012). Family caregiving of older adults. In T. R. Prohaska, L. A. Anderson, & R. H. Binstock (Eds.), *Public health for an aging society* (pp. 181–204). Baltimore, MD: Johns Hopkins University Press.

Gitlin, L. N., Winter, L., Dennis, M. P., Hodgson, N. A., & Hauck, W. W. (2010). A biobehavioral home-based intervention and the well-being of patients with dementia and their caregivers: The COPE randomized trial. *JAMA, 304*(9), 983–991. doi:10.1001/jama.2010.1253

Gitlin, L. N., & Wolff, J. (2011). Family involvement in care transitions of older adults: What do we know and where do we go from here? In P. Dilworth-Anderson (Ed.), *Annual review of gerontology and geriatrics: Pathways through the transitions of care for older adults* (pp. 31–64). New York, NY: Springer Publishing.

Grady, P. A., & Gough, L. L. (2015). Nursing science: Claiming the future. *Journal of Nursing Scholarship, 47*(6), 512–521.

He, W., Goodkind, D., & Kowal, P. (2015). *An aging world* (U.S. Census Bureau, International Population Reports, P95/16-1). Washington, DC: U.S. Government Publishing Office.

Hodgson, N. A., & Gitlin, L. N. (in press). The role of the interprofessional team in the management of speech and language disorders among persons with dementia. In M. Kulshreshtha & A. Neustein (Eds.), *Evaluating the role of speech technology in medical case management*. Boston, MA: Walter De Gruyter.

Hodgson, N. A., Gitlin, L. N., Winter, L., & Czekanski, K. (2011). Undiagnosed illness and neuropsychiatric behaviors in community-residing older adults with dementia. *Alzheimer's Disease and Associated Disorders, 25*(2), 109–115. doi:10.1097/WAD.0b013e3181f8520a

Institute of Medicine, Committee on the Future Health Care Workforce for Older Americans & Board on Health Care Services. (2008). *Retooling for an aging America: Building the health care workforce*. Washington, DC: National Academies Press. doi:10.1097/00006205-200612000-00002

Jutkowitz, E., Kuntz, K. M., Dowd, B., Gaugler, J. E., MacLehose, R. F., & Kane, R. L. (in press). Effects of cognition, function, and behavior on out-of-pocket medical and nursing home expenditures and time spent caregiving for dementia. *Alzheimer's and Dementia*.

Kales, H. C., Gitlin, L. N., Stanislawski, B., Marx, K., Turnwald, M., Watkins, D., & Lyketsos, C. G. (2016). WeCareAdvisor™: The development of a caregiver-focused, web-based program to assess and manage behavioral and psychological symptoms of dementia. *Alzheimer Dementia and Associated Disorders*. Advance online publication. doi:10.1097/WAD.0000000000000177

Kelly, K., Reinhard, S. C., & Brooks-Danso, A. (2008). Professional partners supporting family caregivers. *American Journal of Nursing, 108*(Suppl. 9), 6–12. doi:10.1097/01.NAJ.0000336400.76635.db

Leff, B., & Burton, J. R. (1996). Acute medical care in the home. *Journal of the American Geriatrics Society, 44*(5), 603–605. doi:10.1111/j.1532-5415.1996.tb01452.x

Leff, B., Burton, L., Guido, S., Greenough, W. B., Steinwachs, D., & Burton, J. R. (1999). Home hospital program: A pilot study. *Journal of the American Geriatrics Society, 47*(6), 697–702. doi:10.1111/j.1532-5415.1999.tb01592.x

Marx, K. A., Stanley, I. H., Van Haitsma, K., Moody, J., Alonzi, D., Hansen, B. R., & Gitlin, L. N. (2014). Knowing versus doing: Education and training needs of staff in a chronic care hospital unit for individuals with dementia. *Journal of Gerontological Nursing, 40*(12), 26–34. doi:10.3928/00989134-20140905-01

National Academy of Medicine. (2016). *Families Caring for an Aging America*. Washington, DC: National Academies Press.

National Alliance for Caregiving & AARP. (2009). *Caregiving in the U.S.* Retrieved from http://www.aarp.org/content/dam/aarp/ppi/2015/caregiving-in-the-united-states-2015-report-revised.pdf

National Institute of Aging & Duke University. (2004). *National long-term care survey*. Retrieved from http://www.nltcs.aas.duke.edu

Northouse, L. L., Katapodi, M. C., Song, L., Zhang, L., & Mood, D. W. (2010). Interventions with family caregivers of cancer patients: Meta-analysis of randomized trials. *CA: A Cancer Journal for Clinicians, 60*(5), 317–39. doi:10.3322/caac.20081

Okura, T., & Langa, K. M. (2011). Caregiver burden and neuropsychiatric symptoms in older adults with cognitive impairment: The aging, demographics, and memory study (ADAMS). *Alzheimer Disease and Associated Disorders, 25*(2), 116–21. doi:10.1097/WAD.0b013e318203f208

Ortman, J. M., Velkoff, V. A., & Hogan, H. (2014). *An aging nation: The older population in the United States*. Washington, DC: U.S. Census Bureau.

Ory, M. G., & Hoffman, R. R, III. (1999). Prevalence and impact of caregiving: A detailed comparison between dementia and nondementia. *Gerontologist, 39*(2), 177.

Pruchno, R. A., Brill, J. E., Shands, Y., Gordon, J. R., Genderson, M. W., Rose, M., & Cartwright, F. (2008). Convenience samples and caregiving research: How generalizable are the findings? *The Gerontologist, 48*(6), 820–827.

Pruchno, R. A., & Gitlin, L. N. (2012). Family caregiving in late life: Shifting paradigms. In R. Blieszner & V. H. Bedford (Eds.), *Handbook of families and aging* (pp. 515–541). Santa Barbara, CA: Praeger.

Reinhard, S. C., Feinberg, L. F., Choula, R., & Houser, A. (2015). *Valuing the invaluable: 2015 update*. Washington, DC: AARP Public Policy Institute.

Reinhard, S. C., Levine, C., & Samis, S. (2012). *Home alone: Family caregivers providing complex chronic care*. New York, NY: AARP Policy Institute.

Roth, D. L., Dilworth-Anderson, P., Huang, J., Gross, A. L., & Gitlin, L. N. (2016). Measuring positive aspects of caregiving for persons with dementia: Differential item functioning by race and other characteristics. *Journal of Gerontology: Psychological Sciences, 70*(6), 813–819. doi:10.1093/geronb/gbv034

Schulz, R., O'Brien, A. T., Bookwala, J., & Fleissner, K. (1995). Psychiatric and physical morbidity effects of dementia caregiving: Prevalence, correlates, and causes. *Gerontologist, 35*(6), 771–791.

Schulz, R., & Tompkins, C. A. (2010). *Informal caregivers in the United States: Prevalence, characteristics, and ability to provide care. Human factors in home health care*. Washington, DC: National Academies of Sciences Press.

Solli, H., Hvalvik, S., Bjørk, I. T., & Hellesø, R. (2015). Characteristics of the relationship that develops from nurse-caregiver communication during telecare. *Journal of Clinical Nursing, 24*(13–14), 1995–2004. doi:10.1111/jocn.12786

Spillman, B. C., Wolff, J., Freedman, V. A., & Kasper, J. D. (2014). *Informal caregiving for older Americans: An analysis of the 2011 National Study of Caregiving*. Report prepared for the Office of Disability, Aging and Long-Term Care Policy Office of the Assistant Secretary for Planning and Evaluation, U.S. Department of Health and Human Services.

Stensletten, K., Bruvik, F., Espehaug, B., & Drageset, J. (2014). Burden of care, social support, and sense of coherence in elderly caregivers living with individuals with symptoms of dementia. *Dementia, 15*(6), 1422–1435. doi:10.1177/1471301214563319

Stone, R. I. (2015). Factors affecting the future of family caregiving in the United States. In J. E. Gaugler & R. L. Kane (Eds.), *Family caregiving in the new normal* (pp. 57–77). London, UK: Elsevier.

Vickrey, B. G., Mittman, B. S., Connor, K. I., Pearson, M. L., Della Penna, R. D., Ganiats, T. G., . . . Lee, M. (2006). The effect of a disease management intervention on quality and outcomes of dementia care: A randomized, controlled trial. *Annals of Internal Medicine, 145*(10), 713–726.

Winter, L., & Parks, S. M. (2008). Family discord and proxy decision makers' end-of-life treatment decisions. *Journal of Palliative Medicine, 11*(8), 1109–1114. doi:10.1089/jpm.2008.0039

Wolff, J. L. (2012). Family matters in health care delivery. *JAMA, 308*(15), 1529–1530. doi:10.1001/jama.2012.13366

Wolff, J. L., Boyd, C. M., Gitlin, L. N., Bruce, M. L., & Roter, D. L. (2012). Going it together: Persistence of older adults' accompaniment to physician visits by a family companion. *Journal of the American Geriatrics Society, 60*(1), 106–112. doi:10.1111/j.1532-5415.2011.03770.x

Wolff, J. L., Clayman, M., Rabins, P., Cooke, M., & Roter, D. (2015). An exploration of patient and family engagement in routine primary care visits. *Health Expect, 18*(2), 188–198.

Wolff, J. L., & Roter, D. L. (2008). Hidden in plain sight: Medical visit companions as a resource for vulnerable older adults. *Archives of Internal Medicine, 168*(13), 1409–1415.

Wolff, J. L., Roter, D. L., Barron, J., Boyd, C. M., Leff, B., Finucane, T., . . . Gitlin, L. N. (2014). A tool to strengthen the older patient-companion partnership in primary care: Results from a pilot study forthcoming. *Journal of the American Geriatrics Society, 62*(2), 312–319. doi:10.1111/jgs.12639

Wolff, J. L., & Spillman, B. C. (2014). Older adults receiving assistance with physician visits and prescribed medications and their family caregivers: Prevalence, characteristics, and hours of care. *Journals of Gerontology: Series B, Psychological Sciences and Social Sciences, 69*, S65–S72. doi:10.1093/geronb/gbu119

Wolff, J. L., Spillman, B. C., Freedman, V. A., & Kasper, J. D. (2016). A national profile of family and unpaid caregivers who assist older adults with health care activities. *JAMA Internal Medicine, 176*(3), 372–379. doi:10.1001/jamainternmed.2015.7664

12

Aging in Place: Adapting the Environment

Marilyn J. Rantz, Kari R. Lane, Lori L. Popejoy, Colleen Galambos, Lorraine J. Phillips, Lanis Hicks, Greg Alexander, Laurel Despins, Richelle Koopman, Marjorie Skubic, Mihail Popescu, and James Keller

It was clear to any young nurse, in the 1970s and 1980s, that the looming problem facing our society was the coming "explosion" of the aging population. Predictions in every data source about the U.S. population repeated the impending "crisis" in which increased numbers of older people would simply overload and "implode" the long-term care system. At the same time, health care advances were amazing; many people who previously would have been identified as having "terminal" diagnoses suddenly had a better prognosis both for survival and for a good quality of life for more years than had ever been experienced before.

The predictions were not lost on the federal Health Care Financing Administration (HCFA), now the Centers for Medicare and Medicaid Services (CMS). Concerned about the predictions, they launched several HCFA-sponsored large demonstration pilot projects to test potential approaches for modifying long-term care services in an effort to find potential solutions (Hughes, 1985; Kemper, 1990). These demonstrations preceded state and federal public policy decisions to encourage the development of home- and community-based services and the HCFA-sponsored demonstrations of community nursing organizations of the 1990s (Abt Associates Inc., 2000; Collins, Butler, Gueldner, & Palmer, 1997; Elkan et al., 2001).

Nurses were at the forefront, not only providing direct services to older adults in the community and long-term care settings, but also working to influence the development of new models of care, and encouraging older adults to maintain independence and function, and receive health promotion services where they lived. For instance, the Minnesota Block Nurse Program was started more than 30 years ago. The program combined public health and home care ideas and used the skills of nurses to keep people independent and manage chronic illness; that program is still active today (Living at Home Network of Block Nurse Programs, 2016; Martinson, Jamieson, O'Grady, & Sime, 1985; Metropolitan Council of the Twin Cities Area,

1990). Nurse-run clinics, which are often affiliated with schools of nursing and funded by small grants and demonstrations, have been operating in public housing, nursing homes, rehabilitation centers, and community sites since the early 1980s (Matherlee, 1999).

Local efforts in the 1980s attempted to work through county agencies in some states, not only to build affordable elder housing, but also to offer nursing services within the housing. Stated goals of these efforts were to help people stay healthier, and (it was hoped) avoid nursing home care. In the mid-1990s, the potential solutions to the projected explosion of aging people seemed to be directed at modifying traditional approaches to long-term care, with none of the real revolutionary change that the problem was demanding. Environments were clearly ripe for change—both actual living environments for people to age well and the public policies and political environment that influenced neighborhoods and communities. In this chapter, we present one such example of a program of research and university faculty effort to revolutionize traditional models of long-term care for older adults and influence public policy to disseminate a new model of care delivery promoting independence and function through the end of life.

THE AGING IN PLACE PROJECT AT THE SINCLAIR SCHOOL OF NURSING

In 1996, at the American Academy of Nursing (AAN) meeting, participants were challenged to create a new vision for care and services for the looming surge of elders in the United States. Several faculty and administrators from the school were attending and gathered informally just after the session. We began brainstorming about what we could do at our school of nursing to launch a visionary new approach for serving elders. We realized we had a group of faculty with strengths and expertise in gerontological nursing to provide the critical mass and skills that could launch such a new vision to better meet the needs of elders in the future. The question was, what would that new vision be?

We came home from the academy meeting with some preliminary ideas and convened a large group of interdisciplinary faculty from across the campus. With sage advice and creative ideas, we decided to "blow up" the traditional long-term care system, talk to elders and their families about what they wanted, and start anew (Marek & Rantz, 2000; Rantz et al., 2008). We conducted a series of focus groups, and the message from older people was consistent throughout the process. Seniors wanted to remain independent as long as possible and in the home of their choice, if at all possible, through the end of life. Families, on the other hand, wanted their mom (or dad or other relative) to be safe, above all else. Interesting verbal exchanges among participants ensued during the group discussions, and the seemingly conflicting values emerged during the sessions. Our interdisciplinary team was challenged and continued to meet to create a new vision—Aging in Place (AIP). This AIP vision continues now, 20 years later. Highlights include:

- A dramatic change to the way long-term care is provided in this country through a new approach to care and service delivery
- The foundation of care is RN care coordination/community case management supported by an interdisciplinary team of social workers, activity personnel, rehabilitation specialists, physicians, and aides managed by the RN care coordinator
- Providing seniors with the right services at the right time and early illness detection and intervention to maximize regaining or maintaining health and independence
- Provide research and education opportunities for students and faculty to support and train the next generation of health care workers

To achieve this AIP vision, two complementary parts were designed: an innovative home care agency (Sinclair Home Care) and an innovative independent living environment, TigerPlace, named after the University of Missouri (MU) mascot, the tiger. For the AIP Project to be fully realized in Missouri, legislation was required; the necessary legislation was successfully passed in 1999 and 2001 (Rantz et al., 2008). These two pieces of legislation made the AIP Project an official Missouri demonstration (*without* any state funds); this was our first public policy change. The next large policy change was to work with state regulators to be able to construct and operate TigerPlace under the new visionary approach, which did not match current regulatory requirements; this second change took 3 years. TigerPlace was envisioned to be an ideal AIP independent living environment where people could live through the end of life, with care and services from Sinclair Home Care brought to them in their private homes as needed. It opened and rapidly filled to capacity in 2004.

SINCLAIR HOME CARE

In 1999, prior to the development of TigerPlace and after 3 years of business planning on the AIP vision, the project team successfully applied for a CMS grant to test the concept of AIP for home- and community-based services delivered through a home health and home care agency. A new agency, Sinclair Home Care (initially named Senior Care), was started as a department within the Sinclair School of Nursing. The new agency specialized in services for older adults, was certified for both Medicare and Medicaid clients, and also served those people funded by private insurers and private pay.

With grant funding (1999–2003), we were able to develop a critical research foundation for the AIP work. Our goals were to test the effectiveness and cost-effectiveness of RN care coordination. The project to facilitate AIP in community living sites was funded by the grant, as these nursing services were not reimbursable at the time. Some decisions that were critical to success were:

- Use an electronic health record (EHR) for medical records and charting of services.
- Use a carefully selected set of standardized measures of health with known validity and reliability to use in the care of clients, and also use for assessment

of outcomes and quality of care. These standardized measures enabled comparisons with other groups and state and national databases.

- Collect cost, staffing, and quality outcomes data to monitor the agency operations, as well as the AIP evaluation.

For 10 years, Sinclair Home Care provided Medicare and Medicaid home health services to the older residents in six counties in the mid-Missouri region using RN nursing care coordination, which enabled an excellent evaluation of that AIP service approach for older adults (Marek et al., 2005, 2010; Marek, Popejoy, Petroski, & Rantz, 2006; Marek, Stetzer, Adams, Popejoy, & Rantz, 2012). The team wanted to be able to potentially influence legislators and other public policy makers about the value of RN care coordination to not only older adults and their families, but also to pose possible solutions to the growing demand for traditional long-term care services and the rapid escalation of older adult health care costs. Importantly, we carefully examined outcomes of care and costs using Medicare and Medicaid files, recognizing that both were essential to influencing public policy.

For outcomes, the CMS evaluation (1999–2003) demonstrated that clients who received care from Sinclair Home Care with RN care coordination had improved clinical outcomes (cognition, depression, activities of daily living [ADLs], and incontinence) compared with individuals of similar case mix in nursing homes (Marek et al., 2005). Outcomes (pain, shortness of breath, and ADLs) were also significantly better for clients with RN care coordination than without RN care coordination in a community-based waiver program called Missouri Care Options (MCO; Marek et al., 2006). A later study comparing AIP to traditional home care found that even though AIP clients were significantly older, more likely to be on Medicaid, be cognitively impaired, and be depressed, they had significantly lower rates of decline in ADLs and instrumental activities of daily living (IADLs; Popejoy et al., 2015). Additionally, they experienced significantly fewer rehospitalizations and emergency department visits, but all-cause hospitalization rates were not different (Popejoy et al., 2015).

For costs to Medicare, monthly costs were significantly lower ($686) for MCO clients with RN care coordination compared to those without care coordination (Marek et al., 2010). Finally, total costs to Medicare and Medicaid were $1,592 lower per month in the AIP group than a nursing home comparison group over a 12-month period (Marek et al., 2012). The measurement of significant cost savings and better clinical outcomes has been essential to our efforts, the efforts of other nurses, and the efforts of organizations to change public policy for funding of RN care coordination services. Importantly, Medicare regulations were changed so that limited funding is now available for some of these services (AMA, 2013). This is evidence that yes, indeed, research and practice demonstrations with continuous evaluation and publication of measurable results *can* influence and change public policy.

TIGERPLACE, IDEAL HOUSING FOR AIP, STATE DEMONSTRATION

As explained previously, legislation was required and successfully passed in 1999 and 2001 with the assistance of a group of interdisciplinary stakeholders, including a state legislator, that grew from our original interdisciplinary group initiated in 1996 (Rantz et al., 2008; Rantz, Popejoy, Musterman, & Miller, 2014). The legislation enabled the construction of TigerPlace as the state's first AIP site and officially recognized the Sinclair School of Nursing AIP Project as a Missouri demonstration. The legislation did *not* fund the evaluation or construction, as no funds were associated with its passage, but regulators were directed to work with the AIP site and develop an approach that would enable the construction, operation, and regulation of the demonstration.

Recognizing that additional capital would be needed to fund the project, the school, through a publicly announced Request for Proposals process, sought a partner for the initiative. Americare Systems, Inc., of Sikeston, Missouri, a well-respected long-term care owner/operator of numerous assisted living and nursing homes in several states in the Midwest, stepped forward. The plan was for the school to provide the RN care coordination, as well as health promotion and care services through Sinclair Home Care; Americare would build, own, and operate the building and services related to housing, dining, and hospitality. Key staff of Americare and faculty of the school worked on detailed plans for day-to-day operations, planned with regulators, created architectural plans, and developed detailed operational agreements between the entities. We created a private–public partnership dedicated to the success of TigerPlace as a business, incorporating the AIP research/state demonstration evaluation, and including educational experiences for students of all disciplines at the university.

The foundation for the care delivery system at TigerPlace is RN care coordination, and there is a commitment from all staff to maximize independence and function through the end of life. Just as in the community-based evaluation of AIP, funded by CMS (explained earlier), we made the same three decisions that were critical to success:

1. The continued use of an EHR for all health records
2. Collection of routine health assessment information on admission and every 6 months using standardized health measures (these assessments are used in everyday clinical decision making as well as for continued research about the effectiveness of AIP, and can be used in other related studies)
3. Continuously collecting cost, quality, and staffing data for longitudinal evaluation of AIP for publication of results in order to potentially influence public policy

We also made an important fourth decision:

4. To create a research infrastructure for ongoing development and testing of technology to help older people age well, remaining as independent as possible as long as possible.

Infrastructure for Interdisciplinary Research

All older persons who move into TigerPlace understand and agree that they are participating in a state evaluation of AIP and that their de-identified health information will be used in research. Faculty from the College of Engineering were solicited to join the planning team to design the building's electronic networking infrastructure that would support technology research. The joint team helped plan for appropriate network cabling, a server room, and easy access to each apartment via an attic with walkway and lighting for future retrofitting as needed.

TigerPlace opened in 2004 with 31 well-designed apartments, each with screened porches and easy access via sunlit interior corridors and exterior exits via the screened porch. It was expanded in 2008 to a total of 54 apartments due to demand. Then, in 2011 as planned, Americare built an 85-bed Medicare skilled nursing facility, the Neighborhoods of TigerPlace, with five distinct "neighborhoods" in the facility, on property adjacent to TigerPlace. The rehabilitation focus of this facility has served the general community demand for these services; also, some residents of TigerPlace have used the services episodically for rehabilitation following joint replacement or other health events and then they return to their home at TigerPlace.

All residents who move into TigerPlace agree upon admission (via written informed consent) to actively participate in ongoing wellness activities and complete biannual health assessments. These assessments are used as clinical information by the health care staff and are also considered outcome measures to evaluate the effectiveness of the AIP Project. Assessment measures include: Minimum Data Set, Geriatric Depression Scale (GDS), Mini-Mental State Examination (MMSE), SF12® Health Survey, ADLs, and IADLs, and fall risk assessments. Other functional and health data collected include gait speed, Timed Up and Go (TUG), length of stay, hospitalizations, chronic illnesses, and medications. As in the earlier AIP CMS evaluation, we found that, in addition to these regular assessments, the RN care coordinators were able to make some early illness connections related to subtle changes in a resident's condition (Marek et al., 2005, 2006; Rantz et al., 2005). It was our vision that in addition to testing a new model of care in the AIP Project, there could also be new technological discoveries for early illness detection that could enhance care coordination with ongoing assessments and observation.

Technology Research to Enhance AIP

In 2005, the Center for Eldercare and Rehabilitation Technology (CERT) in the College of Engineering at the MU installed the first version of an environmentally embedded sensor system to potentially measure functional status (Rantz et al., 2005, 2008). Early focus groups of older people revealed that they did not want to *do* anything with the technology, that they did not want to wear anything, and they wanted it to work seamlessly (Courtney, Demiris, Rantz, & Skubic, 2008; Demiris, Hensel, Skubic, & Rantz, 2008; Demiris, Parker-Oliver, Dickey, Skubic, & Rantz, 2008). Years of ongoing research and development have resulted in a sensor system that continuously (24×7) collects data; automated algorithms analyze the data and send care coordinators health alerts *days and even weeks before health status changes are apparent to residents or care coordinators* (Rantz et al., 2012, 2013; Rantz, Skubic et al., 2015; Skubic, Guevara, & Rantz, 2015).

Residents kept asking for reliable fall detection from a sensor that they did *not have to wear*, and the research team developed new methods for privacy-protecting depth image processing for not only fall detection (Figure 12.1), but also automated fall risk assessment (Stone & Skubic, 2013, 2014; Stone, Skubic, Rantz, Abbott, & Miller, 2015). Recent analyses revealed that using automated analysis of in-home gait speed can *predict falls 3–4 weeks before they occur*. In these analyses, the odds of a resident falling within 3 weeks after a cumulative in-home gait speed change of 2.54 cm/sec is 4.22 times the odds of a resident falling within 3 weeks after no change (Phillips et al., 2017). The sensor system can send fall risk alerts, just as it does health alerts, weeks before events, providing adequate time for older people, their family members, and care coordinators to pursue ways to intervene with fall prevention strategies to prevent a fall from occurring (Stone, Skubic, & Back, 2014).

Research results from the Eldertech team have added to the success of the AIP model at TigerPlace. Since 2005, sensor systems have included various sensors: passive infrared motion sensors; a bed sensor that captures pulse, respiration, and restlessness; and gait analysis/fall detection systems using vision, radar, acoustic arrays, and the Microsoft Kinect depth camera (Skubic et al., 2013; Skubic, Alexander, Popescu, Rantz, & Keller, 2009). Sensor systems are installed in the apartments of those residents who elect to participate in the technology research. The current version includes: (a) bed sensor (monitors heart rate, restlessness, and respirations; Rosales, Su, Skubic, & Ho, in press); (b) motion sensors to monitor activity in rooms (Wang, Skubic, & Zhu, 2012); and (c) Kinect depth images to monitor walking, gait parameters, report falls in real time, and automatically assess fall risk (Stone et al., 2015; Stone & Skubic, 2013). The sensors send health, increasing fall risk, and fall alerts in real time to direct care staff (Rantz, Skubic, et al., 2015). Figure 12.2 is an

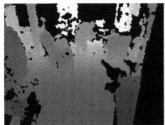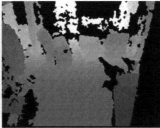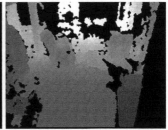

FIGURE 12.1 Images of a fall. A sequence of depth images showing a fall that was captured in a TigerPlace apartment. The depth image captures a distance measure for each pixel. The fall detection and gait analysis systems extract a 3D silhouette of a person moving about in the scene. These are colored in the depth images shown. Blue shows the detected ground plane. The grayscale readings show depth; darker gray is closer and lighter gray is farther away. The black regions are noise, often from glass or metal surfaces (see the color version of this image on the inside back cover).

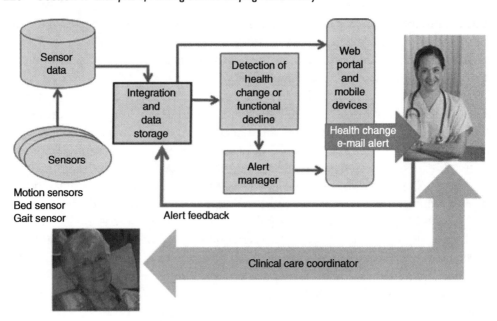

FIGURE 12.2 In-home health sensor system.

illustration of the health sensor system developed by the Eldertech team and used by the care coordinators at TigerPlace.

Since 2010, health alerts have been automatically triggered by computer algorithms designed to detect changes in trends in each resident's sensor data that may indicate a change in health status. The technology with health, fall risk, and fall alerts enhances care coordination effectiveness (Rantz, Skubic, et al., 2010, 2012). Recently, we compared length of stay in TigerPlace between residents ($n = 52$) with environmentally embedded alert-generating sensor systems and residents ($n = 81$) without such sensor systems, all of whom received care coordination services (Rantz, Lane, et al., 2015). Care coordinators receive health alerts for the group living with the sensor system, assess and intervene to determine if the health alert was clinically significant. Strikingly, the group living with sensors had an average length of stay of 4.3 years, whereas length of stay for the comparison group without sensors was 2.6 years. It appears that the embedded sensor technology increases length of stay even further at TigerPlace by another 1.7 years. That being said, the RN care coordination model at TigerPlace appears to have increased the average length of stay by about a year, even for those living without sensors, compared to the national median residential senior housing length of stay of 22 months (i.e., 1.8 years; Caffrey et al., 2012). Cost to residents was analyzed and compared to skilled nursing home costs, which demonstrated a projected cost savings of $29,920 per person (Rantz, Lane, et al., 2015).

Advancements in early illness recognition using environmentally embedded sensors are pushing the envelope to help not only older people living at TigerPlace, but also those individuals living in senior housing and long-term care settings, and at home. Fourteen research projects have been funded by the National Science

Foundation, National Institutes of Health, the Agency for Healthcare Research and Quality, the U.S. Administration on Aging, the RAND/Hartford Foundation, and the Alzheimer's Association, for a total over $10 million. The research infrastructure at TigerPlace, with two groups of residents, with and without the sensor system, living there through the end of life has facilitated research projects and enabled evaluation of the effectiveness of the technology in a real-world setting. Efforts are now under way to commercialize the sensor-based health alert system. This will allow deployment in other types of senior housing and target user groups for scaled-up studies, as well as making the technology available to a wide range of older adults who can benefit.

Policy makers are interested in the results of our technology research. Our research team is committed to dissemination of results and also has assistance from the MU News Bureau to prepare national press releases with new findings in major publications. Keeping the public informed about the work is important, so news articles and film coverage are actively planned. We maintain two websites about the work to share with other researchers, health care providers, students, and the public (www.eldertech.missouri.edu and www.agingmo.com).

In July 2015, Dr. Skubic, the engineering lead for the Eldertech Research team, testified to the federal Senate Committee on Aging about the advancements that could enable elders to remain at home as independent as possible and as long as possible. She was challenged to analyze the cost implications of using the technology to reduce the burden on long-term care services. This analysis led to the cost savings mentioned previously ($29,920 per person). In addition, an analysis was done using a reimbursement model, comparing the average annual cost of long-term care paid by Medicaid (in Missouri) to the cost of reimbursing expenses for the in-home sensor-based health alert system and the nursing care coordination. The cost savings was estimated at $87,000 per person. This finding was of interest to policy makers, and we are hopeful that they will seriously consider technology in the home as an alternative to facility care for elders in the future. Our team will continue working toward additional cost-effective technological advancements in the home, publicizing these results, informing policy makers, and influencing their decisions.

Results of the Missouri Demonstration of AIP at TigerPlace

The AIP results from the state demonstration have been consistent (Rantz, Phillips, et al., 2011; Rantz, Popejoy, Galambos, et al., 2014) and consistent with the Sinclair Home Care CMS evaluation (1999–2003) explained earlier (Marek et al., 2005, 2006, 2010, 2012). Using the health data routinely collected for all residents who have lived at TigerPlace, two 4-year evaluations have been conducted. The first 4 years (2005–2008) at TigerPlace (*n* = 66) revealed that the program was effective in restoring health and maintaining independence while being cost-effective (Rantz, Phillips, et al., 2011).

Similar results were found for the subsequent 4 years (2009–2012) of the program (*n* = 128) (Rantz, Popejoy, Galambos, et al., 2014). Positive health outcomes (fall risk, gait velocity, functional ambulation profile [FAP], handgrips, SF-12 PH, SF-12 MH, GDS), slightly negative ADLs, IADLs, and MMSE, and positive cost-effectiveness results were found. Combined care and housing costs for any resident who was receiving additional care services and qualified for nursing home care ($n = 44$) were about *$20,000 less per year per person than nursing home care*. As discussed previously in the section "Technology Research to Enhance AIP," in a follow-up analysis of length of stay, residents living at TigerPlace without sensors had a length of stay of 2.6 years (Rantz, Lane, et al., 2015). This is nearly a year more than that of the national median of people living in residential senior housing (1.8 years), and may be attributable to the RN care coordination model at TigerPlace. These evaluation results are of interest to public policy makers in our state and other states, as they search for options for their state to address the growing demand for elder housing, assisted living, and other long-term care options.

Notice in the evaluations that outcome data as well as cost data are key elements. They must be planned and measured repeatedly to be able to attract and influence policy decisions. Using these data to publish findings is important; also, disseminating results so that the public knows the potential impact that could benefit them is essential. In 2008, the AAN recognized the AIP Project at the Sinclair School of Nursing as an Edge Runner. As explained on the AAN website,

> *Raise the Voice*: Edge Runners are the practical innovators who have led the way in bringing new thinking and new methods to a wide range of health care challenges. Edge Runners have developed care models and interventions that demonstrate significant, sustained clinical and financial outcomes.

The AAN promotes the Edge Runner programs as potential "answers to the many problems that plague our health system." Our team has maintained our Edge Runner status through the continued evaluation and publication of those results that demonstrate program effectiveness and cost-effectiveness.

There is interest in duplicating TigerPlace and the care coordination delivery model in other states. Our team has developed collaborative relationships with other universities, particularly the University of Arkansas. The technology is generating national and international interest. Visitors from around the world are common at TigerPlace, interacting with residents, families, staff, students, and faculty to learn about the project.

Importance of Interdisciplinary Team for Planning, Operations, and Research

The importance of an interdisciplinary team to get the work done and to engage in thoughtful planning cannot be overemphasized. The use of such an interdisciplinary team ensures that the program is exposed to a diversity of ideas and that a variety of perspectives are represented. With diversity of ideas, better decisions are made for the program and the people it serves. From its inception, interdisciplinary team work has been a foundation for the work in the AIP Project and at Tiger-Place—from the conceptualization of our unique model to the development of our approach to the implementation of our health care and research initiatives. In terms of AIP operations, the nursing component is supported by qualified social workers who address psychosocial issues, work with families, garner community resources, and liaise with agencies and the larger community. Throughout the history of our project, social work services have been provided on both a part-time and a full-time basis. In the original community-based operations of Sinclair Home Care, a full-time social worker was essential to serve the then Medicare- and Medicaid-certified agency. When the agency downsized to accommodate just TigerPlace (as explained earlier), the operations could not fund a full-time position.

However, over the years as TigerPlace expanded, we discovered that a full-time social worker was most beneficial and essential to support the work and activities of the nursing and all staff of TigerPlace. The social worker's focus is on meeting the psychosocial needs of the client and family members, which allows the nursing staff to focus on the physical aspects of care, care planning, and care coordination. With the support of social work staff, all needs of the patient are more fully met (Galambos, Starr, Musterman, & Rantz, 2015).

Sinclair Home Care has also benefited from the presence of social work intern students, which helps to provide new perspectives and approaches to health care operations. These students infuse extra energy, knowledge, and expertise to existing AIP services. Student supervision is carried out by the full-time social worker, which is an important responsibility of this position (Galambos et al., 2015). TigerPlace serves as a learning laboratory for not just social work students, but students from many disciplines, such as nursing, engineering, health information and management, medicine, rehabilitation, and veterinary medicine. Students learn the importance of interdisciplinary problem solving through these experiences.

The interdisciplinary focus of the research team has been essential to that success as well. Conducting complex aging studies requires such a team. With the commitment from faculty in engineering, nursing, social work, health management and informatics, physical therapy, medicine, and other schools and colleges at MU, our productivity as a research team is still growing today. Nearly every Friday afternoon for almost 15 years, members of the team come together to guide studies in progress, plan new ones, and mentor students as well as other faculty. Since the construction of TigerPlace, these meetings are held there, in a classroom. Students and faculty interact with the people who live there each week. Such interactions inform and challenge our next research ideas.

REASONS FOR SUCCESS OF AIP PROJECT

From the beginning, AIP was inspired by nurses with a vision to change the care for older adults. We built an interdisciplinary team that included not only health care professionals, but also consumers, architects, veterinarians, engineers, and information technologists. We partnered with Americare, a high-quality, visionary nursing home corporation, which has supported a radically different vision of care for older adults. We work tirelessly to build relationships with legislators in order to facilitate the changes in public policy needed for the vision to happen. We have stayed closely connected with the regulatory community so that we can continue to achieve high-quality outcomes, while giving care in a different way.

Perhaps our biggest success has been our willingness to be pushed to seek unique solutions to age-old problems. As people age, they often become more frail, and staying in the same environment becomes an increasing challenge. The older adults and their families who are partners with us in this enterprise asked us to think differently about early illness, falls, frailty, and infections. They asked to find ways to monitor changes in their condition but not to tie them down to their rooms, or to a sick role. We have stepped up to that challenge: nurses, social workers, engineers, health information technology professionals, physical therapists, and many others discover new ways to identify early illness through changes in activity and passive vital sign measurement, risk for falls through measurement of stride length, and remediation of future fall risk by using depth image sensors.

Our health care team, including RN care coordinators, social workers, nurses, and aides, works closely with families to develop interdisciplinary plans of care based on the resident/family's needs and wishes. We put services in place judiciously and thoughtfully, to avoid inducing dependence on others. The system of care delivery, including the use of EHRs, allows for quality improvement and early recognition of system problems. We have found that it is essential to the system of care delivery that everyone from the housekeepers to administrators is empowered to think about how to improve care and residents' experiences. We have also found that EHRs are essential elements for program effectiveness, so that health outcomes can be measured, cost of care and services evaluated, and quality of care and services assessed. *Always* measure cost, quality, outcomes, and describe the staffing and services so that others can replicate and learn from what we have done in the AIP Project.

CONCLUSION

Our experience with AIP supports the benefits that can be achieved when physical environments and care models are re-envisioned to more successfully meet the needs of older adults. We have demonstrated that through adapting environments to be more responsive and more relevant to older adults, effectiveness and efficiency can be achieved. A public policy approach that capitalizes on the successes of our project would simultaneously add to the quality of life of older adults while realizing fiscal savings. It is time for our nation to adopt such an approach.

REFERENCES

Abt Associates Inc. (2000). *Evaluation of the community nursing organization demonstration final report*. Cambridge, MA: Author.

American Medical Association. (2013). *CPT codes for evaluation and management.* Retrieved from http://www.ama-assn.org/ama/pub/physician-resources/solutions-managing-your-prac tice/coding-billing-insurance/cpt.page

Caffrey, C., Sengupta, M., Park-Lee, E., Moss, A., Rosenoff, E., & Harris-Kojetin, L. (2012). *United States, 2010. NCHS data brief, no 91. Residents living in residential care facilities: Statistics.* Hyatts- ville, MD: National Center for Health.

Collins, C., Butler, F. R., Gueldner, S. H., & Palmer, M. H. (1997). Models for community base long- term care for the elderly in a changing health system. *Nursing Outlook, 45,* 59–63.

Courtney, K. L., Demiris, G., Rantz, M. J., & Skubic, M. (2008). Needing smart home technologies: The perspective of older adults in continuing care retirement communities. *Informatics in Pri- mary Care, 16*(3), 195–201.

Elkan, R., Kendrick, D., Dewey, M., Hewitt, M., Robinson, J., Blair, M., . . . Brummell, K. (2001). Effectiveness of home based support for older people: Systematic review and meta-analysis. *British Medical Journal, 323,* 1–9.

Demiris, G., Hensel, B. K., Skubic, M., & Rantz, M. J. (2008). Senior residents' perceived need of and preferences for "smart home" sensor technologies. *International Journal of Technology Assessment in Health Care, 24*(1), 120–124.

Demiris, G., Parker Oliver, D., Dickey, G., Skubic, M., & Rantz, M. (2008). Findings from a participatory evaluation of a smart home application for older adults. *Technology and Health Care, 16,* 111–118.

Galambos, C., Starr, J., Musterman, K., & Rantz, M. (2015). Staff perceptions of social work student contributions to home health care services at an independent living facility. *Home HealthCare Now, 33*(4), 206–214.

Hughes, S. L. (1985). Apples and oranges? A review of evaluation of community-based long-term care. *Health Services Research, 20*(4), 461–488.

Kemper, P. (1990). Case management agency systems of administering long-term care: Evidence from the channeling demonstration. *The Gerontologist, 30*(6), 817–824.

Living at Home Network of Block Nurse Programs. (2016). Retrieved from http://lahnetwork .org/about

Marek, K. D., Adams, S. J., Stetzer, F., Popejoy, L., Petroski, G. F., & Rantz, M. (2010). The rela- tionship of community-based nurse care coordination to costs in the Medicare and Medicaid programs. *Research in Nursing & Health, 33,* 235–242.

Marek, K. D., Popejoy, L., Petroski, G., Mehr, D., Rantz, M. J., & Lin, W. (2005). Clinical outcomes of aging in place. *Nursing Research, 54*(3), 202–211.

Marek, K. D., Popejoy, L., Petroski, G., & Rantz, M. J. (2006). Nurse care coordination in community- based long-term care. *Journal of Nursing Scholarship, 38*(1), 80–86.

Marek, K. D., & Rantz, M. J. (2000). Aging in place: A new model for long-term care. *Nursing Administration Quarterly, 24*(3), 1–11.

Marek, K. D., Stetzer, F., Adams, S. J., Popejoy, L., & Rantz, M. (2012). Aging in place versus nurs- ing home care: Comparison of costs to Medicare and Medicaid. *Research in Gerontological Nursing, 5*(2), 123–129.

Martinson, I. M., Jamieson, M. K., O'Grady, B., & Sime, M. (1985). The block nurse program. *Jour- nal of Community Health Nursing, 2*(1), 21–29.

Matherlee, K. (1999). *The nursing center in concept and practice: Delivery and financing issues in serving vulnerable people* (National Health Policy Forum, No. 746). Retrieved from http://www.nhpf .org/library/issue-briefs/IB746_NursCenter_9-13-99.pdf

Metropolitan Council of the Twin Cities Area. (1990). *Living-at-home and block nurse programs: An analysis of client and cost information, 1988–1990.* St. Paul, MN: Metropolitan Council.

Phillips, L. J., DeRoche, C., Rantz, M., Alexander, G. L., Skubic, M., Despins, L., . . . Koopman, R. (2017). Using embedded sensors in independent living to predict gait changes and falls. *Western Journal of Nursing Research, 39*(1), 78–94. doi:10.1177/0193945916662027

Popejoy, L., Stetzer, F., Hicks, L., Rantz, M. J., Galambos, C., Popescu, M., . . . Marek, K. (2015). Comparing aging in place to home health care: Impact of nurse care coordination on utiliza- tion and costs. *Nursing Economics, 33*(6), 306–313.

Rantz, M. J., Lane, K. R., Phillips, L. J., Despins, L. A., Galambos, C., Alexander, G. L., . . . Miller, S. J. (2015). Enhanced RN care coordination with sensor technology: Impact on length of stay and cost in aging in place housing. *Nursing Outlook, 63*, 650–655.

Rantz, M. J., Marek, K. D., Aud, M. A., Tyrer, H. W., Skubic, M., Demiris, G., & Hussam, A. A. (2005). A technology and nursing collaboration to help older adults age in place. *Nursing Outlook, 53*(1), 40–45.

Rantz, M. J., Phillips, L., Aud, M., Marek, K. D., Hicks, L. L., Zaniletti, I., & Miller, S. J. (2011). Evaluation of aging in place model with home care services and registered nurse care coordination in senior housing. *Nursing Outlook, 59*(1), 37–46.

Rantz, M. J., Popejoy, L. L., Galambos, C., Phillips, L. J., Lane, K. R., Marek, K. D., . . . Ge, B. (2014). The continued success of registered nurse care coordination in a state evaluation of aging in place in senior housing. *Nursing Outlook, 62*(4), 237–246.

Rantz, M. J., Popejoy, L., Musterman, K., & Miller, S. J. (2014). Influencing public policy through care coordination research. In G. Lamb (Ed.), *Care coordination: The game changer; how nursing is revolutionizing quality care* (pp. 203–220). Silver Spring, MD: American Nurses Association.

Rantz, M. J., Porter, R., Cheshier, D., Otto, D., Servey, C. H., Johnson, R. A., . . . Taylor, G. (2008). TigerPlace, a state-academic-private project to revolutionize traditional long-term care. *Journal of Housing for the Elderly, 22*(1/2), 66–85.

Rantz, M. J., Skubic, M., Alexander, G., Aud, M., Wakefield, B., Koopman, R., & Miller, S. (2010). Improving nurse care coordination with technology. *Computers, Informatics, Nursing, 28*(6), 325–332.

Rantz, M. J., Skubic, M., Koopman, R. J., Alexander, G., Phillips, L., Musterman, K. I., . . . Miller, S. J. (2012). Automated technology to speed recognition of signs of illness in older adults. *Journal of Gerontological Nursing, 38*(4), 18–23.

Rantz, M. J., Skubic, M., Miller, S. J., Galambos, C., Alexander, G., Keller, J., & Popescu, M. (2013). Sensor technology to support aging in place. *Journal of the American Medical Directors Association, 14*(6), 386–391.

Rantz, M. J., Skubic, M., Popescu, M., Galambos, C., Koopman, R. J., Alexander, G. L., . . . Miller, S. J. (2015). A new paradigm of technology-enabled "vital signs" for early detection of health change for older adults. *Gerontology, 61*(3), 281–290.

Rosales, L., Su, B. Y., Skubic, M., & Ho, K. C. (in press). Heart rate estimation from hydraulic bed sensor ballistocardiogram. *Journal of Ambient Intelligence and Smart Environments, 2012*, 2587–2590.

Skubic, M., Alexander, G., Popescu, M., Rantz, M., & Keller, J. (2009). A smart home application to eldercare: Current status and lessons learned. *Technology and Health Care, 17*(3), 183–201.

Skubic, M., Guevara, R., & Rantz, M. (2015). Automated health alerts using in-home sensor data for embedded health assessment. *IEEE Journal of Translational Engineering in Health and Medicine, 3*, 1–11.

Skubic, M., Rantz, M., Miller, S., Guevara, R. D., Koopman, R., Alexander, G., & Phillips, L. (2013). Non-wearable in-home sensing for early detection of health changes. In R. Schultz (Ed.), *Quality of life technology for the disabled and elderly* (pp. 227–244). Boca Raton, FL: CRC Press.

Stone, E., & Skubic, M. (2013). Unobtrusive, continuous, in-home gait measurement using the Microsoft Kinect. *IEEE Transactions on Biomedical Engineering, 60*(10), 2925–2932.

Stone, E., & Skubic, M. (2014, June 25–27). *Testing real-time in-home fall alerts with embedded depth video hyperlink.* Paper presented at the International Conference on Smart Homes and Health Telematics (ICOST), Denver, CO.

Stone, E., Skubic, M., & Back, J. (2014, August 26–30). Automated health alerts from Kinect-based in-home gait measurements. In *2014 36th Annual International Conference of the IEEE Engineering in Medicine and Biology Society* (pp. 2961–2964). New York, NY: Institute of Electrical and Electronics Engineers.

Stone, E., Skubic, M., Rantz, M. J., Abbott, C., & Miller, S. (2015). Average in-home gait speed: Investigation of a new metric for mobility and fall risk assessment of elders. *Gait & Posture, 41*, 57–62.

Wang, S., Skubic, M., & Zhu, Y. (2012). Activity density map visualization and dis-similarity comparison for eldercare monitoring. *IEEE Journal of Biomedical and Health Informatics, 16*(4), 607–614.

13

Aging in Place: Innovative Teams

Sarah L. Szanton

BACKGROUND

As a nurse practitioner providing house calls, I had one patient I could not get out of my mind. We will call her Annie Lee. She was 100 years old, lived by herself in an apartment, could not read, and could not get her wheelchair through the doorway into her kitchen. This barrier in her environment caused her to crawl from the doorway to her refrigerator. Despite these challenges, she had a wonderful spirit, gave wisdom freely, and was philosophical about what she could and could not do. Her diabetes and hypertension were not well controlled. How could they be? And how could I as a health care provider think that was her most important priority? I provided house calls to low-income residents throughout West Baltimore who found it difficult to leave their homes to see a primary care provider (PCP). One of my patients had to crawl to answer the door. Many could not get up their stairs to sleep in their own beds. And several could only eat snack foods because they were unable to prepare light meals for themselves.

This experience was life-changing for me. I initially approached the visits as a classically trained nurse practitioner. Intent on leveraging my therapeutic relationship with these older adults to help them self-manage their current conditions, I had not been trained to observe their environment and the ways in which it either supported or inhibited them. I had not been trained to observe their overall life goals and how their chronic conditions fit within those.

In this work, it was only too clear that holes in floors, shaky banisters, shelves that were too high to reach, and the mismatch between what people needed and what the environment required of them were inhibiting their health and their ability to age where they wanted to, which for almost everyone was at home. I had not yet studied aging theory, but this experience made me viscerally understand the idea of "person–environment fit," the theory that Powell Lawton developed in the 1970s (Lawton & Nahemow, 1973), which Miss Lee demonstrated well. Her abilities and

227

her kitchen doorway did not fit. This made the home environment for her stressful, which impacted her health and function.

I knew that people like Miss Lee were important because they were my patients. I did not yet understand how much their experiences represent policy histories and opportunities to change current policy. Demographic shifts make these policy decisions that much more important; by 2050, the percentage of the U.S. population over 65 years of age will be double what it is now (Ortman, Velkoff, & Hogan, 2014). The vast majority of older adults prefer to "age in place" in their home community rather than age in an institution. As a society, we will need to develop multiple ways of helping older adults age in place depending on their individual strengths and needs. Because the number of older adults in the United States is projected to continue growing (U.S. Census Bureau, 2013), it is increasingly urgent to identify ways to support aging with independence.

Aging with independence is important for multiple reasons. It affords better quality of life for older individuals and their families (Schwanen & Ziegler, 2011) and is a foundational American value that, when achieved, saves resources for society to use in other ways.

However, for almost everyone, at every income level, aging brings functional challenges that can compromise independence. These functional challenges result from interactions between an individual's health and his or her surrounding environment. Low-income older adults face even greater challenges to independence, as they are likely to have more comorbidities (Green et al., 2003), experience more functional limitations as a result (Fuller-Thomson, Nuru-Jeter, Minkler, & Guralnik, 2009; Minkler, Fuller-Thomson, & Guralnik, 2006), and, by definition, have fewer resources to modify their home environments. This combination places them at even greater risk for reduced activity levels, social isolation, falls, and other adverse events.

I studied and obtained my PhD from Johns Hopkins University to learn the research skills to leverage my clinical insights into policy-relevant research. When the 2007 deep recession hit, the National Institutes of Health put out a call for proposals for innovative team members in areas including those hardest hit by the recession. I thought hard about "handymen" (or women)—home repair specialists who do odd jobs and repairs—and about how much good they could do for the patients I had seen in West Baltimore.

I conceived of combining nurse visits with handyman repair and assistive devices. In fleshing out my ideas, I looked at a program called Advancing Better Living for Elders (ABLE), which had already been proven effective in addressing similar challenges. ABLE had been previously evaluated through a randomized controlled trial of 306 older adults in Philadelphia. The program provided occupational and physical therapy sessions involving home modifications and training in their use, as well as instruction in problem-solving strategies, energy conservation, safe performance of basic and instrumental activities of daily living (ADLs and IADLs), fall recovery techniques, and muscle and balance training. The evaluation of this model provided strong evidence that a program focused on improving community-dwelling older adults' function and control over their circumstances could help to promote aging with independence in these populations and even delay mortality (Gitlin et al., 2006, 2009). I wanted to build on the strengths of ABLE, while also modifying the intervention to address additional threats to aging with independence (such as perilous home environments and their interactions with underlying health issues) more explicitly.

Though not funded at that submission, we received useful critical feedback. I repurposed pilot funding money I had to pilot this new idea, which we called CAPABLE (Community Aging in Place, Advancing Better Living for Elders). This is another lesson in a research trajectory. Sometimes you have to do exactly what you propose and other times (often when working with foundations) if you have a new idea that is compelling to you and the funder, you can gain permission to change what it funds.

CAPABLE augmented ABLE by adding support for actual repairs to unsafe home environments (as opposed to strictly home modifications and adaptive equipment such as grab bars and raised toilet seats) and a nurse to comprehensively assess and address health concerns that could contribute to functional limitations within the home environment, such as pain, depression, medication reconciliation, and PCP advocacy and communication. These realms were added in the service of increasing clients' capacity to perform their basic and IADLs.

Innovative teams can be important and must be guided by your theory of change or of the phenomenon in place. For example, the dominant theory for this work is person–environment fit, and it is about improving function to allow older adults to achieve their goals. This sort of model is a perfect fit for occupational therapists (OTs). OTs help people across the life span participate in the things they need and want to do (American Occupational Therapy Association, 2016). The American Association of Occupational Therapists states that OTs ask "What matters to you?" not "What's the matter with you?" When adding team members from different disciplines, it is necessary to maintain a balance between what is essential and what will not make the program too unwieldy. In adding the OT component to my vision for a program that would aid the patients I had seen, I was influenced by this OT emphasis of "what matters to you?"; this perspective then informed the registered nursing aspect of the program we created, as well.

The CAPABLE intervention involves universal assessment of every client by an RN/OT team, which then allows an interdisciplinary team—including the client, nurse, OT therapist, and a home repair specialist ("handyman")—to tailor an individualized plan that addresses potential threats to aging independence in the home environment while working toward functional goals set by the clients themselves. Table 13.1 summarizes the visits and their sequencing; for a more detailed overview of the nurse's role in CAPABLE, see the article by Pho et al. (2012).

Our team conducted a randomized controlled pilot trial of CAPABLE in 2009–2010. In a sample of 40 low-income older adults, older adults who had been randomly assigned to receive the CAPABLE intervention showed improvement for all primary outcomes when compared to a control group. This resulted in less difficulty with ADLs and IADLs, less pain, and improved fall-avoidance efficacy

TABLE 13.1   *CAPABLE Targeted Areas, Goals, and Treatment Approaches*

Dimension	Target: Approach and Goal
Environment	Housing safety: repair built environment to ↓ fall risk, ↑ mobility, and ADLs/IADLs
	Ability to access primary care and appropriate specialists
Person: **Individual factors**	Self-care: ↑ ability to independently conduct ADLs and IADLs
	Communication with PCP: ↑ patient activation to facilitate better chronic disease management
	Medication management: ↑ ability to adhere to medication regime
Intrinsic: **Physiological factors**	Strength/balance: ↑ ability to stand, balance, and recover from falls, near-falls
	Depression: enhance skills for mood management
	Pain: to decrease pain to facilitate function

ADL, activities of daily living; IADL, instrumental activities of daily living; PCP, primary care provider.
Source: Szanton et al. (2014).

(Szanton et al., 2011). Based on those findings, the CAPABLE team was funded by the National Institutes of Health to conduct a 300-person randomized clinical trial assessing whether the intervention improves function, well-being, and health care costs on a larger scale. Also, through the Center for Medicare and Medicaid Innovation, which was created by the Affordable Care Act, the team received funding to provide the CAPABLE intervention to 500 people and test whether the program delayed nursing home admission and reduced preventable hospital costs.

The remainder of this chapter details how CAPABLE works to improve lives while saving more than it costs; how the innovative delivery team works together, the ways in which it is innovative, and lessons learned; what we learned about changing policy; and policy insights such as taking advantage of the policy moment, leveraging diverse data metrics for diverse stakeholders, and lessons from translating research into policy.

OVERVIEW OF CAPABLE

CAPABLE is based on clinical insight, relevant aging theories, resilience (Szanton & Gill, 2010), person–environment fit (Lawton & Nahemow, 1973), enhancing control (Schulz, Heckhausen, & O'Brien, 1994) and evidence-based practices. CAPABLE uses up to 10 home sessions, each of 60 to 90 minutes duration, over a 4-month period. It draws upon clinical approaches to enhance uptake and adoption of intervention strategies by study participants such as patient-directed care and motivational interviewing (Prochaska & Velicer, 1997; Reuben, 2007; Richards et al., 2007; Von Korff, Gruman, Schaefer, Curry, & Wagner, 1997). Each intervention participant receives every component of the intervention (assessment, education, interactive problem-solving), but nurses and OTs clinically tailor the interactions to each participant's goals, strengths, and challenges. See Table 13.2 for an overview of the intervention.

TABLE 13.2 *Intervention Content by Visit and Discipline*

Session Number	Who	When	Content	Interventionist Follow-Up
1	OT #1	Within 10 days of baseline data collection	Introduction to OT portion of CAPABLE. Issue Intervention folder. Function-focused OT assessment including functional mobility, activities of daily living and instrumental activities of daily living (C-CAP). Determine participant's functional goals. Screen for Physical Therapy referral.	
2	OT #2	1–2 weeks later	Fall risk and recovery education. Conduct home assessment and identify necessary repairs or modifications.	Develop work order for home repairs/modifications and send to liaison who will send to HM.
3	HM #1	After receiving work order	Visit home to assess which materials to purchase for ordered modification and repairs.	Purchase materials.
4	RN #1	One month after baseline data visit	Introduction to RN portion of CAPABLE. Function-focused RN assessment including pain, mood, strength, balance, medication information, need for health care provider (PCP) advocacy/communication.	Make medication calendar for participant. Review participant's medications including side effects, interactions, and possible changes. Consult with pharmacist if on high-alert or > 15 medications.
5	HM #2	Once have supplies	Repair and modify home based on participant-goal prioritized work order.	HM notifies OT when this is complete.
6	OT #3	2–3 weeks after last OT session	Brainstorm and develop Action Plan with participant for participant-identified goal #1 (examples include safely bathing, going upstairs, or preparing food).	
7	RN #2	3–4 weeks after initial RN session	Determine goals in RN domain together, start to brainstorm goal #1 (examples include pain in standing, fall prevention). Demonstrate CAPABLE exercises. Review medication calendar. Discuss participant/PCP communication.	Develop correspondence to PCP if necessary.
8	OT #4	1 month after last session	Review Action Plan #1. Brainstorm and develop Action Plan with participant for participant-identified goal #2. Review HM work and train participant on new assistive devices as able.	Issue assistive devices or medical equipment as available.

(continued)

TABLE 13.2　*Intervention Content by Visit and Discipline (continued)*

Session Number	Who	When	Content	Interventionist Follow-Up
9	RN #3	3–4 weeks after last session	Complete Brainstorming/Problem-solving process. Develop Action Plans for identified goals with participant. Assess PCP response to communication of participant needs. Review/assess/troubleshoot exercise regimen. Issue Health Care Passport to enhance communication and key questions for PCP.	
10	OT #5	1 month after last session	Review Action Plan #2. Brainstorm and develop Action Plan with participant for participant-identified goal #3. Issue AE and DME (if not already done) and train participant on new assistive devices and modifications.	
11	RN #4	3–4 weeks after last session	Review progress and use of strategies for all target areas. Issue and review RN section of Flipbook that summarizes program. Evaluate achievement of goals and readiness to change scale. Help participant generalize brainstorming process for future health issues. Ask if participant has any final questions.	
12	OT #6	3–4 weeks after last session	Review OT section of the Flipbook. Help participant generalize solutions for future problems and problem-solving techniques. Review and sign work order. Review goals and participant's achievement of them. Review readiness score. Ask if participant has any final questions.	

AE, adaptive equipment; CAPABLE, Community Aging in Place, Advancing Better Living for Elders; C-CAP, Client-Clinician Assessment Protocol; DME, durable medical equipment; HM, handyman; OT, occupational therapist; PCP, primary care provider.

Source: Szanton et al. (2014).

Intervention Delivery Characteristics

CAPABLE consists of an assessment-driven, individually tailored package of interventions delivered by an OT (≤ 6 home visits for ≤ 1 hour), an RN (≤ 4 home visits for ≤ 1 hour), and a handyman team (see Table 13.2). The number of visits is usually

10 but can be less if the participant has few goals to address with either the OT or the nurse. Sessions are spaced so that participants have opportunities to practice new strategies or activities with the health professional and then on their own. Communication between the OT, nurse, and handyman is enhanced by a secure share site, which can be remotely logged into by the interventionists and enable electronic documentation that can be reviewed for fidelity and also contribute to understanding intervention costs.

The Occupational Therapist Role

In the **first and second sessions,** the OT meets with participants and conducts a semistructured clinical interview using the Client-Clinician Assessment Protocol (C-CAP; Petersson, Fisher, Hemmingsson, & Lilja, 2007). The C-CAP provides a systematic approach to identify and prioritize areas that are problematic to participants, such as getting into the shower or reaching for items while cooking. For each area the participant prioritizes as important, the OT observes the participant's performance and evaluates safety, efficiency, difficulty, and environmental barriers and supports. The OT provides a CAPABLE notebook to each participant, which contains educational materials, contact information, and a calendar to integrate the sessions by the nurse and handyman interventionists. This also helps with interprofessional communication. Also in the course of this session, the OT assesses the environmental home safety (common safety and mobility risks our team finds include holes in walkways, uneven carpeting, and absent railings or banisters). Based on the environmental assessment, observation of ADL, and identification of the participant's goals, the OT and participant discuss possible environmental modifications or repairs. The OT then provides a list of agreed-upon assistive devices and housing repairs to the handyman coordinator via e-mail. In **OT sessions 3–5,** the OT engages the participant in problem solving to identify behavioral and environmental contributors to performance difficulties and strategies for attaining functional goals. The OT coaches participants to use specific strategies such as conserving energy during tasks, simplifying tasks and the environment, and using assistive devices. Also, the OT provides balance and fall recovery techniques to decrease fear of falling. In each session, the OT reinforces strategy use, reviews problem solving, refines strategies, and provides education and resources to address future needs. Home modifications (grab bars, rails, raised toilet seats) are coordinated with the handyman to ensure that they are provided in a timely manner and meet the needs of the participant. The OT follows up with training in their use. In the **final** (sixth) **OT** session, the OT reviews all techniques, strategies, and devices, and helps the participant to generalize success to other situations.

The Nurse Role

The RN meets with participants for up to four sessions during the same 4 months as the OT sessions. **The first RN session** follows the first OT session within

1 month. In this session, the RN assesses the participant using the C-CAP RN (Pho et al., 2012), in which the RN focuses on how and whether pain, depression, strength and balance, medication management, and ability to communicate with the PCP impact daily function. In this assessment, the RN and the participant identify and prioritize goals, and make plans to achieve those goals. The RN also adds educational resources to the CAPABLE notebook to reinforce its use as a resource. In **RN visits 2 and 3,** the RN and the participant work on the goals identified through the C-CAP RN. To do this, they identify barriers to each goals. For example, if they rush to the bathroom due to incontinence, the RN and the participant would examine the reasons—how much diuretic, timing of diuretic, extent of coffee, have they tried timing toileting, what footwear, is the bathroom on the same level? In each session, the RN reinforces strategy use, reviews problem solving, refines strategies (such as Otago-based exercises or pain management), and provides education and resources to address future needs (e.g., pill box for medication management). Both the RN and the participant usually have homework or tasks they do between sessions. In the **final** (fourth) **session,** the RN reviews the participant's strategies and helps to generalize them to other possible challenges.

The Handyman Role

The handyman portion is contracted with Civic Works (www.civicworks.com), which is a nonprofit AmeriCorps site located in Baltimore. It is a part of a network of many AmeriCorps sites, which can be excellent sources of "handypeople" in other cities. The contractor at Civic Works coordinates the ordering of the assistive devices as well as the repair and modification supplies. The handyman makes as many home visits as it takes to provide the renovations/modifications that the OT orders. Generally there is one visit to assess what supplies will be required to implement the work order and then a full day's work to complete it. The budget for this work is up to $1,300 per household based on real expenditures in the CAPABLE pilot study (Szanton et al., 2011). We found this dollar amount adequate for most renovations necessary to achieve safer, more functional homes.

THREE INNOVATIONS OF THE CAPABLE MODEL IN ACTION

CAPABLE is innovative in three ways. First, it is not just client-centered but client-directed. Second, unlike most forms of home health care, the nurse and OT strive to address the functional goals of the client, not strictly the medical issues. Third, the CAPABLE model treats the home environment as a key influence on health, such that fixing up an older adult's home interior is done for the purpose of achieving health-related goals.

Value Added by the CAPABLE Approach

An older adult like Miss Lee would be likely to be admitted to a hospital or a nursing home over time due to her multimorbidity, taking multiple medications, social isolation, and her frail physical and emotional state (Woods et al., 2005). The CAPABLE team of OT, RN, and handyman seeks to reverse the vicious cycle so many older adults with similar risk profiles as Miss Lee fall into of becoming increasingly deconditioned, depressed, and frail over time. The hope is that consequently, these actions will also decrease future risk for serious medical consequences, injury, or further functional declines that would require costly care (Woods et al., 2005).

Lessons Learned About the Impact of Client-Directed Care

In our experience, prioritizing the clients' goals makes them likely to follow through. When clients say they are worried about falls, and the CAPABLE nurse presents core strengthening exercises to help prevent falls, then the client is very likely to follow through on the exercises because they relate to her goal. Client-directed care can be hard at first for the RN to get used to, as RNs are accustomed to having medical goals and imparting them to the client.

Lessons Learned About Addressing Medical and Functional Issues Through Interdisciplinary Team

Similar to addressing the client's goals, addressing their specific functional goals is the key to motivation. Clients are often not as concerned about their medical disease as they are about the ability to function. When we address both, it is a support for the client to be able to live with independence and dignity and leads to durable uptake of the new strategies.

Lessons Learned About Housing/Environment as Health

The changes to the home environment are durable and serve as visible reminders for clients to address their daily function with their new CAPABLE approaches. After CAPABLE is over, if participants forget to take their pain medications, they will still have repaired holes, raised toilet seats, and sturdy banisters to help them move around the home with increased function. Hopefully, these environmental changes work with their intrinsic changes and new problem-solving strategies to approach inevitable new issues as they age.

POLICY LESSONS LEARNED IN WORKING ON TRANSLATING CAPABLE TO POLICY

Build or Adapt From What Already Works

One can have an innovative program and build from the groundwork of others. One can adapt and make it fit new situations. CAPABLE got an advantaged start by building on the framework of ABLE. We adapted and built from the forms, training, cost-tracking categories, and evidence base. Drawing from Dr. Laura Gitlin's program of research meant our team was building on her years of thought and experience, which solved logistical, training, and grantsmanship problems.

Always Think of Stakeholders in Design

It is much easier to influence policy makers if the outcomes of your research are outcomes that the stakeholder cares about. There is a saying that if you are in the business of changing policy, then you are in the business of solving someone else's problem. For example, an intervention that only measures quality of life will be important to some, but others will want to see how much it costs and potentially saves the stakeholder. Other examples include discovering how much an intervention decreases the admission rate or changes Healthcare Effectiveness Data and Information Set (HEDIS) measures. Understanding this from the beginning is crucial to affecting policy.

Fit Your Interest With What Society Needs

You may have worked clinically with a specialized set of patients, such as people who use a certain kind of device or have one type of cancer. This is an important basis for your ideas on how to change care or policy. However, you must be able to frame your research in terms of a larger population—for example, all cancer patients or at least all cancer survivors or something that is broader—to get real policy interest. Practice being able to explain to colleagues why your work makes sense to prioritize above other work. Policy is always a series of choices that balance some interests over others. Keeping society's urgent needs in mind will help you get funded to do your research and will help you leverage your results into policy change. If you have done your research into a tiny population that has small effect on the health care system, you will not have as many people lined up to put your research findings into action.

Take Advantage of the Policy Moment

In any moment, there are key policy challenges that people who make policy seek to address. If you are thinking about policy in your local institutions, these challenges will be different from the national challenges that federal government institutions seek to address. However, a perennial interest is better care for lower cost. Learning how to frame your research in terms of current conversations such as "bending the cost curve" or moving toward authentically patient-centered care is important. Framing your work in this way is crucial in addressing the needs of your institution, your patient population, your state, or your country—at any level in which you work. It is also important for convincing others of seeing your work as the answer to their problems. Doing this well will enable you to move farther faster; others will be pushing it along if it fits their agenda as well. This is good stewardship of your research. Get others to feel that it solves their challenges.

Different Decision Makers Are Guided by Different Kinds of Data

If you have studied rhetoric or persuasion, you know that good speeches contain ethos, pathos, and logos. As researchers, we clearly establish ethos, which is credibility. Our bios and degrees speak for us. We also are well trained to use logos or logical data. We present our outcomes with p values and explain what they mean. We often ignore the pathos part. That is the story, the emotion, the why of it. This omission is a mistake, as decisions by policy makers (as by all decision makers) are made by interplay between the brain's executive and limbic systems (Morse, 2006). The limbic system is fueled by emotion. What this means is that facts are not the only driver of behavior. Emotion is a deep driver of behavior as well.

Although logic and story are both necessary in communication, it is important to think through a balance based on the goal of each communication. For example, if you write to a reporter, you might want to include personal quotations from your research participants about the impact of your program. In contrast, if you communicate with leaders at Centers for Medicare and Medicaid Services, you will want to have mostly data about costs and quality changes due to your program. It will still be helpful to have some stories or quotations. This is part of the reason clinicians do an especially good job of advocacy: we understand the deep personal impact of what we do. I was a lobbyist before I was a nurse and I partly went to nursing school because the stories the nurses told their congresspersons were so much more compelling than what I was able to tell.

CONCLUSION

Nurses are well equipped to construct innovative teams, and then research and communicate the impact of their projects to policy makers to advance a healthier society. To do this, nurses can frame their ideas in terms of current societal challenges, measure what costs and benefits there will be to stakeholders, and provide both stories and quantitative data to impact decision makers. Often the most interesting ideas are the ones that come from working between several disciplines. Learning to work with teams can allow us to develop these ideas to improve health for all.

REFERENCES

American Occupational Therapy Association. (2016). About occupational therapy. Retrieved from http://www.aota.org/about-occupational-therapy.aspx

Fuller-Thomson, E., Nuru-Jeter, A., Minkler, M., & Guralnik, J. M. (2009). Black-white disparities in disability among older Americans: Further untangling the role of race and socioeconomic status. *Journal of Aging and Health, 21*(5), 677–698. doi:10.1177/0898264309338296

Gitlin, L. N., Hauck, W. W., Dennis, M. P., Winter, L., Hodgson, N., & Schinfeld, S. (2009). Long-term effect on mortality of a home intervention that reduces functional difficulties in older adults: Results from a randomized trial. *Journal of the American Geriatrics Society, 57*(3), 476–481. doi:10.1111/j.1532-5415.2008.02147.x

Gitlin, L. N., Winter, L., Dennis, M. P., Corcoran, M., Schinfeld, S., & Hauck, W. W. (2006). A randomized trial of a multicomponent home intervention to reduce functional difficulties in older adults. *Journal of the American Geriatrics Society, 54*(5), 809–816. doi:10.1111/j.1532-5415.2006.00703.x

Green, C. R., Anderson, K. O., Baker, T. A., Campbell, L. C., Decker, S., Fillingim, R. B., . . . Vallerand, A. H. (2003). The unequal burden of pain: Confronting racial and ethnic disparities in pain. *Pain Medicine (Malden, Mass.), 4*(3), 277–294.

Lawton, M. P., & Nahemow, L. (1973). Ecology and the aging process. In C. Eisdorfer & M. P. Lawton (Eds.), *The psychology of adult development and aging* (pp. 619–674). Washington, DC: American Psychological Association.

Minkler, M., Fuller-Thomson, E., & Guralnik, J. M. (2006). Gradient of disability across the socio-economic spectrum in the United States. *New England Journal of Medicine, 355*(7), 695–703. doi:10.1056/NEJMsa044316

Morse, G. (2006). Decisions and desire. *Harvard Business Review, 84*(1), 42–51.

Ortman, J. M., Velkoff, V. A., & Hogan, H. (2014). *An aging nation: The older population in the United States*. Washington, DC: U.S. Census Bureau.

Petersson, I., Fisher, A. G., Hemmingsson, H., & Lilja, M. (2007). The Client-Clinician Assessment Protocol (C-CAP): Evaluation of its psychometric properties for use with people aging with disabilities in need of home modifications. *OTJR: Occupation, Participation and Health, 27*(4), 140–148.

Pho, A. T., Tanner, E. K., Roth, J., Greeley, M. E., Dorsey, C. D., & Szanton, S. L. (2012). Nursing strategies for promoting and maintaining function among community-living older adults: The CAPABLE intervention. *Geriatric Nursing (New York, NY), 33*(6), 439–445. doi:10.1016/j.gerinurse.2012.04.002

Prochaska, J. O., & Velicer, W. F. (1997). The transtheoretical model of health behavior change. *American Journal of Health Promotion, 12*(1), 38–48.

Reuben, D. B. (2007). Better care for older people with chronic diseases: An emerging vision. *JAMA, 298*(22), 2673–2674. doi:10.1001/jama.298.22.2673

Richards, K. C., Enderlin, C. A., Beck, C., McSweeney, J. C., Jones, T. C., & Roberson, P. K. (2007). Tailored biobehavioral interventions: A literature review and synthesis. *Research and Theory for Nursing Practice, 21*(4), 271–285.

Schulz, R., Heckhausen, J., & O'Brien, A. T. (1994). Control and the disablement process in the elderly. *Journal of Social Behavior and Personality, 9,* 139–152.

Schwanen, T., & Ziegler, F. (2011). Wellbeing, independence, and mobility: An introduction. *Ageing and Society, 31*(5), 719–733. doi:10.1017/S0144686X10001467

Szanton, S. L., & Gill, J. M. (2010). Facilitating resilience using a society-to-cells framework: A theory of nursing essentials applied to research and practice. *Advances in Nursing Science, 33*(4), 329–343. doi:10.1097/ANS.0b013e3181fb2ea2

Szanton, S. L., Wolff, J. W., Leff, B., Thorpe, R. J., Tanner, E. K., Boyd, C., . . . Gitlin, L. N. (2014). CAPABLE trial: A randomized controlled trial of nurse, occupational therapist and handyman to reduce disability among older adults: Rationale and design. *Contemporary Clinical Trials, 38*(1), 102–112.

Szanton, S. L., Thorpe, R. J., Boyd, C., Tanner, E. K., Leff, B., Agree, E., . . . Gitlin, L. N. (2011). Community aging in place, advancing better living for elders: A bio-behavioral-environmental intervention to improve function and health-related quality of life in disabled older adults. *Journal of the American Geriatrics Society, 59*(12), 2314–2320. doi:10.1111/j.1532-5415.2011.03698.x

U.S. Census Bureau. (2013). *American community survey, 2007–2011, detailed tables* (unpublished manuscript). Retrieved from www.socialexplorer.com/home

Von Korff, M., Gruman, J., Schaefer, J., Curry, S. J., & Wagner, E. H. (1997). Collaborative management of chronic illness. *Annals of Internal Medicine, 127*(12), 1097–1102.

Woods, N. F., LaCroix, A. Z., Gray, S. L., Aragaki, A., Cochrane, B. B., Brunner, R. L., . . . Women's Health Initiative. (2005). Frailty: Emergence and consequences in women aged 65 and older in the women's health initiative observational study. *Journal of the American Geriatrics Society, 53*(8), 1321–1330. doi:10.1111/j.1532-5415.2005.53405.x

14

Chronic Illness: Addressing Hypertension and Health Disparities in Communities

Yvonne Commodore-Mensah, Martha Hill, and Cheryl Dennison Himmelfarb

Chronic illnesses, including hypertension (HTN), represent a major global public health challenge, in part because of compelling ethnic and racial disparities in the quality and outcomes of care. Nurse scientists have conducted trials demonstrating the effectiveness of community-based interventions to improve HTN care and control. These trials have generated evidence that has shaped policy and practice to improve HTN care and reduce HTN disparities in communities.

BACKGROUND

Chronic Illnesses: A Global Context

Chronic illnesses, also known as noncommunicable diseases (NCDs), are one of the major public health challenges of the 21st century; they include cardiovascular diseases (CVDs), cancer, chronic respiratory diseases, and diabetes (World Health Organization, 2015). Of the 38 million deaths globally due to NCDs in 2012, more than 40% were premature and preventable (WHO, 2014). NCDs impose a substantial economic burden. They are projected to cost more than $30 trillion and will impoverish millions of people globally over the next 20 years (Bloom et al., 2011). Death from CVD, a major NCD, has been reduced dramatically in high-income countries due to medical advances in the management of CVD and related risk factors, including HTN and smoking. However, in low- and middle-income countries, this favorable shift has not been observed, and a concomitant epidemic of communicable and NCDs is under way (WHO, 2014). Globalization, rapid urbanization, aging of the population, and changes in individual lifestyle behaviors have contributed to the increased prevalence of NCDs. Although addressing medical management through evidence-based strategies is critical, combating the rising trend in NCDs also requires health policies that address social, economic, and behavioral contributors to this phenomenon.

The Global NCD Action Plan was instituted in 2013 by WHO to address the devastating socioeconomic and public health impact of NCDs. Targets include reducing harmful use of alcohol by at least 10%, insufficient physical activity by 10%, sodium intake by 30%, tobacco use by 30%, HTN by 25%; halting the rise of obesity and diabetes; improving coverage of treatment for prevention of heart attacks and strokes by at least 50% and providing 80% access to basic technologies and essential medicines (WHO, 2014). Notably, all nine targets are inextricably linked to HTN outcomes. The action plan also calls for all countries to set national NCD targets and be accountable for attaining them.

In the United States, NCDs, including CVDs, stroke, cancer, type 2 diabetes, and obesity, are the most common and preventable health conditions. Seven of the top 10 causes of death in 2010 were NCDs and together, CVDs and cancer account for nearly half of all deaths. About half of U.S. adults have at least one major CVD risk factor (Fryar, Chen, & Li, 2012), including excessive sodium intake (Cogswell et al., 2012) and physical inactivity (Centers for Disease Control and Prevention, 2014). These modifiable behaviors not only contribute to illness, suffering, and death related to NCDs, but also lead to costly treatment and poor outcomes. It is estimated that 68% of health care spending in the United States in 2010 was for NCDs (Gerteis et al., 2014). Effective interventions and policies to reduce the prevalence and improve management of NCDs are needed.

Hypertension

The positive direct association between HTN and CVD risk is strong, continuous, graded, independent, and predictive. This association has been established across sexes, age groups, racial/ethnic groups, and geographical boundaries (Whelton et al., 2002). Despite decades of progress in detection, treatment, and control of HTN in the United States, it remains a burdensome public health problem. The prevalence of HTN is 33% (Mozaffarian et al., 2016), and it is projected that by 2030, approximately 41% of U.S. adults will have HTN, which reflects an 8.4% increase from 2012 (Mozaffarian et al., 2016). The HTN awareness, treatment, and control rates from the 2009 to 2012 National Health and Nutrition Examination Survey (NHANES) are estimated as 83%, 77%, and 54% respectively (Mozaffarian et al., 2016). According to NHANES data from 2003 to 2004 through 2011 to 2012, awareness increased from 75.2% to 82.1%, treatment improved from 65.0% to 74.5%, and control improved from 39.4% to 51.8% (Mozaffarian et al., 2016). It is of great concern that between 2003 and 2013, the national mortality rate attributable to HTN increased by 8.2% and the number of deaths rose by 35% (Mozaffarian et al., 2016). Of note, awareness, treatment, and control of HTN vary across the country and the highest burden is in the southern United States (Olives, Myerson, Mokdad, Murray, & Lim, 2013).

A tripling of real (2008 dollars) total direct medical costs of CVD has been projected to occur between 2010 and 2030, raising costs from $272.5 billion to $818.1 billion (Heidenreich et al., 2011). HTN is the most expensive component contributing to this economic burden, with annual costs projected to increase by $130.4 billion from 2010 to 2030 (Heidenreich et al., 2011). The mean expenditure per person for HTN treatment was higher for non-Hispanic Blacks ($887) and Hispanics ($981) than for non-Hispanic Whites ($679) in 2010 (Davis, 2013). Effective prevention strategies are needed to limit the growing disease and economic burden related to HTN, particularly where racial and ethnic disparities exist.

In order to reach the WHO target of 25% relative reduction and contain the prevalence of HTN and reduce the associated economic burden, community- and population-based strategies are required to address modifiable risk factors for HTN. HTN can be prevented and managed with complementary primordial, primary, and secondary prevention strategies that target the populace as well as individuals at higher risk. Additionally, current evidence suggests that the most effective strategies to improve cardiovascular health include (a) individually focused approaches that target individual behavior change; (b) health care system approaches that encourage and reward efforts by providers and patients; and (c) population-based approaches that target broader populations (Mozaffarian et al., 2016).

Population-based and clinical studies have highlighted the importance of primordial and primary secondary prevention of HTN. *Primordial prevention* is defined as the prevention of the development of risk factors in the first place, whereas *primary prevention* is defined as interventions to modify adverse levels of risk factors once present to prevent the occurrence of HTN (Kavey et al., 2003; Lenfant, 1996). Primordial and primary preventions of HTN provide a unique opportunity to interrupt the continuous costly cycle of HTN management and associated complications. Healthy lifestyle interventions that are applied earlier in life provide the biggest long-term potential for avoiding the precursors that lead to HTN and ultimately reducing the burden on communities (Whelton et al., 2002). Intensive targeted strategies must be utilized in high-risk groups such as those with social and environmental risks, family history of HTN, African American ancestry, and sedentary lifestyles. Further, these strategies must be culturally acceptable, affordable, and sustainable.

HTN rarely occurs in isolation. Instead, it often occurs with other comorbidities such as diabetes and obesity. Approximately 50% of patients with diabetes have HTN (Barnett, 1994), and approximately 75% of the incidence of HTN is directly related to overweight and obesity (Mozaffarian et al., 2016). The associations between and among HTN, obesity, and diabetes are multifactorial with complex hemodynamic, metabolic, and endocrine pathways involved (Barnett, 1994; Mozaffarian et al., 2016). Numerous clinical trials have shown that HTN treatment and control markedly reduce incident stroke (by 35%–40%), myocardial infarction (by 15%–25%), and heart failure (by up to 64%; Chobanian et al., 2003; Psaty et al., 1997; SPRINT Research Group et al., 2015). In addition to management with antihypertensive medication, intensive lifestyle modification alone or in combination with medication are effective strategies to treat and control HTN and related comorbidities (Ornish et al., 1998; Ratner et al., 2005). Patients must be counseled on the importance of smoking cessation, dietary modification, regular physical activity, and stress management using effective strategies (Artinian et al., 2010; Commodore-Mensah & Himmelfarb, 2012).

Health Disparities

In the landmark report *Unequal Treatment: Confronting Racial and Ethnic Disparities in Health Care*, the Institute of Medicine outlined disparities in health outcomes and quality of care experienced by racial/ethnic minorities (Institute of Medicine [U.S.] Committee on Understanding and Eliminating Racial and Ethnic Disparities in Health Care, 2003). The report defined disparities in health care as racial or ethnic differences in the quality of health care that are not due to access-related factors or clinical needs, preferences, and appropriateness of intervention.

Despite advances in health care in the United States and reduction in CVD mortality since the 1970s, a large body of published research suggests that racial and ethnic minorities experience a lower quality of health services, and are less likely to receive even routine medical procedures than Whites (Agency for Healthcare Research and Quality, 2014; Institute of Medicine (U.S.) Committee on Understanding and Eliminating Racial and Ethnic Disparities in Health Care, 2003). For instance, African Americans are less likely to receive appropriate cardiac medication (Herholz et al., 1996) even when confounders are controlled for.

Studies of racial/ethnic differences in CVDs provide compelling evidence of health disparities. For instance, African American adults have among the highest prevalence of HTN in the world (Mozaffarian et al., 2016). The age-adjusted prevalence of HTN is 44.9% and 46.1% among African American men and women, respectively (Mozaffarian et al., 2016). African Americans are more likely to develop HTN at a younger age, develop CVD and end-stage renal disease, and die from CVD than other racial/ethnic groups. HTN awareness, treatment, and control rates are lowest among Mexican Americans compared with Whites and Blacks (Centers for Disease Control and Prevention, 2012). In addition to socioeconomic, genetic, and behavioral factors that drive these disparities, differences in health care quality are important contributors. African Americans receive worse care than Whites for about 40% of quality measures, including HTN, and worse access to care for 33% of measures, such as insurance coverage and wait times (Agency for Healthcare Research and Quality, 2014).

The sources of HTN and health disparities in communities are complex. They are rooted in historic inequities in the United States and involve health systems, health care professionals, utilization managers, and patients. Racial and ethnic minorities experience a range of barriers to accessing adequate care, even when insured at the same level as Whites, including barriers of language, geography, and cultural familiarity (Institute of Medicine [U.S.] Committee on Understanding and

Eliminating Racial and Ethnic Disparities in Health Care, 2003). The sources of HTN and health disparities may be grouped under patient-level, provider-level, and system-level factors.

At the patient level, racial and ethnic minorities are more likely to refuse provider-recommended services (Sedlis et al., 1997), adhere poorly to treatment regimens, and delay seeking appropriate care (Mitchell & McCormack, 1997). However, differences in refusal rates are small and do not fully account for racial and ethnic disparities in receipt of treatments (Institute of Medicine [U.S.] Committee on Understanding and Eliminating Racial and Ethnic Disparities in Health Care, 2003). These behaviors may be attributed to a cultural mismatch between the patient and provider, mistrust, misunderstanding of provider recommendations, and/or lack of knowledge on how to effectively utilize health services. Although it has been postulated that biological-based racial differences in response to treatment (for instance, enalapril, an antihypertensive used to reduce the risk of heart failure; Exner, Dries, Domanski, & Cohn, 2001) may account for the racial differences in the type and intensity of care provided, these differences are not due to "race" but are attributable to differences in the distribution of polymorphic traits between populations (Wood, 2001).

At the provider level, bias toward racial/ethnic minorities, clinical uncertainty when interacting with minority patients, and beliefs and stereotypes held by the provider about the behavior or health of minorities may contribute to HTN disparities. However, research on how patient race/ethnicity influences provider decision making is limited. In addition, health care providers whether or not racial/ethnic minorities may not recognize expressions of prejudice in their own behavior.

Health care providers' diagnostic and treatment decisions may be influenced by their patient's race/ethnicity. For instance, Schulman et al. (1999) found that physicians referred White male, Black male, and White female hypothetical "patients" for cardiac catheterization at the same rates (approximately 90% for each group), but were significantly less likely to recommend catheterization procedures for Black female patients exhibiting the same symptoms. Minority patients also report a higher perception of racial discrimination in health care than nonminorities (LaVeist, Nickerson, & Bowie, 2000). Although providers may not deliberately provide inequitable care to minorities, several characteristics of the clinical encounter may contribute to these inequities. Providers may make medical decisions under time and resource constraints and with limited information. Time constraints may hamper a provider's ability to accurately assess symptoms of patients when cultural or linguistic barriers exist.

The fragmented nature of the health care system and deficiencies in the availability of culturally appropriate services inevitably contribute to and exacerbate health disparities in minorities. Language barriers pose a problem for the foreign-born in health care systems that lack resources, knowledge, and institutional priority to provide adequate translation services. This is particularly relevant as 41% of Americans have limited English proficiency and 20% of Spanish-speaking Latinos do not seek care due to language barriers (Zong & Batalova, 2015). The lack of or limited navigation services for underserved communities may have a differential impact on racial and ethnic minorities. Moreover, the geographic distribution and access to convenient community-based centers may influence the quality of care ethnic minorities receive, regardless of insurance status.

SUCCESSFUL STRATEGIES TO REDUCE HYPERTENSION AND HEALTH DISPARITIES IN COMMUNITIES

From the 1970s until recently, most federal and professional society initiatives to test models of care and effective treatment for HTN focused on the doctor–patient dyad. A series of national reports issued by the National Heart, Lung, and Blood Institute's National High Blood Pressure Program's Joint National Committees provided guidelines on diagnosis, evaluation, and treatment. These guidelines were written by predominantly physician groups and were based on data from large national multisite trials that tested both lifestyle and medication interventions to lower blood pressure (BP) and on expert opinion. Little, if any attention, was paid to social determinants of health, patient self-care, nonphysician providers, and support systems for ambulatory care management. In the meantime, studies were funded by National Institutes of Health (NIH) to reach out to communities to find and care for individuals with HTN who were not in care or not remaining in care. The findings from these studies increased understanding of psychosocial and behavioral factors in ethnic and racial minority communities that influenced entering and remaining in HTN care. Further, intervention trials of nonpharmacological treatment increased knowledge of cultural and behavioral aspects of CVD risk factors, care, and control. Strategies demonstrated by nursing research to be successful include: community-based participatory research (CBPR), patient-centered care, and new team-based care delivery models incorporating nonphysician providers such as nurses, pharmacists, and community health workers (CHWs). A combination of these strategies was utilized in the studies described in the rest of this chapter.

Exemplars of Nurse-Led Research to Reduce the Hypertension Quality Gap and Disparities

Nurses have been involved in the conduct of clinic and community-based research to improve the HTN quality gap and reduce ethnic disparities in HTN outcomes dating as far back as 1950 (Frant & Groen, 1950). Nurses' roles and contributions to research have since evolved, with nurse scientists leading research teams to examine social, cultural, economic, and behavioral determinants of HTN outcomes and barriers to BP control. In what follows, we highlight studies that exemplify nurses' roles in leading research to reduce HTN and health disparities and influence health policy.

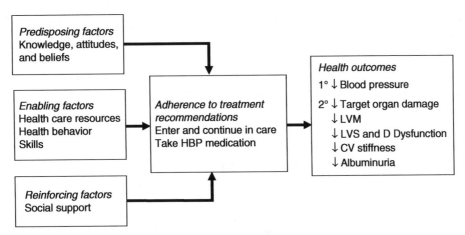

FIGURE 14.1 Conceptual framework from Hill et al. (1999) with main study variables illustrating the relationship of predisposing, enabling, and reinforcing factors to adherence to treatment recommendations and to health outcomes.

CV, cardiovascular; D, diastolic; HBP, high blood pressure; LVM, left ventricular mass; LVS, left ventricular systolic.

Source: Hill et al. (1999). With permission of Oxford University Press.

The series of studies conducted by Hill, Bone, Levine, Dennison, and colleagues, known as The Young Black Male High Blood Pressure Studies, integrated numerous strategies in consecutive clinical trials supported by the National Institute of Nursing Research (NINR). The studies were based on a modification of the Kreuter and Green PRECEDE–PROCEED Model (Green & Kreuter, 2005). See Figure 14.1 for the model that facilitated research examining and addressing determinants of BP control among this high-risk population (Hill et al., 1999; M. T. Kim, Hill, Bone, & Levine, 2000). This model was adapted for subsequent related studies.

The Comprehensive High Blood Pressure Care and Control in Young Urban Black Men Study (Dennison, Post, et al., 2007; Hill et al., 1999, 2003) was a nurse-led, 5-year randomized controlled trial (RCT) of hypertensive urban African American men (*N* = 309). This trial evaluated the effectiveness of a more intensive comprehensive educational–behavioral–pharmacological intervention delivered by a nurse practitioner/community health worker/physician (NP/CHW/MD) team and a less intensive education and referral intervention in controlling BP and minimizing progression of left ventricular hypertrophy (LVH) and renal insufficiency. At the 36-month follow-up, the more intensive intervention resulted in lower BP and decreased progression of LVH. At 5 years, with 91% of the original cohort accounted for, LVH prevalence in the more intensive group was lower compared to the less intensive group (37% vs. 56%, *p* = .02; Dennison, Post, et al., 2007). This study demonstrated that addressing social determinants of BP control, such as providing free medications, and utilizing a multifaceted, individually tailored and multidisciplinary team, is critical in improving BP control.

The HiHi Study (Dennison, Peer, Steyn, Levitt, & Hill, 2007), led by Hill, Dennison, and South African colleagues, was a cross-sectional descriptive study (*N* = 403) of peri-urban Black South Africans, which examined social, behavioral, and physiological factors influencing HTN care and control as a guide to planning for a subsequent community-based intervention trial. With the modified PRECEDE–PROCEED Model (Green & Kreuter, 2005) used in the Baltimore studies as the guiding framework, significant determinants of BP control included fewer anti-hypertensive medications, better compliance to HTN recommendations, younger age, female, higher education, and moderate alcohol consumption (Dennison, Peer, Steyn, et al., 2007). Patient-, provider-, and system-level interventions were identified as important areas to address to reduce HTN disparities in primary health care settings in poor Black South African communities.

As the success of these integrated strategies became evident in the young urban Black male population, Kim, Han, et al. adapted these strategies for a series of studies in a Korean American population. Using a CBPR approach, the Self-Help Intervention Program for High Blood Pressure Care (SHIP-HBP; M. T. Kim et al., 2011; M. T. Kim, Han, Park, Lee, & Kim, 2006) was a 15-month trial ($N = 359$) that consisted of 6-week behavioral education, home telemonitoring of BP, and a 12-month bilingual nurse telephone counseling among Korean immigrants. Evidence-based HTN treatment guidelines and behavioral recommendations were adapted into more culturally relevant education materials for the participants. The intervention resulted in a sharp increase in BP control rates, which was sustained over 12 months. Baseline BP control improved from 30% to 73% after 3 months and this level of control was sustained after 12 months of follow-up (83.2%, $p < .001$).

At the beginning of their program of research, Hill, Bone, and colleagues developed the Hill–Bone Compliance to High Blood Pressure Therapy Scale (M. T. Kim et al., 2000). The 14-item Hill–Bone Compliance Scale assesses patient behaviors for three important behavioral domains of HTN treatment: (a) reduced sodium intake; (b) appointment keeping; and (c) medication taking. The instrument is well validated, with strong evidence for internal consistency and strong positive evidence for reliability, structural validity, hypothesis testing, and criterion validity. It has been translated, culturally adapted, and validated for use in numerous populations and languages, including African Americans in East Baltimore, Korean Americans (Song et al., 2011) in urban and suburban Maryland, and the primary care setting in Portugal (Nogueira-Silva et al., 2016) and South Africa (Dennison, Peer, Lombard, et al., 2007; Dennison, Peer, Steyn, et al., 2007; Lambert et al., 2006). Today, this scale is one of the most frequently used tools assessing self-reported adherence to HTN therapy (C. J. Kim et al., 2016).

One of the key principles of HTN and chronic disease management is the use of multidisciplinary teams, which consist of a variety of health professionals synergistically using their respective skills to improve patient care. The COACH trial (Allen et al., 2011), led by Allen, Dennison, Hill, and colleagues, was a community-based RCT ($N = 525$) examining the effectiveness of a comprehensive program of CVD risk reduction delivered by NP/CHW teams versus enhanced usual care (EUC) to improve BP, lipids, and glycated hemoglobin, in socioeconomically disadvantaged patients in urban community health centers. The NP/CHW intervention included aggressive pharmacological management, tailored low-literacy educational materials, and behavioral counseling for lifestyle modification and problem solving to address barriers to adherence and control. A significantly greater improvement in systolic BP (difference, 6.2 mmHg), diastolic BP (difference, 3.1 mmHg), and perceptions of the quality of chronic illness care was observed in the NP/CHW intervention as compared to the EUC intervention.

To address the common barriers to BP control and self-management, Artinian et al. (2007) designed a nurse-managed BP telemonitoring trial among community-dwelling African Americans. The intervention consisted of weekly telecounseling, self-monitoring of BP, and weekly telecommunication with an intervention nurse. The intervention group experienced both clinically and statistically significant reduction in systolic BP (13.0 mmHg) and clinically significant reduction in diastolic BP (6.3 mmHg) after the 12-month follow-up period.

Key features of these effective nurse-led HTN care models include a team-based approach, using nurses, NPs, and CHWs, that is patient-centered; care tailored to meet patients' needs; a multifaceted approach with systems support for clinical decision making (e.g., treatment algorithms); and patient self-management. Several of these trials employed CBPR methods to include members of the target community in the design of the interventions and in the development of evaluation tools, identification of study participants, and dissemination of study findings to the community. The culturally sensitive and tailored intervention strategies in these nurse-led studies have been demonstrated to be effective in improving HTN care and reducing health disparities by addressing common patient-, provider-, community-, and system-level barriers to care. This body of research has had substantive impact on HTN-related health policy, though critical challenges remain. In the next section, we address how nursing research has supported policy to further improve HTN care and outcomes.

SHAPING POLICY TO REDUCE HYPERTENSION AND HEALTH DISPARITIES IN COMMUNITIES

Today around the globe, particularly in underserved low- and middle-income countries, as the numbers of people with HTN and attention to NCDs increase, the role of nurses in leading multidisciplinary HTN research, policy, and practice advances continues to expand (Dennison Himmelfarb, Commodore-Mensah, & Hill, 2016). The research described earlier and related research have been broadly peer-reviewed and disseminated to audiences of fellow scientists and clinicians, in addition to policy makers. Thus, the science has been debated prior to informing further scientific endeavors and informing consensus on recommendations for policy and practice. Despite obstacles and processes that often are neither linear nor logical, nurse scientists have been successful in influencing HTN policy processes through agenda setting, evidence-based consensus development and decision making, to implementation and evaluation. These nurse scientists maximized the impact of their research by attracting the interest of policy makers and clinicians and utilizing their rigorous science. The irrefutable evidence from their trials convinced these audiences that new policies and different approaches were valuable. These nurse scientists also fostered the behavioral changes necessary to put the new policies into practice. Achieving this has been possible because of active participation in networks, professional societies, and government committees, through which research findings and concepts circulate and are gradually filtered. Think tanks, advocacy coalitions, policy streams, policy communities, and national and regional networks are frequently cited as being important in this regard (Committee on Public Health Priorities to Reduce and Control Hypertension in the U.S. Population, Board on Population Health and Public Health Practice, & Institute of Medicine, 2010). To that end, nurse scientists have provided thoughtful leadership in nursing and interprofessional organizations such as the American College of Cardiology, American Heart Association, American Nurses Association, American Society of Hypertension, International Society of Hypertension in Blacks, and the Preventive Cardiovascular Nurses Association and state and national organizations, among others, to influence evidence-based practice and policy.

Research-based evidence has contributed to policies and practices that have had dramatic impact on peoples' lives. This body of evidence demonstrates the value and impact of nurse-led and team-based strategies including CHWs, telemonitoring, and systems support for clinical decision making in community-based efforts on improvements in HTN care and reduction in disparities. The disseminated methods and findings provide guidance and resources for implementing recommendations to integrate nurse-led and team-based strategies to improve HTN care. Policy advocates use the evidence and resources to advance policy. For example, state and federal legislative action has supported comprehensive polices to build capacity for an integrated and sustainable CHW workforce in the public health arena and state health departments have made progress with establishing CHW programs (Brownstein et al., 2005; Centers for Disease Control and Prevention [CDC], 2015). Further integration of this body of evidence into policy and practice is seen in the American Nurses Association *Cardiovascular Nursing: Scope and Standards of Practice* (Handberg et al., 2015); numerous scientific statements (Brush et al., 2015); clinical guidelines (James et al., 2014); and state and national programs (Bartolome, Chen, Handler, Platt, & Gould, 2016), such as Million Hearts® (Dennison Himmelfarb & Hayman, 2013; Melnyk et al., 2016).

Numerous challenges remain as we endeavor to further reduce HTN disparities. Availability of preventive care and well-trained HTN care teams are needed to manage higher patient volumes through population-based approaches as provided for in the Affordable Care Act. Reimbursement models for team-based care and home monitoring that are outcomes-based and community-based, not visit-based, and other strategies to ensure alignment of incentives are needed (Dennison & Hughes, 2009). It is abundantly clear that further improvements in HTN outcomes and disparities will require policy that supports research funding and health care reimbursement based upon innovative new models for HTN care delivery.

CONCLUSION

Nurse scientists have led rigorous research to improve HTN care quality and reduce disparities by holistically examining social, cultural, economic, and behavioral and medical determinants of HTN outcomes and designing culturally sensitive interventions focused on addressing these factors. These intervention studies have generated evidence that has shaped HTN-related policy and practice over almost two decades.

REFERENCES

Agency for Healthcare Research and Quality. (2014). *National healthcare disparities report.* (AHRQ Publication No. 14-0006). Rockville, MD: Author.

Allen, J. K., Dennison Himmelfarb, C. R., Szanton, S. L., Bone, L., Hill, M. N., Levine, D. M., & Anderson, K. (2011). Community Outreach and Cardiovascular Health (COACH) trial: A randomized, controlled trial of nurse practitioner/community health worker cardiovascular disease risk reduction in urban community health centers. *Circulation Cardiovascular Quality and Outcomes, 4*(6), 595–602. doi:10.1161/CIRCOUTCOMES.111.961573

Artinian, N. T., Flack, J. M., Nordstrom, C. K., Hockman, E. M., Washington, O. G., Jen, K.-L. C, & Fathy, M. (2007). Effects of nurse-managed telemonitoring on blood pressure at 12-month follow-up among urban African Americans. *Nursing Research, 56*(5), 312–322. doi:10.1097/01.NNR.0000289501.45284.6e

Artinian, N. T., Fletcher, G. F., Mozaffarian, D., Kris-Etherton, P., Van Horn, L., Lichtenstein, A. H., . . . American Heart Association Prevention Committee of the Council on Cardiovascular Nursing. (2010). Interventions to promote physical activity and dietary lifestyle changes for cardiovascular risk factor reduction in adults: A scientific statement from the American Heart Association. *Circulation, 122*(4), 406–441. doi:10.1161/CIR.0b013e3181e8edf1

Barnett, A. H. (1994). Diabetes and hypertension. *British Medical Bulletin, 50*(2), 397–407.

Bartolome, R. E., Chen, A., Handler, J., Platt, S. T., & Gould, B. (2016). Population care management and team-based approach to reduce racial disparities among African Americans/blacks with hypertension. *The Permanente Journal, 20*(1), 53–59. doi:10.7812/TPP/15-052

Bloom, D. E., Cafiero, E. T., Jané-Llopis, E., Abrahams-Gessel, S., Bloom, L. R., Fathima, S., . . . Weinstein, C. (2011). *The global economic burden of noncommunicable diseases* (No. 2016). Geneva, Switzerland: World Economic Forum.

Brownstein, J. N., Bone, L. R., Dennison, C. R., Hill, M. N., Kim, M. T., & Levine, D. M. (2005). Community health workers as interventionists in the prevention and control of heart disease and stroke. *American Journal of Preventive Medicine, 29*(5 Suppl. 1), 128–133. doi:10.1016/j.amepre.2005.07.024

Brush, J. E., Jr., Handberg, E. M., Biga, C., Birtcher, K. K., Bove, A. A., Casale, P. N., . . . Wyman, J. F. (2015). 2015 ACC health policy statement on cardiovascular team-based care and the role of advanced practice providers. *Journal of the American College of Cardiology, 65*(19), 2118–2136. doi:10.1016/j.jacc.2015.03.550

Centers for Disease Control and Prevention. (2012). Vital signs: Awareness and treatment of uncontrolled hypertension among adults: United States, 2003–2010. *Morbidity and Mortality Weekly Report, 61*(35), 703–709.

Centers for Disease Control and Prevention. (2014). NCHS FastStats: Deaths and mortality. Retrieved from http://www.cdc.gov/nchs/fastats/deaths.htm

Centers for Disease Control and Prevention. (2015). *Addressing chronic disease through community health workers: A policy and systems-level approach.* Atlanta, GA: Author.

Chobanian, A. V., Bakris, G. L., Black, H. R., Cushman, W. C., Green, L. A., Izzo, J. L., Jr., . . . National High Blood Pressure Education Program Coordinating Committee. (2003). The seventh report of the Joint National Committee on prevention, detection, evaluation, and treatment of high blood pressure: The JNC 7 report. *JAMA, 289*(19), 2560–2572. doi:10.1001/jama.289.19.2560

Cogswell, M. E., Zhang, Z., Carriquiry, A. L., Gunn, J. P., Kuklina, E. V., Saydah, S. H., . . . Moshfegh, A. J. (2012). Sodium and potassium intakes among US adults: NHANES 2003–2008. *American Journal of Clinical Nutrition, 96*(3), 647–657. doi:10.3945/ajcn.112.034413

Committee on Public Health Priorities to Reduce and Control Hypertension in the U.S. Population, Board on Population Health and Public Health Practice, & Institute of Medicine. (2010). Implementing a population-based policy and systems approach to the prevention and control of hypertension. In *A population-based policy and systems change approach to prevent and control hypertension* (pp. 175–197). Washington, DC: National Academies Press. doi:10.17226/12819

Commodore-Mensah, Y., & Himmelfarb, C. R. (2012). Patient education strategies for hospitalized cardiovascular patients: A systematic review. *Journal of Cardiovascular Nursing, 27*(2), 154–174. doi:10.1097/JCN.0b013e318239f60f

Davis, K. (2013). Expenditures for hypertension among adults age 18 and older, 2010: Estimates for the U.S. civilian noninstitutionalized population. Retrieved from https://meps.ahrq.gov/data_files/publications/st404/stat404.shtml

Dennison, C. R., & Hughes, S. (2009). Reforming cardiovascular care: Quality measurement and improvement, and pay-for-performance. *Journal of Cardiovascular Nursing, 24*(5), 341–343. doi:10.1097/JCN.0b013e3181b4346e

Dennison, C. R., Peer, N., Lombard, C. J., Kepe, L., Levitt, N. S., Steyn, K., & Hill, M. N. (2007). Cardiovascular risk and comorbid conditions among black South Africans with hypertension in public and private primary care settings: The HIHI study. *Ethnicity & Disease, 17*(3), 477–483.

Dennison, C. R., Peer, N., Steyn, K., Levitt, N. S., & Hill, M. N. (2007). Determinants of hypertension care and control among peri-urban black South Africans: The HIHI study. *Ethnicity & Disease, 17*(3), 484–491.

Dennison, C. R., Post, W. S., Kim, M. T., Bone, L. R., Cohen, D., Blumenthal, R. S., . . . Hill, M. N. (2007). Underserved urban African American men: Hypertension trial outcomes and mortality during 5 years. *American Journal of Hypertension, 20*(2), 164–171. doi:10.1016/j.amjhyper.2006.08.003

Dennison Himmelfarb, C. R., Commodore-Mensah, Y., & Hill, M. N. (2016). Expanding the role of nurses to improve hypertension care and control globally. *Annals of Global Health, 82*(2), 243–253. doi:10.1016/j.aogh.2016.02.003

Dennison Himmelfarb, C. R., & Hayman, L. L. (2013). Calling all cardiovascular nurses: Be one in a million hearts: Million Hearts initiative. *Journal of Cardiovascular Nursing, 28*(2), 103–105. doi:10.1097/JCN.0b013e3182819dcc

Exner, D. V., Dries, D. L., Domanski, M. J., & Cohn, J. N. (2001). Lesser response to angiotensin-converting-enzyme inhibitor therapy in black as compared with white patients with left ventricular dysfunction. *New England Journal of Medicine, 344*(18), 1351–1357. doi:10.1056/nejm200105033441802

Frant, R., & Groen, J. (1950). Prognosis of vascular hypertension: A 9-year follow-up study of 418 cases. *Archives of Internal Medicine (Chicago, Ill.: 1908), 85*(5), 727–750.

Fryar, C. D., Chen, T., & Li, X. (2012). Prevalence of uncontrolled risk factors for cardiovascular disease: United States, 1999–2010. Retrieved from http://www.cdc.gov/nchs/products/databriefs/db103.htm

Gerteis, J., Izrael, D., Deitz, D., LeRoy, L., Ricciardi, R., Miller, T., & Basu, J. (2014). *Multiple chronic conditions chartbook* (AHRQ Publication No. Q14-0038). Rockville, MD: Agency for Healthcare Research and Quality.

Green, L. W., & Kreuter, M. W. (Eds.). (2005). *Health promotion planning: An educational and ecological approach* (4th ed.). New York, NY: McGraw-Hill.

Handberg, E., Arslanian-Engoren, C., Baas, L., Dennison Himmelfarb, C., Gura, M. T., Klein, D., . . . Zarling, K. K. (2015). *Cardiovascular nursing: Scope and standards of practice* (2nd ed.). Silver Spring, MD: American Nurses Association.

Heidenreich, P. A., Trogdon, J. G., Khavjou, O. A., Butler, J., Dracup, K., Ezekowitz, M. D., . . . Council on Cardiovascular Surgery and Anesthesia, and Interdisciplinary Council on Quality of Care and Outcomes Research. (2011). Forecasting the future of cardiovascular disease in the United States: A policy statement from the American Heart Association. *Circulation, 123*(8), 933–944. doi:10.1161/CIR.0b013e31820a55f5

Herholz, H., Goff, D. C., Ramsey, D. J., Chan, F. A., Ortiz, C., Labarthe, D. R., & Nichaman, M. Z. (1996). Women and Mexican Americans receive fewer cardiovascular drugs following myocardial infarction than men and non-Hispanic whites: The Corpus Christi heart project, 1988–1990. *Journal of Clinical Epidemiology, 49*(3), 279–287. doi:10.1016/0895-4356(95)00572-2

Hill, M. N., Bone, L. R., Hilton, S. C., Roary, M. C., Kelen, G. D., & Levine, D. M. (1999). A clinical trial to improve high blood pressure care in young urban black men: Recruitment, follow-up, and outcomes. *American Journal of Hypertension, 12*(6), 548–554.

Hill, M. N., Bone, L. R., Kim, M. T., Miller, D. J., Dennison, C. R., & Levine, D. M. (1999). Barriers to hypertension care and control in young urban black men. *American Journal of Hypertension, 12*(10 Pt. 1), 951–958. doi:10.1016/s0895-7061(99)00121-1

Hill, M. N., Han, H. R., Dennison, C. R., Kim, M. T., Roary, M. C., Blumenthal, R. S., . . . Post, W. S. (2003). Hypertension care and control in underserved urban African American men: Behavioral and physiologic outcomes at 36 months. *American Journal of Hypertension, 16*(11 Pt. 1), 906–913. doi:10.1016/s0895-7061(03)01034-3

Institute of Medicine (U.S.) Committee on Understanding and Eliminating Racial and Ethnic Disparities in Health Care. (2003). *Unequal treatment: Confronting racial and ethnic disparities in health care*. Washington, DC: National Academies Press.

James, P. A., Oparil, S., Carter, B. L., Cushman, W. C., Dennison Himmelfarb, C., Handler, J., . . . Ortiz, E. (2014). 2014 evidence-based guideline for the management of high blood pressure in adults: Report from the panel members appointed to the eighth joint national committee (JNC 8). *JAMA, 311*(5), 507–520. doi:10.1001/jama.2013.284427

Kavey, R. E., Daniels, S. R., Lauer, R. M., Atkins, D. L., Hayman, L. L., Taubert, K., & American Heart Association. (2003). American Heart Association guidelines for primary prevention of atherosclerotic cardiovascular disease beginning in childhood. *Circulation, 107*(11), 1562–1566.

Kim, C. J., Schlenk, E. A., Ahn, J. A., Kim, M., Park, E., & Park, J. (2016). Evaluation of the measurement properties of self-reported medication adherence instruments among people at risk for metabolic syndrome: A systematic review. *Diabetes Educator, 42*(5), 618–634. doi:10.1177/0145721716655400

Kim, M. T., Han, H. R., Hedlin, H., Kim, J., Song, H. J., Kim, K. B., & Hill, M. N. (2011). Teletransmitted monitoring of blood pressure and bilingual nurse counseling-sustained improvements in blood pressure control during 12 months in hypertensive Korean Americans. *Journal of Clinical Hypertension, 13*(8), 605–612. doi:10.1111/j.1751-7176.2011.00479.x

Kim, M. T., Han, H. R., Park, H. J., Lee, H., & Kim, K. B. (2006). Constructing and testing a self-help intervention program for high blood pressure control in Korean American seniors: A pilot study. *Journal of Cardiovascular Nursing, 21*(2), 77–84. doi:10.1097/00005082-200603000-00002

Kim, M. T., Hill, M. N., Bone, L. R., & Levine, D. M. (2000). Development and testing of the Hill-Bone Compliance to High Blood Pressure Therapy scale. *Progress in Cardiovascular Nursing, 15*(3), 90–96.

Lambert, E. V., Steyn, K., Stender, S., Everage, N., Fourie, J. M., & Hill, M. (2006). Cross-cultural validation of the Hill-Bone Compliance to High Blood Pressure Therapy Scale in a South African, primary healthcare setting. *Ethnicity & Disease, 16*(1), 286–291.

LaVeist, T. A., Nickerson, K. J., & Bowie, J. V. (2000). Attitudes about racism, medical mistrust, and satisfaction with care among African American and white cardiac patients. *Medical Care Research and Review: MCRR, 57*(Suppl. 1), 146–161.

Lenfant, C. (1996). Task force on research in epidemiology and prevention of cardiovascular diseases: A revisit. *Circulation, 93*(9), 1605–1607.

Melnyk, B. M., Orsolini, L., Gawlik, K., Braun, L. T., Chyun, D. A., Conn, V. S., . . . Olin, A. R. (2016). The Million Hearts initiative: Guidelines and best practices. *Nurse Practitioner, 41*(2), 46–53; quiz 53–54. doi:10.1097/01.NPR.0000476372.04620.7a

Mitchell, J. B., & McCormack, L. A. (1997). Time trends in late-stage diagnosis of cervical cancer: Differences by race/ethnicity and income. *Medical Care, 35*(12), 1220–1224.

Mozaffarian, D., Benjamin, E. J., Go, A. S., Arnett, D. K., Blaha, M. J., Cushman, M., . . . Turner, M. B. (2016). Heart disease and stroke statistics—2016 update: A report from the American Heart Association. *Circulation, 133*(4), e38–e360. doi:10.1161/CIR.0000000000000350

Nogueira-Silva, L., Sa-Sousa, A., Lima, M. J., Monteiro, A., Dennison Himmelfarb, C., & Fonseca, J. A. (2016). Translation and cultural adaptation of the Hill-Bone Compliance to High Blood Pressure Therapy scale to Portuguese. *Revista Portuguesa de Cardiologia: Orgao Oficial da Sociedade Portuguesa de Cardiologia = Portuguese Journal of Cardiology: An Official Journal of the Portuguese Society of Cardiology, 35*(2), 93–97. doi:10.1016/j.repc.2015.07.013

Olives, C., Myerson, R., Mokdad, A. H., Murray, C. J., & Lim, S. S. (2013). Prevalence, awareness, treatment, and control of hypertension in United States counties, 2001–2009. *PLOS ONE, 8*(4), e60308. doi:10.1371/journal.pone.0060308

Ornish, D., Scherwitz, L. W., Billings, J. H., Brown, S. E., Gould, K. L., Merritt, T. A., . . . Brand, R. J. (1998). Intensive lifestyle changes for reversal of coronary heart disease. *JAMA, 280*(23), 2001–2007. doi:10.1001/jama.280.23.2001

Psaty, B. M., Smith, N. L., Siscovick, D. S., Koepsell, T. D., Weiss, N. S., Heckbert, S. R., . . . Furberg, C. D. (1997). Health outcomes associated with antihypertensive therapies used as first-line agents: A systematic review and meta-analysis. *JAMA, 277*(9), 739–745.

Ratner, R., Goldberg, R., Haffner, S., Marcovina, S., Orchard, T., Fowler, S., . . . Diabetes Prevention Program Research Group. (2005). Impact of intensive lifestyle and metformin therapy on cardiovascular disease risk factors in the diabetes prevention program. *Diabetes Care, 28*(4), 888–894. doi:10.2337/diacare.28.4.888

Schulman, K. A., Berlin, J. A., Harless, W., Kerner, J. F., Sistrunk, S., Gersh, B. J., . . . Escarce, J. J. (1999). The effect of race and sex on physicians' recommendations for cardiac catheterization. *New England Journal of Medicine, 340*(8), 618–626. doi:10.1056/NEJM199902253400806

Sedlis, S. P., Fisher, V. J., Tice, D., Esposito, R., Madmon, L., & Steinberg, E. H. (1997). Racial differences in performance of invasive cardiac procedures in a Department of Veterans Affairs medical center. *Journal of Clinical Epidemiology, 50*(8), 899–901. doi:10.1016/s0895-4356(97)00089-9

Song, Y., Han, H. R., Song, H. J., Nam, S., Nguyen, T., & Kim, M. T. (2011). Psychometric evaluation of Hill-Bone medication adherence subscale. *Asian Nursing Research, 5*(3), 183–188. doi:10.1016/j.anr.2011.09.007

SPRINT Research Group, Wright, J. T., Jr., Williamson, J. D., Whelton, P. K., Snyder, J. K., Sink, K. M., . . . Ambrosius, W. T. (2015). A randomized trial of intensive versus standard blood-pressure control. *New England Journal of Medicine, 373*(22), 2103–2116. doi:10.1056/NEJMoa1511939

Whelton, P. K., He, J., Appel, L. J., Cutler, J. A., Havas, S., Kotchen, T. A., . . . National High Blood Pressure Education Program Coordinating Committee. (2002). Primary prevention of hypertension: Clinical and public health advisory from the national high blood pressure education program. *JAMA, 288*(15), 1882–1888. doi:10.1001/jama.288.15.1882

World Health Organization. (2014). Global status report on noncommunicable diseases 2014. Retrieved from http://www.who.int/nmh/publications/ncd-status-report-2014/en

World Health Organization. (2015). Noncommunicable diseases. Retrieved from http://www .who.int/mediacentre/factsheets/fs355/en

Wood, A. J. (2001). Racial differences in the response to drugs: Pointers to genetic differences. *New England Journal of Medicine, 344*(18), 1394–1396. doi:10.1056/NEJM200105033441811

Zong, J., & Batalova, J. (2015). The limited English proficient population in the United States. Retrieved from http://www.migrationpolicy.org/article/limited-english-proficient -population-united-states

15

Chronic Illness: Promoting Cardiovascular Health in Socioeconomically Austere Rural Areas

Debra K. Moser

About 60 million Americans (20% of the population) live in rural areas, and sadly, the cardiovascular health of rural America is in crisis (Knudson, Meit, & Popat, 2014). In most rural areas of the country, particularly in the South, mortality rates, major acute cardiac event rates, and the prevalence and incidence of cardiovascular disease (CVD) and associated CVD risk factors are substantially and persistently higher than in nonrural areas (Kulshreshtha, Goyal, Dabhadkar, Veledar, & Vaccarino, 2014; McConnell et al., 2010; O'Connor & Wellenius, 2012). Although there is little intervention research in rural areas in the United States to improve cardiovascular health (Gruca, Pyo, & Nelson, 2016), there have been a few successful CVD risk reduction studies (Khare, Koch, Zimmermann, Moehring, & Geller, 2014; Tideman et al., 2014). Although initially effective in most cases, the changes at the individual level have not been maintained once the research is over, and the interventions have not been sustained locally or at the community level (Khare et al., 2014).

Failure to see a sustained effect from CVD risk reduction efforts in rural areas is common, particularly when there are no provisions by the research team for continuing an effective intervention and the support it entails. Participants often feel abandoned when researchers withdraw an intervention that has successfully engaged them (Fletcher, Burley, Thomas, & Mitchell, 2014). Such participants are less likely to maintain changes in CVD risk factors that they have made, and to participate in future studies. At times, the entire rural community develops feelings of mistrust toward researchers, to the extent that participation by the entire community in studies is decreased (Mudd-Martin et al., 2014).

For CVD risk reduction research to have any long-term effect in rural communities, clearly, its effects must be maintained after the researchers leave, and the intervention must be disseminated and used in other parts of the community, the region, the state, and even the nation. Policy changes from small local initiatives to widespread state policy implementation can have an appreciable effect on sustaining interventions from successful research projects, and ultimately reducing the marked CVD disparities seen in rural America. The purpose of this chapter is to describe a group of community-based CVD risk reduction interventions and the efforts made to sustain the intervention and its effects through a variety of policy changes. This work was (and is being) conducted in central Appalachian Kentucky, one of the most socioeconomically austere rural areas in the country with some of the most unhealthy counties. Measures of quality adjusted life expectancy (a composite measure of quality of life and mortality) put Kentucky in the bottom five of the United States based on the poor quality of life reported by residents and their shorter life expectancy (Jia, Zack, & Thompson, 2011).

APPALACHIAN KENTUCKY

Cardiovascular Health of the Region

CVD, a chronic condition, remains the number one killer of people in the United States (Mozaffarian et al., 2016; Roger et al., 2012), but there are marked disparities in CVD and CVD risk factor prevalence throughout the nation (Appalachian Regional Commission, 2016; Chowdhury et al., 2016; Go et al., 2013; Liburd, Giles, & Mensah, 2006; Mensah, Mokdad, Ford, Greenlund, & Croft, 2005). Individuals who reside in rural areas have disproportionately higher rates of CVD risk factors, CVD, and CVD mortality (Kulshreshtha et al., 2014; McConnell et al., 2010; O'Connor & Wellenius, 2012; United States Census Bureau, n.d.). Rural Appalachia has higher rates of heart disease mortality than any other area of the nation for all race/ethnicities, both genders, and all age groups (Halverson, Barnett, & Casper, 2002). Of all of Appalachia, Appalachian Kentucky has the worst cardiovascular health in the 13-state Appalachian region, and has a long legacy of substantial, unaddressed CVD health disparities (City-Data.Com, 2014; Kentucky Institute of Medicine, 2007).

The Kentucky Institute of Medicine provides objective data about risk factors and disease outcomes at the county level, which is heavily weighted by CVD risk factors and mortality. Of the 120 counties in Kentucky, the 15 least healthy counties in the state are located in the Appalachian region of Kentucky, and the county with the worst mortality rate in the entire nation is in this region.

Distressed rural environments are characterized by poor access to preventive health care, inadequate insurance, persistent poverty, and low educational attainment, along with reduced access to healthy foods and areas in which to engage in physical activity, all of which contribute to CVD health disparities (Amarasinghe, D'Souza, Brown, Oh, & Borisova, 2009; Halverson & Bischak, 2008, 2010, 2012; Barker et al., 2010). Appalachian Kentucky is noted for having the worst socioeconomic and health conditions in the United States (Appalachian Community Fund, 2014). High rates of persistent poverty and unemployment, low educational level, poor access to health care, and high rates of un- or underinsured individuals are characteristic of the region even after the Affordable Care Act (Kentucky Institute of Medicine, 2007; United States Department of Agriculture [USDA], 2012). Other factors in the community social environment and infrastructure, such as lack of public transportation, food deserts, limited community services, and shortages of health care providers, further exacerbate the health challenges and set the stage for extremely poor cardiovascular health (Kentucky Institute of Medicine, 2007).

Persistent Poverty

Twenty-nine of the 100 poorest and most distressed counties in all of America are in Kentucky. "Distressed" refers to the lowest 10% of the nation's counties in terms of unemployment, per capita income, and poverty. For fiscal year 2012, 41 counties in Appalachian Kentucky were classified as economically distressed (rated on a scale ranging from the best = "attainment," next best = "competitive," followed by "transitional," then "at risk," and the worst = "distressed"), 7 are "at risk," and the remainder are "transitional" (Appalachian Regional Commission, 2012). No county in Appalachian Kentucky was "attainment" or "competitive." Almost half of the distressed counties in all of the 13-state region that contains Appalachia are in Eastern Kentucky (Appalachian Regional Commission, 2012). In addition, they are designated as persistent-poverty counties by the USDA based on the presence of poverty in more than 20% of the residents in the past four censuses (Appalachian Regional Commission, 2008; USDA, 2012). Poor socioeconomic status is associated with high rates of CVD risk factors and CVD (Amarasinghe, D'Souza, Brown, Oh, & Borisova, 2009; Appalachian Regional Commission, 2008; Borak, Salipante-Zaidel, Slade, & Fields, 2012; Liburd et al., 2006; Shaw, Theis, Self-Brown, Roblin, & Barker, 2016), and distressed counties have higher rates of heart disease mortality than nondistressed (Appalachian Regional Commission, 2008; Halverson et al., 2002; Mensah et al., 2005).

Low Educational Attainment

Appalachian Kentucky is ranked 50th (worst) with regard to the number of illiterate adults and has the lowest rates of educational attainment in America (Appalachian Regional Commission, 2016). Low educational attainment contributes to the austerity of resources in this area. Within rural Kentucky, 51.9% of the working-age population met criteria for low literacy, compared to the state rate of 38%. Low levels of education are (a) a risk factor for CVD, (b) associated with a higher risk for all modifiable CVD risk factors (Strand & Tverdal, 2004, 2006), and (c) associated with poorer uptake of CVD-reducing recommendations (Strand & Tverdal, 2006).

Poor Access to Health Care

In Appalachian Kentucky, 50% of counties have only one hospital and 20% have none. The areas targeted by our projects are rural, low-income counties defined as medically underserved areas and/or federally designated health professions shortage areas. Many counties have no health care providers, and most have fewer than half the rate of what is considered acceptable (Kentucky Institute of Medicine, 2007). About 28% of Appalachian Kentucky report that cost is a barrier to health care, compared to 12.8% nationwide (Hacker, 2008). High numbers of residents in Appalachian Kentucky (38.4%, the highest rate in Kentucky) report fair or poor health, no visit to a health professional in the prior year, and no confidence in getting needed health care services (Hacker, 2008). In Appalachian Kentucky, 15% to 21% of individuals lack health care coverage, while another 35% of the Appalachian Kentucky population have Medicare (Social Security Administration, 2014). At least 80% of counties experience service shortages. Lack of health insurance is associated with lower use of preventive services and higher rates of hospitalization for CVD.

Cardiovascular Disease Health Disparities

Appalachian Kentucky is in the "heart and stroke belt" of the United States, so named because of the disproportionately higher rates of heart disease and stroke, and related risk factors (Appalachian Regional Commission, 2008; Department for Public Health, 2014; Keyserling et al., 2016). It has the highest number of heart disease related deaths in the state, with an age-adjusted rate double that of that state overall (Kentucky Institute of Medicine, 2007). About 7.8% to 8.6% (depending on county) of Appalachian Kentucky adults report having coronary heart disease compared to 4.2% nationwide; 7.7% to 10.1% report having had a heart attack compared to 4.4% nationwide (Department for Public Health, 2014; Hacker, 2008). Appalachian Kentucky is in the top first percentile for poor CVD outcomes (Kentucky Department of Public Health, 2009; Kulshreshtha et al., 2014; Lloyd-Jones et al., 2009; Writing Group Members et al., 2016).

The Kentucky Behavioral Risk Factor Surveillance System (BRFSS) and others have noted disproportionately high levels of CVD risk factors in Kentucky and a substantially higher level of multiple CVD comorbidities (Rugg, Bailey, & Browning, 2008). About 44% of Appalachian adults report having high cholesterol levels (Department for Public Health, 2014; Hacker, 2008). People in Appalachian Kentucky report the highest rates of activity limitations due to health problems (Department for Public Health, 2014). About 81% of adults in the area report eating less than five fruits and vegetables per day, and 70.5% do not receive the recommended amount of moderate physical activity per week, while the obesity rate in the area has skyrocketed and more than 71% of adults are overweight or obese (Department for Public Health, 2014).

To summarize, rural Appalachian Kentucky residents face enormous health challenges. Life in these underserved and economically distressed environments contributes to marked CVD health disparities. These rural areas are among the highest for prevalence of multiple CVD risk factors in the 50 states. Given the bleak economic situation in these areas, preventative cardiovascular care has not been a priority. Prevention of CVD, however, must be integrated into these rural communities to improve the CVD risk profile of the population and to reduce the incidence of CVD.

IMPROVING THE CARDIOVASCULAR HEALTH OF APPALACHIA

Improving Cardiovascular Disease Outcomes

Implementation of lifestyle CVD risk factor reduction interventions is effective in reducing CVD risk (Appel et al., 2003, 2006; Kottke et al., 2009; L. F. Lien et al., 2007; Lin et al., 2007; Maruthur, Wang, & Appel, 2009; Mensah & Brown, 2007; Stampfer, Hu, Manson, Rimm, & Willett, 2000; Yusuf et al., 2004). In a groundbreaking study, the INTERHEART investigators demonstrated that nine preventable risk factors explained 90% and 94% of the incidence of myocardial infarction in men and women, respectively, independent of age or culture (Yusuf et al., 2004). Simply improving three risk factors led to an 80% reduction in risk of a cardiac event. These results were similar to those from the Nurses' Health Study, which demonstrated in a prospective cohort study that 75% of the risk for myocardial infarction or stroke would be removed by adherence to lifestyle guidelines (Stampfer et al., 2000). Others have provided equally compelling data demonstrating the power of lifestyle risk modification to prevent events versus "perfect" treatment of a person after an event has occurred (Kottke et al., 2009). Management of CVD risk factors before an event could prevent or postpone 33% of deaths, compared to prevention of only 8% of deaths if "perfect care" was used during an acute event. These data provide strong support for the importance of lifestyle change (i.e., CVD risk factor management) in preventing CVD and further events.

Despite the evidence that lifestyle interventions to reduce CVD risk are successful, they are not widely used in clinical practice, and their use is extremely rare in distressed, underserved rural areas. Moreover, we (Bentley, De Jong, Moser, & Peden, 2005; Dekker, Moser, Peden, & Lennie, 2012; Welsh et al., 2012; Wu, Corley, Lennie, & Moser, 2012) and others (Au et al., 2010; Schoenberg, Bardach, Manchikanti, & Goodenow, 2011) have shown that lifestyle interventions must take into account the unique needs and strengths of individuals being targeted to be effective, must consider the limitations imposed by the environment, and must have a self-care focus in order for individuals to be able to maintain change.

In developing and testing an intervention to target a specific population, particularly one with marked health disparities, it is crucial to develop an intervention relevant to the individuals and community being targeted. Although this seems obvious, it is common for clinicians and investigators to impose interventions or strategies without input from the targeted population. Moreover, for an intervention to be sustained it is critical that buy-in be received from the community before beginning a CVD risk reduction program.

Our investigative team used community-engaged research principles to develop, test, evaluate, disseminate, and sustain our intervention: the HeartHealth intervention. These principles include developing strong community–academic partnerships, engendering equitable power and responsibility for community members, working on capacity building, and developing effective dissemination of plans (Ahmed & Palermo, 2010). In introductory work, we assembled a community advisory board, and conducted multiple focus groups that consisted of local lay people, health care providers, and community leaders to identify strengths and barriers that required attention in order to make the intervention appropriate for the population, and to address the relevant barriers to self-care (Mudd-Martin et al., 2014).

Rural Strengths and Barriers to CVD Risk Reduction

In addition to the factors outlined earlier (poverty, low education, lack of access to health care), there are other environmental barriers to CVD risk reduction in rural, distressed areas that we considered in developing the HeartHealth intervention. With regard to the environment, rural Appalachian Kentucky has multiple "food deserts," areas where affordable, fresh, healthy food is not available (Beaulac, Kristjansson, & Cummins, 2009; The Conservation Fund, 2014; Thomson, 2011). Food deserts and poverty go hand in hand, and contribute to the negative CVD risk profile in these rural areas (Beaulac et al., 2009; The Conservation Fund, 2014; Thomson, 2011). Participants in our focus groups stated that it was often difficult to obtain fresh fruit and vegetables or healthier food options given the lack of easily accessible markets that carried such items. Another environmental concern is lack of access to safe places to exercise. Participants in our focus groups stated this concern, and the concern that the changing job situation (move from physically demanding coal mining, logging, and agricultural jobs to service jobs) has produced a sedentary generation. These themes are mirrored in studies by others (Schoenberg et al., 2011; Schoenberg, Hatcher, & Dignan, 2008).

Community members in our focus groups were concerned about their own cardiovascular health and the cardiovascular health of the entire community (Mudd-Martin et al., 2014). Improving CVD risk was a major priority. A common theme expressed to us was growing concern for the health of the community after participants heard in news reports that rural Kentuckians were the most obese, inactive, and unhealthy group in the nation. Accompanying this concern was anxiety over the seemingly overwhelming nature of the problem and lack of knowledge and resources (Mudd-Martin et al., 2014). Lack of motivation to change given a fatalistic attitude about chronic illness has been reported as a barrier to preventative behavior change (Deskins et al., 2006; Mudd-Martin et al., 2014). Preventative care has not been a priority for residents who have financial barriers to receiving health care (Deskins et al., 2006; Strickland & Strickland, 1996). Lack of knowledge about

CVD risk factors or CVD prevention has been reported by others (Deskins et al., 2006; Schoenberg et al., 2008, 2011). Thus, a self-care intervention is ideal to address these concerns.

We and others (Reilly et al., 2016) have found that a major barrier to CVD risk reduction in the area is distrust of health care providers, who are largely not from the community, and who (as stated by several participants in the focus groups), "have no idea how hard it is to change your life, who don't understand or care about this area, and who just say 'lose weight' and give no advice about how to do it." Participants in our studies and in studies by others (Koniak-Griffin et al., 2015; Reilly et al., 2016; Tian et al., 2015) who were recruited by, and received the intervention from, community health workers (also known as indigenous health workers) were highly pleased with this approach, very accepting, and became highly engaged in the studies, and the community health workers were highly effective in promoting lifestyle change.

Another important barrier to CVD risk reduction in rural areas is the high rate of poor mental health, specifically depressive symptoms. Advisory board members noted the problem of poor mental health in the community. This is an important observation because depressive symptoms (a) negatively impact behavior change (Leiferman & Pheley, 2006) and (b) are associated with development of CVD risk factors, CVD, and CVD mortality (Rozanski, Blumenthal, Davidson, Saab, & Kubzansky, 2005).

Although distressed rural areas are commonly portrayed negatively, people living in such communities have a number of strengths that position them to undertake the changes needed to improve their health. Strengths include a strong tradition of community mobilization when awareness of a local problem occurs, and the potential for "home-grown change" (Schoenberg et al., 2008). People are noted for their sense of neighborliness and concern for neighbors, friends, family, and community (Lohri-Posey, 2006; Schoenberg et al., 2008).

Advisory board and focus group members talked about their concern for the health of their community and their willingness to promote lifestyle change in themselves, their family, friends, and community, if necessary resources are available (Mudd-Martin et al., 2014). They identified heart disease as a major issue in the community to tackle. They wanted to be provided with skills and knowledge to reduce CVD risk factors and improve their well-being given the challenges in the community. Most felt that reliance on a health care provider alone to improve one's health would not be effective and that individuals must take responsibility for their own health. Given this belief, most individuals still felt that they did not have the skills or knowledge needed to properly improve their cardiovascular health. For that reason, the idea of engaging in group learning sessions that promoted self-care and "empowered" them to take charge of their health in a group environment was appealing. In developing the HeartHealth intervention, we developed components to address barriers to CVD risk reduction and to take advantage of strengths in the region.

To summarize, individuals living in socioeconomically distressed rural areas are subject to startling disparities in CVD risk factors and CVD expression. For example, Perry County (one of our target communities) in rural Appalachian Kentucky has the worst life expectancy in the entire United States, due largely to excess CVD mortality—in fact, life expectancy there is worse than in Vietnam, Russia, and many other developing countries. Despite these substantial CVD disparities, very little research has been done promoting CVD risk reduction in austere rural areas using a self-care approach to reducing multiple, comorbid CVD risk factors (Hayes, Greenlund, Denny, Croft, & Keenan, 2005).

Although the notion of self-care and its importance to chronic disease management is gaining acceptance in the United States, the reality of self-care among people with chronic conditions is bleak. We have demonstrated, in individuals with heart disease and heart failure, that the vast majority do not practice effective self-care, most providers do not teach effective self-care, and that most individuals are not aware of the need for self-care (Moser et al., 2012; Moser, Doering, & Chung, 2005; Riegel et al., 2009; Riegel, Moser, Powell, Rector, & Havranek, 2006). Our project is highly relevant to rural Kentucky because the intervention is based on promotion of effective self-care in a population with the need for multiple self-care activities (e.g., eating a heart-healthy diet, getting exercise, controlling weight, managing diabetes and hypertension, taking medications if prescribed), who must contend with poor access to health care, long distances to travel to care providers, and lack of preventative services to support CVD risk reduction efforts.

Finally, we and others have demonstrated that depressive symptoms have a substantial and negative impact on (a) self-care activities, including adherence and lifestyle behavior changes (Romanelli, Fauerbach, Bush, & Ziegelstein, 2002; Rozanski et al., 2005; Ziegelstein et al., 2000); and (b) on CVD outcomes (Doering et al., 2010; Rozanski et al., 2005; Song et al., 2010). Failure to address depressive symptoms when attempting to promote adoption of CVD risk reduction sets the stage for failure of the intervention (Jaarsma et al., 2010; McGrady, McGinnis, Badenhop, Bentle, & Rajput, 2009), yet management of depressive symptoms as part of CVD risk reduction interventions is rare. In the populations targeted, where the prevalence of depressive symptoms is high (Moriarty, Zack, Holt, Chapman, & Safran, 2009), it is essential to include management of depressive symptoms. Thus, we integrated depressive symptom management into the intervention.

Description of the HeartHealth Intervention

Based on extensive input from lay people and health care providers in the community, the prevalence of multiple CVD risk factors, the distressed nature of the environment, the barriers to CVD risk reduction, and the strengths inherent in the rural community, we designed, tested, and demonstrated the feasibility and effectiveness of the HeartHealth intervention. The HeartHealth intervention consists of group-based education and counseling delivered using principles known to promote behavior change: use of motivation interviewing; active engagement of participants during all stages of delivery; skills teaching; and individualization of strategies to each participant's specific risk factors and barriers. The intervention was delivered by community health workers extensively trained in all aspects relevant to conceptual underpinnings, delivery, content, and skills taught in the intervention. Community health workers are an integral aspect of the study, given their efficiency, acceptability by the communities, and effectiveness (Adair et al., 2012; Battaglia et al., 2012; Reynolds et al., 2012). These workers are employed from the affected areas and trained to act as liaisons for their communities. They are trusted members of the community, and have access to some of the most distressed areas, well beyond the access of researchers and clinicians. Potential participants usually are willing to take part in the study and commit to finishing once they discuss the project with community health workers.

The following six interactive modules are delivered to participants: (a) principles of self-care and CVD risk reduction; (b) nutrition (includes portion control, eating a diet high in fruits and vegetable and whole grains, reducing saturated and trans fats, reducing sodium intake, reducing total fat intake, clearing up the "good fat vs. bad fat" issue); (c) physical activity; (d) depression control and stress reduction; (e) managing multiple comorbid risk factors; and (f) smoking cessation and/or medication adherence. These modules were delivered over a 6- to 8-week period (there is variability to account for canceled sessions due to snow or other bad weather conditions) by registered nurse community health workers who were trained extensively by our team. The sessions were delivered every 2 weeks to groups of 10 people over a 2-hour period using the principles outlined in Tables 15.1 and 15.2.

TABLE 15.1 *Barriers to Successful CVD Risk Reduction in Rural Appalachia and How the HeartHealth Intervention Addresses Them*

Barriers to CVD Risk Reduction in Appalachia	HeartHealth Intervention
Poverty	Program provided free; gas cards or transportation provided to get to service; problem solving and other skills provided for managing CVD risk factors on limited income; low-literacy materials used (given the interplay of poverty and low income); materials relevant for low-income individuals; physical activity and food options for low-income individuals highlighted
Poor access to health care and lack of health insurance	Program provided free; all materials and demonstrations, including meals, are free; teaching how to engage in self-care reduces need for health care service use
Low levels of education	All materials and delivery methods adapted to address low literacy and low health literacy; materials available for those at all levels of literacy to accommodate those with lowest and highest literacy
Lack of easy access to healthy, affordable foods and safe places to exercise	Detailed walking maps and activity plans developed with each participant to accommodate environment; eating heart-healthy diet by modifying usual diet taught; introduced to markets (some unknown to individuals) and farmers' markets, and healthy eating guides relevant to the community provided
Lack of trust in researchers	Community health workers recruit, collect data, and provide the intervention; research team forms a team with local community members via advisory boards, dissemination of information to entire community about heart health and about study findings
Overwhelming nature of CVD health disparities	Self-care intervention focuses on a "whole health" approach to CVD health; single plan provided that effectively addresses all CVD risk factors (e.g., not separate "low fat" or "diabetic" or "weight loss" plans); motivational approaches provided about high effectiveness of lifestyle change

TABLE 15.2 *HeartHealth Intervention Principles and Relationship to Rural, Distressed Kentucky*

Intervention Component	Addresses CVD Disparities in Rural Kentucky	Community Appropriate	Reduces Barriers to CVD Risk Reduction	Builds on Strengths in Rural Kentucky
Recruitment to study by community workers; intervention done by team that includes local community health workers	Promotes recruitment, retention, and engagement in project of those with most severe health disparities	Increases recruitment, retention, and commitment to the intervention based on the relationship between participant and local community workers; shows respect for community	Promotes recruitment and retention of those most in need, who often do not respond to appeals from "outside" providers or researchers	Respect for local community workers who understand the region
Individualized; promotes self-care (Lorig & Holman, 2003) within the context of the distressed environment (Johnson & Lorig, 2011; Lorig, Laurent, Plant, Krishnan, & Ritter, 2014)	Directly addresses each participant's unique needs and goals; self-care fundamental to effective lifestyle change in people with multiple morbidities	Shows respect and engagement at personal level; participant not just seen as "local KY problem"; provides self-care-unique skills applicable to environment	Provides each participant the skills and knowledge needed to overcome his or her specific and unique barriers	Promotes independence and self-reliance
Motivational interviewing techniques (Brodie & Inoue, 2005; Greaves et al., 2008; Thompson et al., 2011)	Highly effective for promoting behavior change	Nonjudgmental approach driven by participant goals; demonstrates respect for participants and their prior experiences	Breaks down fatalism, denial, and lack of interest in prevention	Shows respect for participants and gives them confidence to make change
Group setting for intervention	Increased effectiveness for behavior change in this population	Provides social support, neighborliness, and opportunity to help others	Participants learn from each other how to overcome barriers	Supports sense of neighborliness
Addresses multiple risk factors	Major source of health disparities	Addresses issues of direct concern to community members	Provides solutions to barriers to reducing multiple risk factors	Community recognizes this problem and wants to work on it
Depression management	Major source of health disparities	Addresses issues of direct concern to people of this society	Depression is a major barrier to successful risk reduction	Reduction of poor mental health is a major focus of the community
Interactive	Increased adoption of behavior change	Shows respect for contributions of participants and for their existing knowledge	Solutions to barriers are offered by participants if their views are solicited and respected	Participants have much to offer to improve sessions
Gas cards for travel; meals served at sessions; times for sessions chosen by participants	Increases retention and engagement in the intervention	Demonstrates respect for participants' time and financial situation while promoting sense of community	Reduces barriers to coming to intervention	Willingness to make change if given the resources

The intervention takes a "whole health" approach to improving the CVD risk factor profile of individuals by promoting self-care of multiple CVD risk factors, underpinned by the Theory of Planned Behavior (Bentley, Lennie, Biddle, Chung, & Moser, 2009; Conn, Tripp-Reimer, & Maas, 2003; Conner, Norman, & Bell, 2002; Deskins et al., 2006; Masalu & Astrom, 2003; N. Lien, Lytle, & Komro, 2002; Povey, Conner, Sparks, James, & Shepherd, 2000). The whole health approach involves adoption of basic healthy lifestyle choices using self-care to influence a number of negative health behaviors. The approach is advocated for life for all people. In contrast to most approaches where a single risk factor is targeted with risk-factor-specific intervention, we target multiple CVD risk factors. Using this approach, the confusion faced by individuals attempting lifestyle change is reduced, as the same whole health approach is advocated for management of multiple CVD risk factors. Such an approach is advocated for lifelong health and reduction of risk from all chronic diseases (Kottke et al., 2009). The modules were created to accommodate those of low health literacy and are written at a sixth grade or lower reading level. Each module includes knowledge provision and skill building. Each module comes with supplementary materials to accommodate those who desire more complex materials.

The Theory of Planned Behavior is commonly used successfully to organize lifestyle modification interventions that require behavior change (Bentley et al., 2009; Conn et al., 2003; Conner et al., 2002; Deskins et al., 2006; Masalu & Astrom, 2003; N. Lien et al., 2002; Povey et al., 2000). We have developed and tested other successful self-care interventions using the Theory of Planned Behavior (Dekker et al., 2012; Welsh et al., 2012; Wu et al., 2012). The Theory of Planned Behavior states that the determinants of behavior change are attitudes, subjective norm, and perceived behavioral control. Attitudes are determined by the individual's beliefs about outcomes of performing the behavior. One who holds strong beliefs that a positively valued outcome will result from a behavior will have a positive attitude toward changing that behavior. The intervention encourages positive attitudes and behavioral beliefs by explaining, simplistically, the pathophysiology of CVD and its relationship to development of CVD risk factors, CVD, and CVD progression. A clear relationship between risk factors and outcomes is established. The benefits of reducing risk factors are emphasized. An individual's subjective norm is determined by his or her normative beliefs—whether important significant others approve or disapprove of the behavior. Someone who believes that certain significant others think she or he should perform a behavior, and who is motivated to meet the expectation of those referents, will hold a positive subjective norm. The program is supported by community health workers, who act as positive role models and subjective norm referents. Perceived behavioral control is the third element of the Theory of Planned Behavior. Perceived control is determined by beliefs about the presence of resources for, and impediments to, behavioral performance. Resources and impediments to lifestyle change are identified in the program, and we work with participants to overcome them and increase sense of control.

Examples of how we achieved the principles of individualization, self-care, and reduction of barriers to following CVD risk reduction practices are as follows.

- *Individualization.* At each intervention session, the entire research team attends and there is time set aside for individual counseling sessions in private (although most people opt to share their risk factors and their struggles with the group, it is possible for participants to keep their values private). At the first session, we discuss all results from baseline data collection, indicate what they mean for the individual, and work to set up individual, realistic goals for CVD risk reduction. We also discuss individual barriers to risk reduction and use motivational interviewing techniques to begin to reduce some of these barriers.
- *Self-care.* We concentrate in each module on providing skills and using demonstration of these skills (e.g., using exercise bands and pedometer—which we give participants—to increase and monitor activity; healthy cooking). Self-care principles are incorporated into each module.
- *Reducing barriers.* We interview each participant and then discuss, with the group, personal and environmental barriers to risk reduction. All sessions include barrier-reducing skills and problem solving. For example, we provide a meal at each session that we cook using locally bought groceries, demonstrating how to use what is available to cook a heart-healthy meal; we map, for each community and each individual, a walking route that is accessible to them; we provide information on eating out and on increasing the heart health of home-cooked foods—in one session, we take a recipe of one of the participants and modify it using heart-healthy principles.

We began our research in this area by employing community health workers to recruit and collect data while the research team delivered the intervention. To increase acceptability and sustainability of the intervention, we transitioned to teaching the community health workers how to deliver the intervention so that eventually all of the research activities were performed by community health workers and the rural Appalachian team.

Intervention Outcomes

We have included more than 1,100 individuals (mean age 58 ± 16 years; 62% women) living in Appalachian Kentucky and at high risk for CVD (by virtue of having two or more modifiable CVD risk factors) in our program to date. These individuals come from counties throughout Appalachian Kentucky and most of our recruitment has come by word of mouth after initial advertising and personal contacts by community health workers. Recruitment goals were met early. Acceptability of the intervention was extremely high and attendance at all data collection and intervention sessions was high.

We are currently conducting a formal randomized controlled trial of this intervention that is funded by the Patient-Centered Outcomes Research Institute ($n = 300$).

Early analyses support the efficacy and effectiveness we have seen in our prior studies. For example, pooled data from a wait list control period (efficacy trial) and a pre–post design (effectiveness trial) demonstrated there were no changes in body mass index, lipid profile, HgA1c in diabetics, or physical activity among individuals in this group. Compared to this, during the active intervention period, the following clinically and statistically significant changes were seen at 1 month postintervention: (a) low density lipoprotein decreased from a pre-intervention level of 110.5 ± 34.5 mg/dL to 95.8 ± 32.6 mg/dL ($p = .01$); (b) high density lipoprotein increased from a pre-intervention level in men of 34.5 ± 13.2 mg/dL to 39.8 ± 12.9 mg/dL ($p = .03$) and in women, increased from a pre-intervention level of 49.6 ± 15.1 mg/dL to a postintervention level of 55.7 ± 15.0 ($p < .001$); (c) total cholesterol decreased from 190 ± 38 mg/dL to 180 ± 36 mg/dL ($p < .001$); (d) pre-intervention, only 21% of participants engaged in moderate activity for 30 minutes per day at least 4 days a week, while postintervention 60% did ($p < .001$); (e) body mass index pre-intervention was 32.6 ± 7.7 down to a postintervention level of 28.4 ± 7.9 ($p < .001$). In a subset of patients, long-term follow-up data (9–12 months) demonstrate that these changes were maintained.

Sustaining the Intervention

Across the Appalachian Kentucky region where we have conducted our studies, a number of local and regional policy changes resulted in sustainment of the intervention. Rural nurse members of the research team adopted or modified the intervention as their standard of care for management of CVD risk factors in their community practices. For example, one advanced practice nurse who ran the community outreach and parish nursing practice for a local rural hospital adopted the intervention and uses the CVD risk prevention strategy in her services. She also received funding from Centers for Medicare and Medicaid Services (CMS) to conduct a study of CVD risk factor screening and effectiveness of nursing advice at the time of screening based on our methods.

Our research partner in central Appalachia directs the Center for Excellence in Rural Health there and oversees a health care service for indigent individuals in the area, Home Place. This service is funded by the state and the University of Kentucky as well as through multiple contracts and service grants. In the Home Place service, in a given year, more than 3,200 adults are served and provided with basic health care. The characteristics of the people seen in this service are striking: 62.5% did not have a physician, 4% had never received health care of any kind, 54.3% were below federal poverty level (compared to 17.7% for the state and 13.8% for the nation), and the remainder were above the federal poverty level, but indigent. Twenty-three percent of clients were overweight and 68.5% were obese, while 31% percent had diabetes. Thus, this is clearly a high-risk patient population. Our intervention was tested in this population, and as a consequence of its effectiveness, the intervention has been adopted by the service and is used for CVD risk reduction.

In efforts to further sustain the intervention, we have taught directors and providers at a variety of community service settings to deliver the intervention or deliver it on request. These service settings include senior centers, schools, health fairs, agricultural centers, churches, sorority organizations, a large health care organization, local clinics and pharmacies, and local businesses. Our intervention has been adopted by some local businesses, health care organizations, police, and firefighters as their required yearly health screening. In some cases, individuals receive a reduction in their health insurance fees for using the intervention.

Members of our community advisory group have also made changes based on their involvement with us as team members and after seeing the popularity and success of the intervention. For example, one of our members is the director of a rural Chamber of Commerce and, inspired by her work with us, she wrote and received a service grant to put in walking paths throughout a small rural town with few safe areas to walk. Others have organized local heart-healthy support groups to sustain our work.

CONCLUSION

Rural health disparities are widening (Singh & Siahpush, 2014) and it is essential that we address these disparities. We provided a needed CVD risk reduction intervention to a major at-risk population living in distressed rural Appalachian Kentucky where CVD risk reduction is difficult. The intervention is sustainable and holds the potential to produce major improvements in public health and decrease rates of CVD risk factors, CVD, and CVD mortality in some of the most high-risk populations in the nation. There are 25 million people living in all of Appalachia who could benefit immediately from this intervention. In addition, a total of 41% of Kentucky residents, and about 20% of the U.S. population, live in rural areas. Thus, the potential for generalizability of our findings to other distressed rural environments is high, particularly if it continues to be sustainable using local and regional policy change methods.

ACKNOWLEDGMENTS

Funding was provided through Patient-Centered Outcomes Research Institute Contract Number, 850-001, and the Department of Health and Human Resources, grant number, D1ARH20134-01-00.

REFERENCES

Adair, R., Christianson, J., Wholey, D. R., White, K., Town, R., Lee, S., . . . Elumba, D. (2012). Care guides: Employing nonclinical laypersons to help primary care teams manage chronic disease. *Journal of Ambulatory Care Management, 35*(1), 27–37. doi:10.1097/JAC.0b013e31823b0fbe

Ahmed, S. M., & Palermo, A. G. (2010). Community engagement in research: Frameworks for education and peer review. *American Journal of Public Health, 100*(8), 1380–1387. doi:10.2105/AJPH.2009.178137

Amarasinghe, A., D'Souza, G., Brown, C., Oh, H., & Borisova, T. (2009). The influence of socioeconomic and environmental determinants on health and obesity: A West Virginia case study. *International Journal of Environmental Research and Public Health, 6*(8), 2271–2287. doi:10.3390/ijerph6082271

Appalachian Community Fund. (2014). Central Appalachia. Retrieved from http://www.appalachiancommunityfund.org/central-appalachia

Appalachian Regional Commission. (2012). County economic status and distressed areas. Retrieved from http://www.arc.gov/appalachian_region/CountyEconomicStatusandDistressedAreasinAppalachia.asp

Appalachian Regional Commission. (2016). Economic assessment of Appalachia: An Appalachian regional development assessment report. Retrieved from https://www.arc.gov/data

Appel, L. J., Brands, M. W., Daniels, S. R., Karanja, N., Elmer, P. J., & Sacks, F. M. (2006). Dietary approaches to prevent and treat hypertension: A scientific statement from the American Heart Association. *Hypertension, 47*(2), 296–308.

Appel, L. J., Champagne, C. M., Harsha, D. W., Cooper, L. S., Obarzanek, E., Elmer, P. J., . . . Young, D. R. (2003). Effects of comprehensive lifestyle modification on blood pressure control: Main results of the PREMIER clinical trial. *JAMA, 289*(16), 2083–2093.

Au, M. G., Cornett, S. J., Nick, T. G., Wallace, J., Wang, Y., Warren, N. S., & Myers, M. F. (2010). Familial risk for chronic disease and intent to share family history with a health care provider among urban Appalachian women, southwestern Ohio, 2007. *Preventing Chronic Disease, 7*(1), A07.

Barker, L., Crespo, R., Gerzoff, R. B., Denham, S., Shrewsberry, M., & Cornelius-Averhart, D. (2010). Residence in a distressed county in Appalachia as a risk factor for diabetes: Behavioral risk factor surveillance system, 2006–2007. *Preventing Chronic Disease, 7*(5).

Battaglia, T. A., McCloskey, L., Caron, S. E., Murrell, S. S., Bernstein, E., Childs, A., . . . Bernstein, J. (2012). Feasibility of chronic disease patient navigation in an urban primary care practice. *Journal of Ambulatory Care Management, 35*(1), 38–49. doi:10.1097/JAC.0b013e31822cbd7c

Beaulac, J., Kristjansson, E., & Cummins, S. (2009). A systematic review of food deserts, 1966–2007. *Preventing Chronic Disease, 6*(3), A105.

Bentley, B., De Jong, M. J., Moser, D. K., & Peden, A. R. (2005). Factors related to nonadherence to low sodium diet recommendations in heart failure patients. *European Journal of Cardiovascular Nursing, 4*(4), 331–336.

Bentley, B., Lennie, T. A., Biddle, M., Chung, M. L., & Moser, D. K. (2009). Demonstration of psychometric soundness of the dietary sodium restriction questionnaire in patients with heart failure. *Heart & Lung: The Journal of Acute and Critical Care, 38*(2), 121–128. doi:10.1016/j.hrtlng.2008.05.006

Borak, J., Salipante-Zaidel, C., Slade, M. D., & Fields, C. A. (2012). Mortality disparities in Appalachia: Reassessment of major risk factors. *Journal of Occupational and Environmental Medicine, 54*(2), 146–156. doi:10.1097/JOM.0b013e318246f395

Brodie, D. A., & Inoue, A. (2005). Motivational interviewing to promote physical activity for people with chronic heart failure. *Journal of Advanced Nursing, 50*, 518–527.

Chowdhury, P. P., Mawokomatanda, T., Xu, F., Gamble, S., Flegel, D., Pierannunzi, C., . . . Town, M. (2016). Surveillance for certain health behaviors, chronic diseases, and conditions, access to health care, and use of preventive health services among states and selected local areas: Behavioral risk factor surveillance system, United States, 2012. *MMWR Surveillance Summary, 65*(4), 1–142. doi:10.15585/mmwr.ss6504a1

City-Data.Com. (2014). Roscommon County, Michigan (MI). Retrieved from http://www.city-data.com/county/Roscommon_County-MI.html

Conn, V. S., Tripp-Reimer, T., & Maas, M. L. (2003). Older women and exercise: Theory of planned behavior beliefs. *Public Health Nursing, 20*(2), 153–163.

Conner, M., Norman, P., & Bell, R. (2002). The theory of planned behavior and healthy eating. *Health Psychology, 21*(2), 194–201.

The Conservation Fund. (2014). Tackling food deserts in Michigan. Retrieved from http://www.conservationfund.org/projects/tackling-food-deserts-in-michigan

Dekker, R. L., Moser, D. K., Peden, A. R., & Lennie, T. A. (2012). Cognitive therapy improves three-month outcomes in hospitalized patients with heart failure. *Journal of Cardiac Failure, 18*(1), 10–20. doi:10.1016/j.cardfail.2011.09.008

Department for Public Health. (2014). *Kentucky behavioral risk factor surveillance system survey data.* Frankfort, Kentucky: Kentucky Department of Public Health. Retrieved from http://chfs.ky.gov/NR/rdonlyres/CC7425CB-575C-4C47-8B80-E499FCBE9CC2/0/2015BRFSSProfiles.pdf

Deskins, S., Harris, C. V., Bradlyn, A. S., Cottrell, L., Coffman, J. W., Olexa, J., & Neal, W. (2006). Preventive care in Appalachia: Use of the theory of planned behavior to identify barriers to participation in cholesterol screenings among West Virginians. *Journal of Rural Health, 22*(4), 367–374. doi:10.1111/j.1748-0361.2006.00060.x

Doering, L. V., Moser, D. K., Riegel, B., McKinley, S., Davidson, P., Baker, H., . . . Dracup, K. (2010). Persistent comorbid symptoms of depression and anxiety predict mortality in heart disease. *International Journal of Cardiology, 145*(2), 188–192. doi:10.1016/j.ijcard.2009.05.025

Fletcher, S. M., Burley, M. B., Thomas, K. E., & Mitchell, E. K. (2014). Feeling supported and abandoned: Mixed messages from attendance at a rural community cardiac rehabilitation program in Australia. *Journal of Cardiopulmonary Rehabilitation and Prevention, 34*(1), 29–33. doi:10.1097/HCR.0b013e3182a52734

Go, A. S., Mozaffarian, D., Roger, V. L., Benjamin, E. J., Berry, J. D., Borden, W. B., . . . Turner, M. B. (2013). Heart disease and stroke statistics—2013 update: A report from the American Heart Association. *Circulation, 127*(1), e6–e245. doi:10.1161/CIR.0b013e31828124ad

Greaves, C. J., Middlebrooke, A., O'Loughlin, L., Holland, S., Piper, J., Steele, A., . . . Daly, M. (2008). Motivational interviewing for modifying diabetes risk: A randomised controlled trial. *British Journal of General Practice, 58*, 535–540.

Gruca, T. S., Pyo, T. H., & Nelson, G. C. (2016). Providing cardiology care in rural areas through visiting consultant clinics. *Journal of the American Heart Association, 5*(7), e002909. doi:10.1161/JAHA.115.002909

Hacker, W. D. (2008). *Kentucky behavioral risk factor surveillance system, 2003–2004 report.* Retrieved from http://chfs.ky.gov/NR/rdonlyres/AEB91F77-072F-4379-ADFE-2789B78DEC09/0/200304Final.pdf

Halverson, J. A., Barnett, E., & Casper, M. (2002). Geographic disparities in heart disease and stroke mortality among black and white populations in the Appalachian region. *Ethnicity & Disease, 12*(4), S3–82–91.

Halverson, J. A., & Bischak, G. (2008). Underlying socioeconomic factors influencing health disparities in the Appalachian region. Retrieved from https://www.arc.gov/research/researchreportdetails.asp?REPORT_ID=9

Hayes, D. K., Greenlund, K. J., Denny, C. H., Croft, J. B., & Keenan, N. L. (2005). Racial/ethnic and socioeconomic disparities in multiple risk factors for heart disease and stroke. *Morbidity & Mortality Weekly Report, 55*(05), 113–117.

Jaarsma, T., Lesman-Leegte, I., Hillege, H. L., Veeger, N. J., Sanderman, R., van Veldhuisen, D. J., & COACH Investigators. (2010). Depression and the usefulness of a disease management program in heart failure: Insights from the COACH (Coordinating study evaluating Outcomes of Advising and Counseling in Heart failure) study. *Journal of the American College of Cardiology, 55*(17), 1837–1843. doi:10.1016/j.jacc.2009.11.082

Jia, H., Zack, M. M., & Thompson, W. W. (2011). State quality-adjusted life expectancy for U.S. adults from 1993 to 2008. *Quality of Life Research, 20*(6), 853–863. doi:10.1007/s11136-010-9826-y

Johnson, V. B., & Lorig, K. (2011). The internet diabetes self-management workshop for American Indians and Alaska Natives. *Health Promotion Practice, 12*, 261–270.

Kentucky Department of Public Health. (2009). Kentucky cardiovascular disease fact sheet. Retrieved from http://chfs.ky.gov/NR/rdonlyres/738A1FCB-4F89-4C25-A6E1-548D3E36BE29/0/KyCVDFactSheet_Aug081.pdf

Kentucky Institute of Medicine. (2007). *The health of Kentucky: A county assessment*. Retrieved from http://www.kyiom.org/pdf/healthy2007a.pdf

Keyserling, T. C., Samuel-Hodge, C. D., Pitts, S. J., Garcia, B. A., Johnston, L. F., Gizlice, Z., . . . Ammerman, A. S. (2016). A community-based lifestyle and weight loss intervention promoting a Mediterranean-style diet pattern evaluated in the stroke belt of North Carolina: The heart healthy Lenoir project. *BMC Public Health, 16*, 732. doi:10.1186/s12889-016-3370-9

Khare, M. M., Koch, A., Zimmermann, K., Moehring, P. A., & Geller, S. E. (2014). Heart smart for women: A community-based lifestyle change intervention to reduce cardiovascular risk in rural women. *Journal of Rural Health, 30*(4), 359–368. doi:10.1111/jrh.12066

Knudson, A., Meit, M., & Popat, S. (2014). *Rural-urban disparities in heart disease*. (Policy Brief #1 from the 2014 update of the *Rural-Urban Chartbook*). Grand Forks: Center for Rural Health, University of North Dakota School of Medicine and Health Sciences.

Koniak-Griffin, D., Brecht, M. L., Takayanagi, S., Villegas, J., Melendrez, M., & Balcazar, H. (2015). A community health worker-led lifestyle behavior intervention for Latina (Hispanic) women: Feasibility and outcomes of a randomized controlled trial. *International Journal of Nursing Studies, 52*(1), 75–87. doi:10.1016/j.ijnurstu.2014.09.005

Kottke, T. E., Faith, D. A., Jordan, C. O., Pronk, N. P., Thomas, R. J., & Capewell, S. (2009). The comparative effectiveness of heart disease prevention and treatment strategies. *American Journal of Preventive Medicine, 36*(1), 82–88. doi:10.1016/j.amepre.2008.09.010

Kulshreshtha, A., Goyal, A., Dabhadkar, K., Veledar, E., & Vaccarino, V. (2014). Urban-rural differences in coronary heart disease mortality in the United States: 1999-2009. *Public Health Report, 129*(1), 19–29.

Leiferman, J. A., & Pheley, A. M. (2006). The effect of mental distress on women's preventive health behaviors. *American Journal of Health Promotion, 20*(3), 196-199.

Liburd, L. C., Giles, H. W., & Mensah, G. A. (2006). Looking through a glass, darkly: Eliminating health disparities. *Preventing Chronic Disease, 3*(3), A72.

Lien, L. F., Brown, A. J., Ard, J. D., Loria, C., Erlinger, T. P., Feldstein, A. C., . . . Svetkey, L. P. (2007). Effects of PREMIER lifestyle modifications on participants with and without the metabolic syndrome. *Hypertension, 50*(4), 609–616.

Lien, N., Lytle, L. A., & Komro, K. A. (2002). Applying theory of planned behavior to fruit and vegetable consumption of young adolescents. *American Journal of Health Promotion, 16*(4), 189–197.

Lin, P. H., Appel, L. J., Funk, K., Craddick, S., Chen, C., Elmer, P., . . . Champagne, C. (2007). The PREMIER intervention helps participants follow the dietary approaches to stop hypertension dietary pattern and the current dietary reference intakes recommendations. *Journal of the American Dietetic Association, 107*(9), 1541–1551.

Lloyd-Jones, D., Adams, R., Carnethon, M., De Simone, G., Ferguson, T. B., Flegal, K., . . . Hong, Y. (2009). Heart disease and stroke statistics: 2009 update. *Circulation, 119*(3), e21-181.

Lohri-Posey, B. (2006). Middle-aged Appalachians living with diabetes mellitus: A family affair. *Family & Community Health, 29*(3), 214–220.

Lorig, K. R., & Holman, H. (2003). Self-management education: History, definition, outcomes, and mechanisms. *Annals of Behavioral Medicine, 26*, 1–7.

Lorig, K., Laurent, D. D., Plant, K., Krishnan, E., & Ritter, P. L. (2014). The components of action planning and their associations with behavior and health outcomes. *Chronic Illness, 10*, 50–59.

Maruthur, N. M., Wang, N. Y., & Appel, L. J. (2009). Lifestyle interventions reduce coronary heart disease risk: Results from the PREMIER trial. *Circulation, 119*(15), 2026–2031. doi:10.1161/CIRCULATIONAHA.108.809491

Masalu, J. R., & Astrom, A. N. (2003). The use of the theory of planned behavior to explore beliefs about sugar restriction. *American Journal of Health Behavior, 27*(1), 15–24.

McConnell, T. R., Santamore, W. P., Larson, S. L., Homko, C. J., Kashem, M., Cross, R. C., & Bove, A. A. (2010). Rural and urban characteristics impact cardiovascular risk reduction. *Journal of Cardiopulmonary Rehabilitation and Prevention, 30*(5), 299-308. doi:10.1097/HCR.0b013e3181d6fb82

McGrady, A., McGinnis, R., Badenhop, D., Bentle, M., & Rajput, M. (2009). Effects of depression and anxiety on adherence to cardiac rehabilitation. *Journal of Cardiopulmonary Rehabilitation and Prevention, 29*(6), 358–364. doi:10.1097/HCR.0b013e3181be7a8f

Mensah, G. A., & Brown, D. W. (2007). An overview of cardiovascular disease burden in the United States. *Health Affairs (Millwood), 26*(1), 38–48.

Mensah, G. A., Mokdad, A. H., Ford, E. S., Greenlund, K. J., & Croft, J. B. (2005). State of disparities in cardiovascular health in the United States. *Circulation, 111*(10), 1233–1241.

Moriarty, D. G., Zack, M. M., Holt, J. B., Chapman, D. P., & Safran, M. A. (2009). Geographic patterns of frequent mental distress. *American Journal of Preventive Medicine, 36*(6), 497–505.

Moser, D. K., Dickson, V., Jaarsma, T., Lee, C., Stromberg, A., & Riegel, B. (2012). Role of self-care in the patient with heart failure. *Current Cardiology Reports, 14*(3), 265–275. doi:10.1007/s11886-012-0267-9

Moser, D. K., Doering, L. V., & Chung, M. L. (2005). Vulnerabilities of patients recovering from an exacerbation of chronic heart failure. *American Heart Journal, 150*(5), 984. doi:10.1016/j.ahj.2005.07.028

Mozaffarian, D., Benjamin, E. J., Go, A. S., Arnett, D. K., Blaha, M. J., Cushman, M. . . . Turner, M. B. (2016). Heart disease and stroke statistics—2016 update: A report from the American Heart Association. *Circulation, 133*(4), e38–e360. doi:10.1161/CIR.0000000000000350

Mudd-Martin, G., Biddle, M. J., Chung, M. L., Lennie, T. A., Bailey, A. L., Casey, B. R., . . . Moser, D. K. (2014). Rural Appalachian perspectives on heart health: Social ecological contexts. *American Journal of Health Behavior, 38*(1), 134–143. doi:10.5993/AJHB.38.1.14

O'Connor, A., & Wellenius, G. (2012). Rural-urban disparities in the prevalence of diabetes and coronary heart disease. *Public Health, 126*(10), 813–820. doi:10.1016/j.puhe.2012.05.029

Povey, R., Conner, M., Sparks, P., James, R., & Shepherd, R. (2000). The theory of planned behaviour and healthy eating: Examining additive and moderating effects of social influence variables. *Psychology & Health, 14*(6), 991–1006. doi:10.1080/08870440008407363

Reilly, R., Evans, K., Gomersall, J., Gorham, G., Peters, M. D., Warren, S., . . . Brown, A. (2016). Effectiveness, cost effectiveness, acceptability and implementation barriers/enablers of chronic kidney disease management programs for indigenous people in Australia, New Zealand and Canada: A systematic review of mixed evidence. *BMC Health Services Research, 16*(1), 119. doi:10.1186/s12913-016-1363-0

Reynolds, C. F., 3rd, Cuijpers, P., Patel, V., Cohen, A., Dias, A., Chowdhary, N., . . . Albert, S. M. (2012). Early intervention to reduce the global health and economic burden of major depression in older adults. *Annual Review of Public Health, 33*, 123–135. doi:10.1146/annurev-publhealth-031811-124544

Riegel, B., Moser, D. K., Anker, S. D., Appel, L. J., Dunbar, S. B., Grady, K. L., . . . Whellan, D. J. (2009). State of the science: Promoting self-care in persons with heart failure: A scientific statement from the American Heart Association. *Circulation, 120*(12), 1141–1163. doi:10.1161/CIRCULATIONAHA.109.192628

Riegel, B., Moser, D. K., Powell, M., Rector, T. S., & Havranek, E. P. (2006). Nonpharmacologic care by heart failure experts. *Journal of Cardiac Failure, 12*(2), 149–153. doi:10.1016/j.cardfail.2005.10.004

Roger, V. L., Go, A. S., Lloyd-Jones, D. M., Benjamin, E. J., Berry, J. D., Borden, W. B., . . . Turner, M. B. (2012). Heart disease and stroke statistics—2012 update: A report from the American Heart Association. *Circulation, 125*(1), e2–e220. doi:10.1161/CIR.0b013e31823ac046

Romanelli, J., Fauerbach, J. A., Bush, D. E., & Ziegelstein, R. C. (2002). The significance of depression in older patients after myocardial infarction. *Journal of the American Geriatrics Society, 50*(5), 817–822.

Rozanski, A., Blumenthal, J. A., Davidson, K. W., Saab, P. G., & Kubzansky, L. (2005). The epidemiology, pathophysiology, and management of psychosocial risk factors in cardiac practice: The emerging field of behavioral cardiology. *Journal of the American College of Cardiology, 45*(5), 637–651.

Rugg, S. S., Bailey, A. L., & Browning, S. R. (2008). Preventing cardiovascular disease in Kentucky: Epidemiology, trends, and strategies for the future. *Journal of the Kentucky Medical Association, 106*(4), 149–161; quiz 149, 162–143.

Schoenberg, N. E., Bardach, S. H., Manchikanti, K. N., & Goodenow, A. C. (2011). Appalachian residents' experiences with and management of multiple morbidity. *Qualitative Health Research, 21*(5), 601–611. doi:10.1177/1049732310395779

Schoenberg, N. E., Hatcher, J., & Dignan, M. B. (2008). Appalachian women's perceptions of their community's health threats. *Journal of Rural Health, 24*(1), 75–83. doi:10.1111/j.1748 -0361.2008.00140.x

Shaw, K. M., Theis, K. A., Self-Brown, S., Roblin, D. W., & Barker, L. (2016). Chronic disease disparities by county economic status and metropolitan classification: Behavioral risk factor surveillance system, 2013. *Preventing Chronic Disease, 13*, E119. doi:10.5888/pcd13.160088

Singh, G. K., & Siahpush, M. (2014). Widening rural-urban disparities in life expectancy, U.S., 1969–2009. *American Journal of Preventive Medicine, 46*(2), e19–e29. doi:10.1016/j.amepre.2013.10.017

Social Security Administration. (2014). Quickfacts. Retrieved from http://www.ssa.gov/policy/ docs/quickfacts/stat_snapshot

Song, E. K., Moser, D. K., Frazier, S. K., Heo, S., Chung, M. L., & Lennie, T. A. (2010). Depressive symptoms affect the relationship of N-terminal pro B-type natriuretic peptide to cardiac event-free survival in patients with heart failure. *Journal of Cardiac Failure, 16*(7), 572–578. doi:10.1016/j.cardfail.2010.01.006

Stampfer, M. J., Hu, F. B., Manson, J. E., Rimm, E. B., & Willett, W. C. (2000). Primary prevention of coronary heart disease in women through diet and lifestyle. *New England Journal of Medicine, 343*(1), 16–22.

Strand, B. H., & Tverdal, A. (2004). Can cardiovascular risk factors and lifestyle explain the educational inequalities in mortality from ischaemic heart disease and from other heart diseases? 26 year follow up of 50,000 Norwegian men and women. *Journal of Epidemiology & Community Health, 58*(8), 705–709. doi:10.1136/jech.2003.014563

Strand, B. H., & Tverdal, A. (2006). Trends in educational inequalities in cardiovascular risk factors: A longitudinal study among 48,000 middle-aged Norwegian men and women. *European Journal of Epidemiology, 21*(10), 731–739. doi:10.1007/s10654-006-9046-5

Strickland, J., & Strickland, D. L. (1996). Barriers to preventive health services for minority households in the rural south. *Journal of Rural Health, 12*(3), 206–217.

Thompson, D. R., Chair, S. Y., Chan, S. W., Astin, F., Davidson, P.M., & Ski, C. F. (2011). Motivational interviewing: A useful approach to improving cardiovascular health? *Journal of Clinical Nursing, 20*, 1236–1244.

Thomson, S. C. (2011). Food deserts: Where poor nutrition thrives. *Health Progress, 92*(6), 8–9.

Tian, M., Ajay, V. S., Dunzhu, D., Hameed, S. S., Li, X., Liu, Z., . . . Yan, L. L. (2015). A cluster-randomized, controlled trial of a simplified multifaceted management program for individuals at high cardiovascular risk (SimCard Trial) in rural Tibet, China, and Haryana, India. *Circulation, 132*(9), 815–824. doi:10.1161/CIRCULATIONAHA.115.015373

Tideman, P. A., Tirimacco, R., Senior, D. P., Setchell, J. J., Huynh, L. T., Tavella, R., . . . Chew, D. P. (2014). Impact of a regionalised clinical cardiac support network on mortality among rural patients with myocardial infarction. *Medical Journal of Australia, 200*(3), 157–160.

U. S. Census Bureau. (n.d.). Quick facts. Retrieved from http://quickfacts.census.gov/qfd/states/ 26/26143.html

U. S. Department of Agriculture. (2012). USDA Economic Research Service. Retrieved from http:// www.ers.usda.gov/data-products/state-fact-sheets.aspx

Welsh, D., Lennie, T. A., Marcinek, R., Biddle, M. J., Abshire, D., Bentley, B., & Moser, D. K. (2012). Low-sodium diet self-management intervention in heart failure: Pilot study results. *European Journal of Cardiovascular Nursing*. doi:10.1177/1474515111435604

Wu, J. R., Corley, D. J., Lennie, T. A., & Moser, D. K. (2012). Effect of a medication-taking behavior feedback theory-based intervention on outcomes in patients with heart failure. *Journal of Cardiac Failure, 18*(1), 1–9. doi:10.1016/j.cardfail.2011.09.006

Yusuf, S., Hawken, S., Ounpuu, S., Dans, T., Avezum, A., Lanas, F., . . . Lisheng, L. (2004). Effect of potentially modifiable risk factors associated with myocardial infarction in 52 countries (the INTERHEART study): Case-control study. *Lancet, 364*(9438), 937–952.

Ziegelstein, R. C., Fauerbach, J. A., Stevens, S. S., Romanelli, J., Richter, D. P., & Bush, D. E. (2000). Patients with depression are less likely to follow recommendations to reduce cardiac risk during recovery from a myocardial infarction. *Archives of Internal Medicine, 160*(12), 1818–1823.

16

Chronic Illness: Telehealth Approaches to Wellness

Stanley Finkelstein and Rhonda Cady

The underlying goal of health reform in the United States (Office of the Legislative Counsel, U.S. House of Representatives, 2010) is achievement of the Institute for Healthcare Improvement's (IHI) Triple Aim (2015), which encompasses improved health and improved experience of care with reduced cost. The digital health technology that is considered fundamental to achieving this goal includes technologies such as mobile health, health information technology, big data analytics, wearable computing, and telehealth (Ostrovsky, Deen, Simon, & Mate, 2014). This chapter focuses on the evidence base for telehealth and how this evidence advances the Triple Aim by influencing policy decisions by clinicians, health systems, and payers (private and government).

Telehealth encompasses the diagnosis and management of health, along with the education of health professionals and consumers. Rapidly replacing the original but restrictive term of *telemedicine*, telehealth reflects a movement from clinician-to-clinician interactions to clinician–consumer interactions. Technology used to support these interactions falls into four domains: live video, store and forward, remote patient monitoring, and mobile health (Center for Connected Health Policy, 2016). The primary potential for telehealth systems is to provide the necessary infrastructure for health delivery systems to move from acute facility-based episodic care provision to remote or virtual wellness and chronic care management. Home telehealth provides the continuity of care often lacking when a person is diagnosed with a new condition or discharged from a prolonged hospitalization.

Home telehealth systems support care delivery between clinicians and consumers regardless of physical location. The rapid emergence of home telehealth systems is a direct result of miniature devices and mobile computing. Relatively inexpensive, ubiquitous, and easy to use, these systems include wearable technologies like fitness trackers, smart watches, smartphones, wearable cameras and smart clothing, and movement monitoring and sensor devices. Mobile computing allows wireless connection between these systems and the Internet, and supports seamless transmission of data between devices.

A consideration of mobile computing is the speed, or bandwidth, of the mobile wireless connection. Typically classified as 3G and 4G, a 4G connection can be 10 times faster than 3G. Whether 3G, 4G, or long-term evolution (LTE), these mobile wireless connections utilize two types of connection speeds: upload and download. The download speed is the rate at which data is received from another source, whereas the upload speed is the rate at which data is sent to another source. Because the majority of mobile computing activity involves downloading data (e-mail, video and audio streaming), download speed is often three to four times faster than upload speed. This difference is an important consideration for home telehealth interactive video applications. A minimum upload speed of 384 kilobytes per second (kbps) is needed for both quality audio and video clarity with a proprietary video application (Cady, Kelly, & Finkelstein, 2008), and similar speed requirements have been identified for Skype video calls (Choi et al., 2014).

Can home telehealth accelerate achievement of the IHI Triple Aim? A recent report analyzed health technology interventions to determine which has the greatest value toward achieving the IHI Triple Aim. Of the 87 technologies evaluated, 23% were evidence-based and the majority of these technologies were aimed at providers (Ostrovsky et al., 2014). Developing an evidence base for home telehealth is paramount to reform and requires a focused and rigorous research agenda. Our research group has investigated the use of remote patient monitoring and home telehealth technologies in diverse populations for the past 35 years. These studies paralleled the development of instrumentation, computers, and communication systems that made the growth, acceptance, and utilization of home telehealth possible. The goals for these studies have been to improve access while providing quality care with cost-effective systems that are satisfactory to consumers and clinicians. In most studies, a randomized, controlled trial methodology has been used so that home telehealth results are evidence-based and can be compared with standard care when policy decisions that affect the transition from the research laboratory to the community setting are considered. Participants in all described studies provided informed consent, following the recommendations of our institutional review board.

CHRONOLOGICAL MILEPOSTS IN HOME TELEHEALTH

Cystic Fibrosis Monitoring Program—Low Tech Data Collection and Communication

An early home measurement monitoring system was developed for assessing progress and planning changes in care for patients with cystic fibrosis (CF; Finkelstein et al., 1986). Study participants kept a paper diary to record daily relevant clinical measurements, symptoms, and free text. Participants were instructed to send their diary to the study data center each week, using the U.S. Postal Service. Diary data was then entered into the study database. Daily measurements made at home were lung capacity, body weight, breathing rate, and pulse. The kind and frequency of coughing and wheezing were included on the list of possible symptoms. Lung capacity was measured with an exercise inspirometer; respiratory rate and pulse were measured by participant caregivers by observation and by counting. During the first 2 years of participation, the 111 subjects maintained a consistent 75% to 80% diary response rate, demonstrating that subjects/caregivers could and would utilize the equipment package, instructions, and protocol to successfully provide clinically useful data from home without the assistance of clinically trained personnel. It presented the possibility of detecting adverse health trends earlier in their development, so that patients could be treated before serious complications developed, thereby preventing the large fluctuations in health status that often accompany CF. This study was a precursor to subsequent remote monitoring developments, which evolved with the emergence of low-cost personal computers (PCs), electronic spirometers and other miniaturized devices, and advanced communication systems.

Overall lessons learned from the CF home monitoring were that patients and caregivers could make and transmit measures from home, and that this home data could be clinically useful. These findings added to the emerging body of evidence regarding successful use of manual observations of home monitoring data to identify changes in clinical status, and the development of computer decision systems to automate this process (Slagle, Finkelstein, Leung, & Warwick, 1989). As with most remote monitoring telehealth programs at that time, a sustainable funding source did not exist and the CF program ended with the completion of the research program.

Lung Transplant Home Monitoring Program— Electronic Data Collection, Miniaturization of Devices, Landline Communication

The lung transplant program at the University of Minnesota has performed more than 900 lung transplants since its inception in 1986. The lung transplant home monitoring research program, which was active from 1992 through 2014, provided a framework for conducting telehealth research that facilitated clinical translation. The underlying premise of remote home monitoring was, and still is, that timely information from clinically informative variables that are remotely acquired could lead to early detection and thus early intervention before problems become more intractable. For lung transplantation, home monitoring was designed to provide early indications of the onset of infection or rejection episodes in the transplanted lung. Ideally, this early intervention would improve the patient's health status and increase survival while containing cost (Finkelstein et al., 1996). Some key questions related to remote monitoring emerged as the program progressed, including patient and clinician acceptance, quality of patient-measured physiological variables, home-to-clinic communications, and data overload.

In the initial home monitoring study, a specially designed electronic spirometer/diary instrument was used by subjects at home to record full spirometry, vital signs (blood pressure, pulse, weight, temperature), and symptoms (coughing, sputum, shortness of breath, exercise). Data was stored in the device until downloaded over each subject's regular landline to the study data center. Subjects were requested to do this download weekly. Possible bronchopulmonary events that needed follow-up clinical evaluation were identified by the study nurse coordinators during weekly data review. Validity analysis confirmed that home spirometry provided reliable estimates of clinic-measured spirometry (Finkelstein et al., 1993; Lindgren et al., 1997). These results helped to overcome the initial concerns about the clinical quality of home data regarding both instrument quality and the ability of study subjects to perform clinical quality measurements at home. When the Centers for Medicare and Medicaid Services (CMS) established the reimbursement policy for home spirometry for asthma and lung transplant recipients, they cited several articles from this study as providing the scientific rationale for their decision.

Further studies in this program utilized new advances in telecommunications, making it easier for subjects to complete the monitoring protocol, such as automated timed downloads every night. The development of clinical decision support tools (Finkelstein, Scudiero, Lindgren, Snyder, & Hertz, 2005) could address economic and clinical factors related to chronic disease management, such as the data overload resulting from frequent monitoring, lessening the need for clinic visits, and the growing shortage of skilled nurses caring for the rapidly growing aging and chronic disease population.

THE TELEHOMECARE PROGRAM— INTERNET ACCESS, VIRTUAL VISITS, ELDERLY SUBJECTS

The TeleHomeCare project was a randomized controlled trial to assess the effectiveness of virtual visits, Internet access, and remote physiological monitoring between a participant's home and home health care (HHC) agencies (Finkelstein et al., 2004). Four rural and one urban HHC agencies participated in the study. TeleHomeCare combined actual and virtual HHC visits with the goal of delivering quality care at acceptable cost for patients receiving skilled nursing care at home. Sixty-eight patients with congestive heart failure (CHF), chronic obstructive pulmonary disease (COPD), or chronic wound care were randomized as subjects in the three arms of the study. The control group received standard HHC as determined by their underlying condition. Two intervention groups received varying levels of telehealth. One intervention group received standard HHC supplemented with virtual visits and Internet access. A second intervention group received standard HHC, supplemented with virtual visits, Internet access, and remote physiological monitoring. Subjects in the second intervention group received pulse oximeters (for oxygen saturation), electronic spirometers (for pulmonary function), and blood pressure cuffs depending on their underlying condition. Virtual visits consisted of two-way audio and video interactions between a health care provider at a central site and the patient at home, transmitted over standard telephone landlines. The overall objectives were to demonstrate that such a program can improve the quality and reduce or contain costs of skilled HHC, while increasing patient access to care and satisfaction with the HHC intervention

Study outcome measures indicated that home telehealth increased satisfaction of both nurses and clients, was less costly than in-person HHC visits, and may reduce the need for increasing levels of care after discharge from the HHC program (Finkelstein, Speedie, & Potthoff, 2006). The TeleHomeCare Program demonstrated the technical feasibility of extending telehealth services to homebound older adults; illustrated new avenues for socialization between elderly, homebound patients and their home care nurses; and showed the potential for improved clinical outcomes at a lower cost. However, policy that reimburses HHC nurses for interactive audio and video communication within a beneficiary's home was ineligible for Medicare reimbursement. Lacking a sustainable payment mechanism, programs such as the TeleHomeCare Program could not continue after research support ended.

THE VIRTUAL ASSISTED LIVING UMBRELLA FOR THE ELDERLY (VALUE) PROGRAM: VIRTUAL VISITS, WEB-BASED SERVICE PORTAL, AGING IN PLACE ELDERLY SUBJECTS

The VALUE project evaluated the impact of a home telehealth program on extending the ability of frail elderly individuals to remain living independently in their home environment. It was a two-armed randomized controlled trial conducted at the University of Minnesota, a rural health care agency, and an urban health care agency. VALUE provided virtual visits with a home care nurse, physiological remote monitoring and a web-based portal for ordering health-related services, messaging between client and health provider, and Internet access, all via a broadband connection (Finkelstein, Speedie, Zhou, Ratner, & Potthoff, 2006).

A total of 99 individuals participated in the study. Control group subjects continued with their regular living accommodations, obtaining supportive services as they did ordinarily, by telephone or visits to senior and community centers. Intervention group subjects received the VALUE workstation consisting of a PC platform with broadband (digital subscriber line [DSL] or cable) connectivity, Health Insurance Portability and Accountability Act (HIPAA) compliant interactive video software, and a web camera. Intervention group subjects also received physiological monitoring devices appropriate to their underlying health condition or continued using monitoring devices they were already utilizing as part of their standard care. A web portal customized for each intervention group subject facilitated access to web-based health education resources, a telehealth nurse, and electronic ordering of various health and community services. It was designed for improved accessibility by older adults and thus included large fonts, simple colors, and easy navigation by mouse pointer of arrow keys (Demiris, Finkelstein, & Speedie, 2001).

Study results indicated that frail older adults could successfully utilize a telehealth platform if it is properly designed to accommodate the usual constraints imposed by aging. Intervention subjects were very satisfied with the VALUE technology, virtual visits, and nurse interactions (Finkelstein et al., 2007). They indicated that VALUE met their expectations and they would recommend VALUE to others.

Compared to control group subjects, the intervention group subjects had significantly fewer emergency department visits, higher use of pharmacy delivery services, and lower use of transportation services. As in earlier studies, lack of continued funding made these advances unsustainable in the economic environment of that time.

THE U SPECIAL KIDS PROGRAM: APRN CARE COORDINATION, TELEPHONE COMMUNICATION, CHILDREN WITH MEDICAL COMPLEXITY

The U Special Kids (USK) program at the University of Minnesota utilized "low-tech" telehealth modalities that included telephone, fax, and e-mail to deliver care coordination to children with medical complexity (CMC; Cohen et al., 2011). Within the USK Medical Home Center (Kelly, Golnik, & Cady, 2008), a team of two advanced practice nurses and a pediatrician delivered telehealth care coordination to more than 100 CMC living throughout the state of Minnesota. CMC have multiple chronic health conditions, receive care from multiple specialists, require numerous medications or rare pharmaceuticals, often have repeated hospitalizations and/or emergency room visits, and are dependent on life-sustaining technology (i.e., feeding tube, tracheotomy, central line, or oxygen; Cohen et al., 2011).

An evaluation of the USK program reviewed hospitalizations within the affiliated health system during the first 5 years of USK enrollment (Cady, Finkelstein, & Kelly, 2009). Findings indicated a significant reduction in unplanned hospitalizations (e.g., acute illness or injury, complications from underlying conditions) from year 1 to year 2, and stabilization over the subsequent 3 years, while planned hospitalizations (e.g., scheduled device insertion/replacement) remained relatively stable over the 5-year period (Cady et al., 2009).

Until recently, the primary model of reimbursement for health care services was fee-for-service (FFS). In this model, reimbursement is tied to "in-person" service use such as clinic visits, emergency department visits, and hospitalizations. Programs like USK that provided telehealth care coordination services were not considered reimbursable by Medicaid and third-party payers and (more importantly) by reducing hospital utilization, reduced FFS reimbursement. Despite the positive evaluation findings, the economic climate of 2008 and FFS reimbursement made funding for the program unsustainable and USK was eliminated.

Nearly 10 years later, a total cost of care (TCC) reimbursement model has flipped the paradigm and is rapidly replacing the FFS model. Within the TCC model, reductions in unplanned high-cost hospitalizations are "rewarded" by sharing of cost savings between the health system and payer. In this new paradigm, health system revenue is linked to the provision of high-quality, cost-effective care, and the value of telehealth care coordination programs like USK is becoming readily apparent.

THE TELEFAMILIES PROGRAM: APRN CARE COORDINATION, TELEPHONE AND VIDEO INTERVENTIONS, CHILDREN WITH MEDICAL COMPLEXITY

The TeleFamilies project was a randomized controlled trial conducted from 2010 to 2014. The primary aim of TeleFamilies was testing the effectiveness of advanced practice registered nurse (APRN) care coordination, delivered via increasing levels of telehealth, for CMC receiving primary care within a traditional health care home (HCH). One hundred sixty-three families of CMC participated in the 30-month trial and were randomized into the control (usual care) or one of two intervention groups. The control group received care coordination through the existing HCH model, which included a medical assistant care coordinator and telephone triage service provided by registered nurses. The intervention groups received APRN care coordination modeled on the USK program, and provided primarily through telephone and video telehealth (Cady et al., 2015).

The TeleFamilies APRN care coordinator was a certified experienced pediatric nurse practitioner who was available via telehealth (telephone and videoconferencing) during office hours. The APRN served as a single point of contact and collaboration for families and addressed care coordination needs within and across settings of care. The APRN's expanded scope of practice and clinical autonomy facilitated assessment of acute changes in a child's conditions via telehealth and (depending on the severity of assessment) management via telehealth, a next-day office visit, or emergency department visit. Video telehealth supported the APRN in physical assessment of the child, "meeting" with the child, family members, and home care providers in the home environment to discuss, assess, and provide feedback on "hands-on" aspects of the child's plan of care.

Effectiveness of the TeleFamilies model of care coordination was measured by changes in child and family outcomes and health care service utilization. Analysis of family satisfaction data measured by key questions from the Consumer Assessment of Health Plans Survey (CAHPS) indicated that the TeleFamilies model was successful in increasing intervention families' perceptions of their providers, their overall health care experience, and provider communication (Looman et al., 2015). Analysis of family outcome data, measured by questions from the National Survey of Children with Special Health Needs (n.d.), indicated that TeleFamilies was successful in improving the adequacy of care coordination received by families in both intervention groups (Cady et al., 2015).

Initial exploration of health care service utilization data compared the number and type of clinical visits for CMC randomized to the control and intervention groups. Clinical visits were categorized as planned or unplanned. A planned clinical visit is scheduled in advance and focuses on maintaining wellness (e.g., planned surgery, preoperative physical, well-child check), whereas an unplanned clinical visit results from an acute change in the child's health and focuses on fixing a problem (e.g., acute illness, complication of life-sustaining technology, or emergency surgery). An increase in planned visits indicates proactive monitoring of a child's condition and early detection of changes in health, whereas a decrease in unplanned visits indicates reduced sickness and/or condition instability. Analysis showed no significant change in unplanned visits across time or groups (control vs. intervention), but the change in planned visits over time significantly increased for the intervention groups. The lack of change in unplanned visits across groups could be attributed to organization-wide quality initiatives aiming at reducing emergency department visits and hospitalizations and changing treatment protocols.

The TeleFamilies project ended in 2014, and unlike the USK program, a shift in the reimbursement landscape supported sustainability of the model. The health system that housed TeleFamilies entered into a TCC demonstration project and the APRN model of care coordination was translated to support a larger number of CMC.

CURRENT STATE OF HOME TELEHEALTH

Studies on the application of home telehealth systems have expanded greatly in the past several years. These include the continued expansion of remote physiological monitoring in tracking and treating chronic disease, and the use of monitoring and video in rehabilitation and educational applications and assisted living settings, the expansion of health-smart homes, and the demands on the nursing role in these programs. What remains relatively unchanged is the reporting on systemic barriers and facilitators, which demonstrates that despite the continued growth in telehealth applications, little has changed in the underlying issues of adoption and sustainability of these systems.

CHRONIC DISEASE MONITORING AND INTERVENTION

Recent trials with COPD and cardiac patients have demonstrated improved outcomes for subjects in the telehealth intervention groups or their equivalence with standard care when compared to control groups following standard care. A randomized controlled trial in Denmark compared the effect of home-based telehealth hospitalization with conventional hospitalization for exacerbations in severe COPD (Jakobsen et al., 2015). Subjects in the intervention group used oximeters and spirometers at home, an oxygen compressor, medication box, and a touch screen with a webcam to communicate with hospital staff during preappointed times for virtual daily ward rounds. Their analysis showed that a subgroup of patients with severe COPD can be treated for acute exacerbations at home, without health professionals being physically present. In a pre–post study in Canada, the effect of telerehabilitation on exercise tolerance and quality of life was tested in a group of patients with moderate to very severe COPD (Marquis, Larivee, Saey, Dubois, & Tousignant, 2015). Patients used a wireless oximeter and heart rate sensor to provide real-time physiological data to the study clinician via encrypted transmission over the Internet. Subjects followed an 8-week exercise program using a commercially available videoconferencing system over a high-speed Internet connection. Exercise tolerance and quality-of-life measures improved after the intervention. Subjects reported very high satisfaction scores for the telerehabilitation program, and adherence to this exercise training was higher than that reported in the literature for conventional on-site training.

In a randomized controlled trial from Finland, investigators studied the use of home telemonitoring to support multidisciplinary care of heart failure patients (Vuorinen et al., 2014). Intervention group patients measured body weight, blood pressure, and pulse, and answered symptom-related questions weekly. Measurements and symptom reports were uploaded to the study nurse using a preinstalled mobile telephone application. Subjects received automatic machine-based feedback on whether or not their measurements were within their personal targets set by their nurse. Control group subjects followed usual care, consisting of a similar multidisciplinary approach, but information exchange took place primarily during clinic visits. Adherence to study protocol was close to 90%, and there were no significant differences in subjects' clinical health or self-care behavior between intervention and control subjects. Telemonitoring increased the nurse's workload by increasing the number of reception visits and telephone contacts.

A cost–benefit analysis for technology-enabled, home-based cardiac rehabilitation in Australia showed that rehabilitation delivered by telehealth was less costly than the conventional on-site program for the service provider, and eliminated the travel costs associated with the on-site program for the participants (Whittaker & Wade, 2014). Both study groups received comprehensive rehabilitative care utilizing exercise, risk modification, and mentoring. Intervention subjects used a mobile phone, a wellness diary, and a wellness web portal with daily text messaging. Clinical outcomes were equivalent for both groups.

ACCEPTANCE AND ADOPTION; FACILITATORS AND BARRIERS

The acceptance and adoption of telehealth programs is a continuing concern to researchers, health care providers, and public and private health care policy makers. A study in the United Kingdom examined the factors affecting the acceptance and adoption of telehealth monitoring for COPD and heart failure by frontline nursing staff (Taylor et al., 2015). They found five main themes that influenced staff acceptance: working in a changing unfamiliar setting, how telehealth is introduced to the nursing staff, how staff experienced and understood telehealth use, working out the technology and services provided prior to widespread clinical introduction, and the integration of telehealth into routine clinical practice. These can serve as facilitators or barriers, depending on how they are developed and achieved in the workplace. Training, accurate and stable telehealth equipment, addressing anticipated workload concerns, and having a local telehealth champion can all contribute to a positive experience and greater staff acceptance.

Farrar explored the impact of telehealth technology on the role of home health nurses caring for patients with mental health concerns (Farrar, 2015). Legal considerations, including licensure and scope of practice, are works in progress addressed by multiple government agencies and boards at the state and federal levels, as well as professional associations such as the American Telemedicine Association. Facilitators and barriers identified in this report include device concerns, data transmission, audio and visual guidance needs, display colors, font size and excessive motion, and cultural changes within the nursing and patient communities. These and earlier reports (Sabati, Snyder, Edin-Stibbe, Lindgren, & Finkelstein, 2001) demonstrate that the same facilitators and barriers to home telehealth acceptance and adoption cross most telehealth applications and that we have made little progress addressing these issues in the past 15 years.

Despite the continued existence of these barriers to adoption and utilization of home telehealth programs, progress has been made on reimbursement and potential viability of these programs in clinical practice. Reimbursement varies from state to state, but increasing state support has impacted federal action on this front, particularly within the Medicare programs (Neufeld, Doarn, & Aly, 2016). Hospital and health system adoption of telehealth faces many of the barriers cited earlier, but the focus remains on the sustainability of programs started with federal, local, and private grant support after start-up funding comes to an end (Merchant, Ward, Mueller, Rural Health Research & Policy Centers, & Rural Policy Research Institute, RUPRI Center for Rural Health Policy Analysis, University of Iowa College of Public Health, Department of Health Management and Policy, 2015; Wicklund, 2016). Policy changes in reimbursement, licensing, and credentialing, as well as clinician buy-in and utilization, remain major concerns. However, despite the slow progress on these issues, the private sector is moving ahead in support of telehealth adoption. In a recent news release, UnitedHealthcare, the largest health insurer in the United States, announced support for virtual care physician visits as a way to "expand consumer access to affordable health care options" (United HealthCare Services, 2015). Many local health care systems have also adopted locally developed virtual visits within their network to promote their belief in the cost-saving potential of this technology.

HEALTH-SMART HOMES

Another exciting application of remote monitoring and home telehealth focuses on a successful "aging in place" environment for the burgeoning population of older individuals in the United States and worldwide. The Centers for Disease Control and Prevention defines *aging in place* as the ability to live in one's own home and community safely, independently, and comfortably, regardless of age, income, or ability level (www.cdc.gov/healthyplaces/terminology.htm). A *smart home* is a residence wired with technology features that monitor the well-being and activities of the residents to improve overall quality of life, increase independence, and prevent emergencies (Demiris & Hensel, 2008). Specially designed homes within a community setting can provide an alternative to adding monitoring and additional communication capability to existing individual residences. For example, Tiger Place on the University of Missouri campus was developed to address the Aging in Place needs within a community setting (Tyrer et al., 2006).

In addition to many of the smart home conveniences and time and money saving systems for heating and cooling, entertainment, and security, *health-smart homes* contain activity and motion sensors that assist elderly residents with many of the tasks needed to remain independent while living in a noninstitutional environment. These may include physiological monitors, activity sensors, appliance monitors, fall detectors, and personal communication applications that continue to advance the concept of aging in place as one approach to address the common desire of the growing population of older individuals to remain in their familiar residences as long as possible. According to Demiris and Hensel (2008), typical physiological monitoring may include pulse, respiration, temperature, blood pressure; activity sensing of walking, cooking, turning lights on/off; security sensing to detect intruders; and safety sensing to detect gas leaks, fires, cooking appliances left on and unattended. More recently, programs to monitor and increase social engagement have been added to the list of desirable applications. Early versions of health-smart homes included monitors and sensors either built into the original construction or utilized electrical wiring running between sensor locations and power sources in retrofitting existing sites. The advances in wireless technologies and miniaturization of sensing devices have made it easier and more economical to retrofit existing seniors' homes and to develop community-based homes, expanding the potential availability of health-smart home benefits. An active research area in health-smart home development is the development of methods to prevent and detect falls. Falls are a major impediment to aging in place, leading to injury, disability, and possibly death. Researchers are developing unobtrusive sensors and algorithms that can monitor residents continuously to assess risk of falling and detect actual falls (Rantz et al., 2015).

The Evangelical Lutheran Good Samaritan Society (GSS) implemented a health-smart home program in 2010 called LivingWell@Home (LW@H). The program incorporates remote biometric and nonbiometric monitoring by nurse specialists and in-person HHC to support Aging in Place (Grant, Rockwood, & Stennes, 2014). Nurse specialists located in Sioux Falls, South Dakota, use data from biometric telehealth monitors such as cardiac, pulmonary, and diabetes monitoring devices and data from nonbiometric motion, sleep, and stove temperature sensors to remotely assess triggering events, which are changes from normal or "baseline" patterns. Depending on the severity or urgency of the event, the nurse specialist notifies the client, HHC agency, or local GSS staff for additional follow-up.

The role of nurse specialist was new to the LW@H program and an evaluation was conducted to understand how these nurses use the telehealth system to support at-risk adults in community-based settings. The evaluation consisted of 4 focus groups conducted over a 29-month time frame, at 6, 12, 18, and 35 months postdeployment of LW@H. Findings from the focus groups (Grant et al., 2014) illustrate the importance of assessing adoption and acceptance of new roles as part of an overall telehealth evaluation. The findings encompassed challenges that included learning the new telehealth systems and "making sense" of large volumes of biometric and nonbiometric data, developing a logical workflow with local sites, and training local personnel on how to install and use the telehealth monitors. Collection and transmission of the biometric and nonbiometric data occurred at different times and made assessment and interpretation of the data challenging. Synchronizing transmission times reduced this challenge and helped nurses developed algorithms for understanding the data. The initial workflow for a "triggering" event (Grant et al., 2014) started with contacting the local HHC agency, which then sent personnel to the client location. The time and effort required for this workflow made nurse specialists apprehensive of false positives and false negatives. Implementation of a "direct-to-client" model, where nurse specialists contact clients directly via telephone for real-time assessment, allowed LW@H to better identify clients needing immediate home care or other support. Most important was that despite challenges of the new role, nurse specialists found their work valuable to clients and home care agencies.

The findings from this study reflect those from the study of Dutch nurses' willingness to use technology, which found "perceived usefulness of home telehealth for the client was the most important predictor of nurses' willingness to use the technology" (van Houwelingen et al., 2015, p. 54). Although the evaluation was conducted from 2011 to 2014, adoption barriers such as insufficient training and technological issues identified by Taylor et al. (2015) were reflected by the early focus group participants. Adoption facilitators such as time to work with and understand the technology, clear workflows, and successful care resulting from telehealth identified by Taylor et al. (2015) were reflected in later focus groups. Actionable use of early findings reduced the barriers and increased the facilitators for adoption, and improved overall functioning of the LW@H system.

Findings from the VALUE study, described earlier, can provide additional capability to a health-smart home. A web-based portal for ordering health and community services, messaging between the resident and health provider or family and friends, and Internet access can enhance a resident's ability to successfully age in place.

Despite the technological advances and potential health-related benefits of health-smart homes, there are still significant concerns that can impact adoption and continued use of the technology. Close monitoring of daily activities can be perceived as an invasion of privacy, and balance between the benefits of monitoring and the need for privacy is a problem for many of us—it is not limited to the aging population. The obtrusiveness of older monitoring devices in health-smart homes often stigmatized the resident and reduced beneficial socialization activities. The increased miniaturization, wireless connectivity, and judicial placement of the monitor devices have helped to reduce this problem.

NURSING COMPETENCIES FOR HOME TELEHEALTH

In recognition of the important nursing roles in the current and future success of home telehealth programs within the health care universe, planners at the University of Minnesota School of Nursing incorporated a telehealth learning environment in their recently launched Bentson Healthy Communities Center (www.nursing .umn.edu/about/our-facilities/bentson-healthy-communities-innovation-center). The center was designed to reflect the future of health care delivery and nursing science. State-of-the-art technology includes the use of electronic health records and supportive technologies such as mobile record systems and the integration of telehealth technologies. Its simulated environments span the continuum of care, including acute, critical, skilled, ambulatory, and home care settings. A major theme of the educational program is the identification of nursing competencies needed to successfully incorporate home telehealth into clinical practice, particularly as the technology moves from the research setting to clinical care.

The group identified specific telehealth activities that nurses currently perform, and then determined several core competencies that nurses needed to master in order to best perform these activities. To be competent in working with telehealth technologies, nurses must understand how telehealth can be used to care for patients at a distance in a variety of settings, must recognize the benefits and limitations of telehealth strategies, and must recognize the value of these technologies to engage and empower patients as partners in managing their own care. They must also be able to use these technologies to develop a plan of care with the patient; these skills include recommendations for care, call-back instructions, and education so that the technology is used properly, progressively, and beneficially during the course of home care. Understanding basic telehealth terminology and the legal and regulatory issues related to telehealth nursing practice will reduce these potential barriers and further the competency of nurses practicing in these settings. As videoconferencing captures a larger amount of home telehealth nursing activity, the nurse must understand the principles of effective videoconference communication and be able to put them into practice in order to provide a competent link between patient, provider, and technology. Finally the nurse must be able to analyze and interpret incoming biometric data from remote patient monitoring devices and be sufficiently skilled in utilizing clinical algorithms to assess patient needs and symptoms.

Developing these competencies to enable successful home telehealth nursing involvement will address many of the barriers cited for poor levels of acceptance and adoption, particularly those focused on nurse–patient interaction, local nurse governance, and technological issues. Barriers involving licensure, institutional issues, local champions, and reimbursement cannot, of course, be resolved by these educational initiatives, but will require policy initiatives at the institutional, state, and federal levels to finally address the barriers to a broader acceptance and adoption of home telehealth as an equal player in caring for patients in a noninstitutional setting.

CONCLUSION

Is the time right for home telehealth? Evidence indicating equivalent or better outcomes when compared to in-person or standard care has been established for numerous populations and technologies. Cost and access considerations have diminished with miniaturization and mobile computing. From a consumer or patient perspective, research has shifted from "can and will they use the technology" to "how do they use the technology to increase engagement" and reflects maturation within the Technology Acceptance Model (Venkatesh & Davis, 2000). While these factors indicate that the time is right for telehealth, a number of barriers continue to plague the health delivery system.

Topping the list of barriers is willingness to use health information technology by nurses. Studies in the Netherlands (van Houwelingen et al., 2015), the United Kingdom, and the United States (Grant et al., 2014) reflect difficulty integrating telehealth into clinical workflows and understanding the value of telehealth for clients. These studies suggest incorporating telehealth education into nursing curriculums and developing training scenarios that highlight how successful telehealth care could remove these barriers, as seen in the University of Minnesota initiatives cited earlier.

In the United States, licensure has created barriers to telehealth use. Nurse licensure is based on the state where a nurse practices. In 1998, the National Council of State Boards of Nursing recognized the need for nurses to practice across state lines, both physically and via technology. The Nurse Licensure Compact (NLC or Compact) allows nurses in Compact states to practice in other Compact states without obtaining an additional license (NCSBN: National Council of State Boards of Nursing, 2016). Since 2000, 25 states have adopted the Compact legislation. For nurses working with telehealth, their practice location is considered the patient's location and licensure must match. Nurses with licensure in a Compact state and practicing (or working with patients) in a Compact state require no additional licensure. Nurses residing in a non-Compact state must obtain licensure in each practice state (or patient location), which creates a barrier to telehealth use.

The final and most formidable barrier to home telehealth is long-term sustainability. The research of our group and others changed reimbursement policy to include hospital-to-hospital, clinic-to-clinic, and clinic-to-nursing home telehealth consultations, but has not moved the dial significantly on clinic-to-home telehealth reimbursement. Reimbursement of home telemonitoring for specific conditions exists, but the limited amount rarely covers the cost of home monitoring equipment and personnel. Successful outcomes of home telehealth include reduced clinic and emergency department visits and unplanned hospital admissions. In an FFS reimbursement environment that rewards in-person care, it is not surprising that home telehealth has not achieved its potential.

A fundamental shift in health care delivery financing is under way and holds promise not only for home telehealth, but also for achievement of the IHI Triple Aim. Medicare, Medicaid, and private payers are increasingly testing TCC payment models. Across the United States, demonstration projects have implemented novel solutions that decrease the cost of care while increasing patient experience and health. Nurses utilizing digital health technologies, including home telehealth, are instrumental in the success of these projects. The transformation of health care delivery depends on increasing use and usefulness of digital and telehealth technologies. Nurses are poised to lead this change and deliver the promise of the IHI Triple Aim.

REFERENCES

Cady, R. G., Erickson, M., Lunos, S., Finkelstein, S. M., Looman, W., Celebreeze, M., & Garwick, A. (2015). Meeting the needs of children with medical complexity using a telehealth advanced practice registered nurse care coordination model. *Maternal and Child Health Journal, 19*(7), 1497–1506. doi:10.1007/s10995-014-1654-1

Cady, R. G., Finkelstein, S. M., & Kelly, A. (2009). A telehealth nursing intervention reduces hospitalizations in children with complex health conditions. *Journal of Telemedicine & Telecare, 15*(6), 317–320.

Cady, R. G., Kelly, A., & Finkelstein, S. M. (2008). Home telehealth for children with special healthcare needs. *Journal of Telemedicine & Telecare, 14*(4), 173–177.

Center for Connected Health Policy. (2016). What is telehealth? Retrieved from http://cchpca.org/what-is-telehealth

Choi, N. G., Hegel, M. T., Marti, C. N., Marinucci, M. L., Sirrianni, L., & Bruce, M. L. (2014). Telehealth problem-solving therapy for depressed low-income homebound older adults. *American Journal of Geriatric Psychiatry, 22*(3), 263–271. doi:10.1016/j.jagp.2013.01.037

Cohen, E., Kuo, D., Agrawal, R., Berry, J., Bhagat, S., Simon, T., & Srivastava, R. (2011). Children with medical complexity: An emerging population for clinical and research initiatives. *Pediatrics, 127*(3), 529–538.

Demiris, G., Finkelstein, S. M., & Speedie, S. M. (2001). Considerations for the design of a web-based clinical monitoring and educational system for elderly patients. *Journal of the American Medical Informatics Association, 8*(5), 468–472.

Demiris, G., & Hensel, B. K. (2008). Technologies for an aging society: A systematic review of "smart home" applications. *IMIA Yearbook of Medical Informatics, 47*(Suppl. 1), 33–40.

Farrar, F. C. (2015). Transforming home health nursing with telehealth technology. *Nursing Clinics of North America, 50*(2), 269–281. doi:10.1016/j.cnur.2015.03.004

Finkelstein, S. M., Budd, J. R., Warwick, W. J., Kujawa, S. J., Wielinski, C. L., & Ewing, L. B. (1986). Feasibility and compliance studies of a home measurement monitoring program for cystic fibrosis. *Journal of Chronic Diseases, 39*(3), 195–205.

Finkelstein, S. M., Lindgren, B., Prasad, B., Snyder, M., Edin, C., Wielinski, C., & Hertz, M. (1993). Reliability and validity of spirometry measurements in a paperless home monitoring diary program for lung transplantation. *Heart Lung, 22*(6), 523–533.

Finkelstein, S. M., Potthoff, S., LeMire, T., Valley, K., Dahle, L., Ratner, E., & Speedie, S. M. (2007). VALUE (Virtual Assisted Living Umbrella for the Elderly) user perceptions. *Telemedicine Journal & E-Health, 13*, 182.

Finkelstein, S. M., Scudiero, A., Lindgren, B., Snyder, M., & Hertz, M. I. (2005). Decision support for the triage of lung transplant recipients on the basis of home-monitoring spirometry and symptom reporting. *Heart & Lung, 34*(3), 201–208.

Finkelstein, S. M., Snyder, M., Edin-Stibbe, C., Chlan, L., Prasad, B., Dutta, P., . . . Hertz, M. I. (1996). Monitoring progress after lung transplantation from home-patient adherence. *Journal of Medical Engineering & Technology, 20*(6), 203–210.

Finkelstein, S. M., Speedie, S. M., Demiris, G., Veen, M., Lundgren, J. M., & Potthoff, S. (2004). Tele-homecare: Quality, perception, satisfaction. *Telemedicine Journal & E-Health, 10*(2), 122–128.

Finkelstein, S. M., Speedie, S. M., & Potthoff, S. (2006). Home telehealth improves clinical outcomes at lower cost for home healthcare. *Telemedicine Journal & E-Health, 12*(2), 128–136.

Finkelstein, S. M., Speedie, S. M., Zhou, X., Ratner, E., & Potthoff, S. (2006). VALUE: Virtual Assisted Living Umbrella for the Elderly: User patterns. In *Engineering in Medicine and Biology Society, 2006. EMBS '06. 28th Annual International Conference of the IEEE* (pp. 3294–3296). New York, NY: Institute of Electrical and Electronics Engineers.

Grant, L. A., Rockwood, T., & Stennes, L. (2014). Testing telehealth using technology-enhanced nurse monitoring. *Journal of Gerontological Nursing, 40*(10), 15–23. doi:10.3928/00989134 -20140808-01

Institute for Healthcare Improvement. (2015). The IHI triple aim. Retrieved from http://www.ihi .org/Engage/Initiatives/TripleAim/Pages/default.aspx

Jakobsen, A. S., Laursen, L. C., Rydahl-Hansen, S., Ostergaard, B., Gerds, T. A., Emme, C., . . . Phanareth, K. (2015). Home-based telehealth hospitalization for exacerbation of chronic obstructive pulmonary disease: Findings from "the virtual hospital" trial. *Telemedicine Journal and e-Health, 21*(5), 364–373. doi:10.1089/tmj.2014.0098

Kelly, A., Golnik, A., & Cady, R. (2008). A medical home center: Specializing in the care of children with special health care needs of high intensity. *Maternal & Child Health Journal, 12*(5), 633–640.

Lindgren, B. R., Finkelstein, S. M., Prasad, B., Dutta, P., Killoren, T., Scherber, J., . . . Hertz, M. I. (1997). Determination of reliability and validity in home monitoring data of pulmonary function tests following lung transplantation. *Research in Nursing & Health, 20*(6), 539–550.

Looman, W. S., Antolick, M., Cady, R. G., Lunos, S. A., Garwick, A. E., & Finkelstein, S. M. (2015). Effects of a telehealth care coordination intervention on perceptions of health care by caregivers of children with medical complexity: A randomized controlled trial. *Journal of Pediatric Health Care, 29*(4), 352–363. doi:10.1016/j.pedhc.2015.01.007

Marquis, N., Larivee, P., Saey, D., Dubois, M. F., & Tousignant, M. (2015). In-home pulmonary tele-rehabilitation for patients with chronic obstructive pulmonary disease: A pre-experimental study on effectiveness, satisfaction, and adherence. *Telemedicine Journal and e-Health, 21*(11), 870–879. doi:10.1089/tmj.2014.0198

Merchant, K. A., Ward, M. M., Mueller, K. J., Rural Health Research & Policy Centers, & Rural Policy Research Institute, RUPRI Center for Rural Health Policy Analysis, University of Iowa College of Public Health, Department of Health Management and Policy. (2015). Hospital views of factors affecting telemedicine use. *Rural Policy Brief, 2015*(5), 1–4.

National Survey of Children with Special Health Care Needs. (n.d.). Data resource center. Retrieved from http://www.childhealthdata.org/learn/NS-CSHCN

National Council of State Boards of Nursing. (2016). Nurse licensure compact. Retrieved from https://www.ncsbn.org/nurse-licensure-compact.htm

Neufeld, J. D., Doarn, C. R., & Aly, R. (2016). State policies influence medicare telemedicine utilization. *Telemedicine Journal and e-Health, 22*(1), 70–74. doi:10.1089/tmj.2015.0044

Office of the Legislative Counsel, U.S. House of Representatives. (2010). Compilation of patient protection and Affordable Care Act. Retrieved from http://www.hhs.gov/healthcare/ rights/law/index.html

Ostrovsky, A., Deen, N., Simon, A., & Mate, K. (2014, June). A framework for selecting digital health technology: IHI innovation report. Retrieved from www.ihi.org

Rantz, M., Skubic, M., Abbott, C., Galambos, C., Popescu, M., Keller, J., . . . Petroski, G. F. (2015). Automated in-home fall risk assessment and detection sensor system for elders. *The Gerontologist, 55*(Suppl. 1), S78–S87. doi:10.1093/geront/gnv044

Sabati, N., Snyder, M., Edin-Stibbe, C., Lindgren, B., & Finkelstein, S. (2001). Facilitators and barriers to adherence with home monitoring using electronic spirometry. *AACN Clinical Issues, 12*, 178–185.

Slagle, J. R., Finkelstein, S. M., Leung, L. A., & Warwick, W. J. (1989). Monitor: An expert system that validates and interprets time-dependent partial data based on a cystic fibrosis home monitoring program. *IEEE Transactions on Bio-Medical Engineering, 36*(5), 552–558. doi:10.1109/10.24258

Taylor, J., Coates, E., Brewster, L., Mountain, G., Wessels, B., & Hawley, M. S. (2015). Examining the use of telehealth in community nursing: Identifying the factors affecting frontline staff acceptance and telehealth adoption. *Journal of Advanced Nursing, 71*(2), 326–337. doi:10.1111/jan.12480

Tyrer, H. W., Alwan, M., Demiris, G., He, Z., Keller, J., Skubic, M., & Rantz, M. (2006). Technology for successful aging. In *Engineering in Medicine and Biology Society, 2006. EMBS '06. 28th Annual International Conference of the IEEE* (pp. 3290–3293). New York, NY: Institute of Electrical and Electronics Engineers. doi:10.1109/IEMBS.2006.259617

United HealthCare Services. (2015). United Healthcare covers virtual care physician visits, expanding consumers' access to affordable health care options. Retrieved from https://www.uhc.com/news-room/2015-news-release-archive/unitedhealthcare-covers-virtual-care-physician-visits

van Houwelingen, C. T., Barakat, A., Best, R., Boot, W. R., Charness, N., & Kort, H. S. (2015). Dutch nurses' willingness to use home telehealth: Implications for practice and education. *Journal of Gerontological Nursing, 41*(4), 47–56. doi:10.3928/00989134-20141203-01

Venkatesh, V., & Davis, F. D. (2000). A theoretical extension of the technology acceptance model: Four longitudinal field studies. *Management Science, 46*(2), 186–204.

Vuorinen, A. L., Leppanen, J., Kaijanranta, H., Kulju, M., Helio, T., van Gils, M., & Lahteenmaki, J. (2014). Use of home telemonitoring to support multidisciplinary care of heart failure patients in Finland: Randomized controlled trial. *Journal of Medical Internet Research, 16*(12), e282. doi:10.2196/jmir.3651

Whittaker, F., & Wade, V. (2014). The costs and benefits of technology-enabled, home-based cardiac rehabilitation measured in a randomised controlled trial. *Journal of Telemedicine and Telecare, 20*(7), 419–422. doi:10.1177/1357633X14552376

Wicklund, E. (2016). Making the most out of telehealth. Retrieved from http://mhealthintelligence.com/news/making-the-most-out-of-telehealth

17

Palliative and End-of-Life Care Issues in Adults: The Physician Orders for Life-Sustaining Treatment (POLST) Program

Susan E. Hickman

Palliative and end-of-life care has received increasing attention from researchers and policy makers over the past 25 years. The Institute of Medicine's (IOM) 2014 report, *Dying in America: Improving Quality and Honoring Individual Preferences*, provides a comprehensive review of the multitude of problems that complicate caring for patients near the end of life. A fragmented and uncoordinated health care system often leads to care that is inconsistent with patient values and goals. Families are poorly integrated into care, yet are expected to take on increasing responsibility for caregiving. Conversations about values, goals, and preferences are essential to providing patient-centered care and supporting high-quality decisions, but these conversations often do not occur or are poorly conducted because of a lack of clinician training. Policy changes and payment reform are needed to support and incentivize high-quality care (IOM, 2014).

The process of discussing patient goals, values, and preferences for care is an important strategy for improving care of the dying. The advance care planning process involves conversations that ideally occur over time between the patient, family members, and treating clinicians. To help ensure that resulting decisions are known and honored in the event that the patient loses decisional capacity, treatment preferences should be recorded and readily accessible (IOM, 2014).

Traditionally, the *living will* has been used to document patient preferences for care at the very end of life. However, living wills are largely ineffective at altering treatments (Fagerlin & Schneider, 2004; Silveira, Wiitala, & Piette, 2014; Wilkinson, Wenger, & Shugarman, 2007) unless they are part of a broader community-based advance care planning system (Hammes, Rooney, & Gundrum, 2010; Hammes, Rooney, Gundrum, Hickman, & Hager, 2012). The language contained in living wills is often vague, requiring interpretation by a physician before the wishes can be acted upon. It can also be challenging for healthy adults to predict their treatment preferences in the future when faced with some unknown health problem. Only a minority of adults have living wills, and the documents are frequently unavailable when needed for those who do (Fagerlin & Schneider, 2004).

Cardiopulmonary resuscitation (CPR) code status orders are an alternative strategy to document patient treatment preferences for care at the end of life. The options are *full code* (attempt resuscitation) or *do not resuscitate* (DNR). However, this approach is problematic as well. A focus on CPR falsely dichotomizes and over-simplifies choices about end-of-life care and palliation (Happ et al., 2002). Patients and family members face numerous decisions in the final months and weeks of life before code status decisions become relevant. The presence of a DNR order is not specific to other life-sustaining treatments or immediately applicable in most situations. However, this is often the only piece of information available about the over-all goals of care. Code status orders may be overgeneralized and assumed to reflect preferences for the broader plan of care, resulting in limitations on treatments that may not necessarily reflect patient preferences (Beach & Morrison, 2002; Holtzman, Pheley, & Lurie, 1994; Zweig, Kruse, Binder, Szafara, & Mehr, 2004).

The Physician Orders for Life-Sustaining Treatment (POLST) program was designed to overcome the limitations of traditional advance care planning tools (Hickman, Hammes, Moss, & Tolle, 2005). The centerpiece of the program is a form used to record treatment preferences as medical orders. It is designed for use with patients with advanced illness or frailty who are nearing the end of life. The POLST form orders are contained in sections: Section A—resuscitation code status; Section B—level of medical interventions (including hospitalization); Section C—antibiotics; and Section D—artificially administered nutrition. The form is completed by a health care professional based on a discussion with the patient or his or her decision maker. It is then signed by a physician, nurse practitioner, or physician assistant, thus recording the patient's treatment preferences as actionable medical orders that can be honored throughout the health care system (Hickman et al., 2005).

The POLST was initially developed in Oregon in the early 1990s, and its use has since spread. The POLST program caught the attention of clinicians and policy makers around the United States, aided in part by the Robert Wood Johnson Foundation Community-State Partnerships Program (Christopher & Bain, 2003; Christopher & Spann, 1999) and the IOM report (Field & Cassel, 1997). The first community outside of Oregon to adopt the POLST was La Crosse, Wisconsin, where POLST use began in 1996. The National POLST Advisory Panel was formed in 2004 with initial members including representatives from the five states using POLST at that time (Oregon, Washington, Wisconsin, West Virginia, and New York) as well as the American Bar Association; later the group expanded to include Pennsylvania. New bylaws were issued in 2007, creating the National POLST Paradigm Task Force. This group provides interested states with educational resources, guidance, and consultation services to support development. As of 2016, almost half the states in the country have an active POLST program endorsed by the National POLST Paradigm

Task Force, and almost every other state has a similar program at varying stages of development. Models based on the POLST paradigm are now being used in the care of tens of thousands of seriously ill patients across the country. Although the name of these programs varies by state, the programs share the same core elements (www .polst.org).

RESEARCH ON THE POLST PARADIGM

Research has played an important role in the development of the POLST paradigm from the beginning. In addition to formative research that led to the development of the POLST (Dunn et al., 1996), researchers have always been actively involved in the national program. A growing body of research provides data to guide implementation and quality improvement as well as drive policy change through evaluations of POLST use. A 2015 review of the literature identified 23 studies on the use of POLST in the clinical context (Hickman, Keevern, & Hammes, 2015) and eight additional studies were published in the subsequent year. A summary of key research findings is provided here.

Patient Characteristics

Patient characteristics, including age, race, and primary disease, influence whether and how the POLST form is used. Older patients are more likely to have POLST (Fromme, Zive, Schmidt, Cook, & Tolle, 2014; Fromme, Zive, Schmidt, Olszewski, & Tolle, 2012; Hammes et al., 2012; Schmidt, Zive, Fromme, Cook, & Tolle, 2014) and orders to limit treatments are more common in older patients than in younger patients (Hickman, Tolle, Brummel-Smith, & Carley, 2004; Schmidt et al., 2014). Non-White patients use POLST less frequently (Hickman, Nelson, Perrin, Moss, Hammes, & Tolle, 2010) and have orders for more aggressive interventions in Section B than White patients (Hickman et al., 2010; Rahman, Bressette, Gassoumis, & Enguidanos, 2015). Diagnosis may influence whether POLST is used. Research on Oregon decedents suggests that patients with cancer are more likely to have POLST at the time of death than patients with heart disease (Fromme et al., 2014).

Setting of Care

The way in which POLST is used also varies by setting. For example, the frequency of different resuscitation code status orders documented on POLST differs depending on the population. In one hospice sample, 99% of patients had a DNR order at the time of death (Hickman et al., 2009). In a mixed community sample drawn from the Oregon POLST registry, only 72% of patients had an order for DNR (Fromme et al., 2012). Overall, the pattern of orders varies, with orders for more curative treatment in populations where there is more variability in prognosis and health status, and orders for more comfort-focused treatment in populations where prognosis and health status are more uniformly poor (Hammes et al., 2012; Hickman et al., 2004, 2009, 2010; Fromme et al., 2012).

Timing of POLST Orders

POLST is intended for patients who are nearing the end of life (www.polst.org). Recent research suggests that POLST is completed a median of 6.4 weeks before death (Zive, Fromme, Schmidt, Cook, & Tolle, 2015). New and revised POLST forms are more common for patients near the end of life (Hickman et al., 2011; Zive et al., 2015). Typically, when POLST forms are revised, it is to document orders for less aggressive treatment (Hickman et al., 2011; Zive et al., 2015). Almost half of forms are written within the final 4 weeks of life (Zive et al., 2015).

Associations Between POLST Form Orders and Outcomes

Section B of the POLST is the form's most unique feature because it provides medical orders for the desired level of medical intervention. Multiple studies have found associations between treatments and Section B orders. Patients with comfort care orders are less likely to receive life-sustaining treatments such as hospitalization than patients with orders for full treatment (Hammes et al., 2012; Hickman et al., 2004, 2009, 2010). The only study to date comparing POLST users with a randomly selected sample of non-POLST users was funded by the National Institute of Nursing Research (NINR; NR009784). Chart review data was abstracted for residents with and without POLST forms at a random sample of facilities in Oregon, Wisconsin, and West Virginia. Multilevel modeling, including facility characteristics and patient characteristics, suggested that patients with comfort care orders were less likely to receive life-sustaining treatments than patients without a POLST form (Hickman et al., 2010). Given that patients with comfort care orders are less likely to go to the hospital, it is unsurprising that additional research suggests patients with orders for comfort care are less likely to die at the hospital (Fromme et al., 2014; Hammes et al., 2012; Pedraza, Culp, Falkenstine, & Moss, 2016; Tuck et al., 2015).

Treatments provided to patients are generally consistent with the orders documented on POLST (Hickman et al., 2011; Lee, Brummel-Smith, Meyer, Drew, & London, 2000). Section A orders about resuscitation are the only section where it is possible make a determination about whether an indicated treatment was *not* provided, because it is clear that CPR was indicated if a patient is deceased and there is no record of a CPR attempt or explanation about why the treatment was not provided (e.g., rigor mortis). In a multistate study, detailed chart reviews yielded data suggesting that treatments were consistent with Section A orders 98% (300/306) of the time. In Sections B, C, and D of the POLST, it is only possible to look at whether the treatment provided is consistent with the order as written. If the treatment is not provided, it is unclear if it was indicated and not provided because of POLST or just not ever indicated. In the multistate study, treatments were consistent with Section B orders 91% (102/112) of the time. A majority of the treatments provided to patients with orders for comfort care were comfort-focused, such as hospitalizations for uncontrolled pain, and only a small number were inconsistent with the order to provide comfort care. Antibiotic use was consistent with orders about antibiotic use 93% (224/241) of the time (Hickman et al., 2011), though there were no differences in antibiotic use between residents with and without POLST (Hickman et al., 2010). Consistency was lowest between treatment and orders about feeding tube use. Feeding tube use was consistent with orders 64% (12/22) of the time. However, the 10 discrepancies were due largely to situations in which the order reflected a preference for a trial period of feeding tube use. Feeding tube use was categorized as inconsistent because a trial had been started and never discontinued or revisited. The small number of cases involved makes it problematic to generalize about the utility of this order.

Clinician Experiences With POLST

Clinician reports about the use of POLST are largely positive. Hospice staff report that POLST helps initiate conversation, guides treatment decisions, and provides clear instructions (Hickman et al., 2004). Emergency medical services (EMS) personnel report that POLST orders often result in changes to the treatments provided when they arrive at the scene, such as withholding CPR (Schmidt, Hickman, Tolle, & Brooks, 2004; Schmidt, Olszewski, Zive, Fromme, & Tolle, 2013). However, there are challenges in implementing POLST, including education gaps resulting in difficulty understanding and explaining the form (Hickman et al., 2009; Sugiyama et al., 2013; Vo et al., 2011; Waldrop, Clemency, Maguin, & Lindstrom, 2014), discomfort with the problems the form raises (Hickman et al., 2009; Sugiyama et al., 2013), and difficulty interpreting the orders (Mirarchi, Cammarata, et al., 2015; Mirarchi, Doshi, Zerkle, & Cooney, 2015). A variety of logistical problems have also been identified, including concerns about the amount of time involved in discussing POLST, challenges in obtaining clinician signatures, problems transferring the form across settings, and family disagreements. Notably, a majority of these problems are not specific to POLST. The frequency, duration, and impact of these problems are unknown. Efforts to implement POLST may draw increased attention to the broader cultural and systems problems described in the recent IOM report (IOM, 2014).

Legal Issues and POLST

A related area of research focuses on the legal issues central to use of the POLST tool. In 2008, investigators at the Oregon Health & Science University School of Nursing, the American Bar Association, and the West Virginia Center for Health, Law, and

Ethics collaborated on a study evaluating potential state legal barriers to POLST implementation (Hickman, Sabatino, Moss, & Nester-Wherle, 2008). Interviews were conducted with key legal informants in each state, and a review of laws was conducted to supplement the interviews. Although some states are able to develop programs based on the POLST model within the language of existing state laws and regulations, most require legislative change (Sabatino & Karp, 2011). Several key areas of the law were identified as representing potential legal barriers, including limitations on consent to forgo life-sustaining treatment, medical preconditions and witnessing requirements, default surrogate provisions, and out-of-hospital DNR (OHDNR) protocol barriers (Hickman et al., 2008). A second study evaluated the factors that facilitated or hindered states with active POLST programs (Sabatino & Karp, 2011). Findings include variability in legislative and regulatory approaches, the identification of facilitators, and delineation of almost 40 issues and barriers encountered during all phases of development (Sabatino & Karp, 2011).

Limitations of Existing POLST Research

There are significant limitations of the existing research on POLST, including potential bias in study samples (Hickman et al., 2015). A large number of studies have been conducted in Oregon where the form was originally developed. It is unclear whether the findings from Oregon are generalizable to other settings (Hickman et al., 2015; Moore, Rubin, & Halpern, 2016). Low response rates and a reliance on hypothetical scenarios raise doubts about the validity and generalizability of some survey findings, such as one study reporting a response rate of 18% (Mirarchi, Cammarata, et al., 2015). A significant unanswered question is how well POLST orders reflect the values-based preferences of informed patients or surrogates. A few small studies have explored this issue, but small sample sizes and methodological limitations limit generalizability (Hickman, Nelson, Smith-Howell, & Hammes, 2014; Meyers, Moore, McGrory, Sparr, & Ahern, 2004; Schmidt et al., 2013). Finally, a majority of these studies are descriptive and nonrandom, making comparisons difficult (Hickman et al., 2015; Moore et al., 2016). For example, a comparison of POLST orders and location of death found significant associations between POLST comfort care orders and death at home in comparison to POLST full treatment orders. However, potential confounders (e.g., hospice) could not be accounted for due to sampling limitations. There were also no comparisons between decedents with and without POLST forms (Fromme et al., 2014).

The only study conducted to date with a rigorous comparison sample was funded by the NINR, the National Institutes of Health leading institute for palliative and end-of-life care research. This 2005 multistate study of POLST in Oregon, Wisconsin, and West Virginia (described earlier) resulted in data about the treatments provided to 1,792 randomly selected long-stay nursing facility residents with and without POLST (NR009784; Hickman et al., 2009, 2010). Multilevel modeling was used in the analysis to account for both facility and patient-level characteristics (Hickman et al., 2010). In a 2014 systematic review of research on the effect of advance care planning on end-of-life care, this NINR-funded project was assigned the highest grade possible for an observational study (Brinkman-Stoppelenburg, Rietjens, & van der Heider, 2014). NINR's support for this kind of research is essential, both because of the high bar set by the scientific review process and the capacity to fund research at the level necessary to support rigorous science. The development of the NINR Office of End-of-Life and Palliative Care Research reflects NINR's commitment to continuing support of this research, which is critical to build the evidence base about POLST and end-of-life care more broadly.

TRANSLATING RESEARCH INTO POLICY

Although the evidence is still emerging and there are still many unanswered questions, the strength of the existing data on POLST has motivated many policy leaders and advocates to move forward with implementation. Data about the POLST model has been important in supporting policy change in states around the country, such as Virginia, Oregon, California, and West Virginia. In 2013, the IOM invited testimony on the evidence supporting POLST as well as legal issues related to POLST use, resulting in a recommendation that all states work toward the implementation of a POLST Paradigm program (IOM, 2014).

INDIANA: A CASE STUDY

The Indiana experience is instructive in demonstrating both how research can be used to drive policy changes at the state level and the complexity of this process. As is reflected by legal research on POLST, state-level policy change is complex (Hickman et al., 2008; Sabatino & Karp, 2011). Strong data are requisite as the starting point for policy change, and an additional investment of time and commitment will also be needed.

The Indiana Physician Orders for Scope of Treatment (POST), Indiana's version of POLST, has its roots firmly planted in research. The Indiana POST form is available online from the Indiana State Department of Health (n.d.; Figure 17.1). The founding members of the Indiana Patient Preferences Coalition (IPPC) met first in 2010 following a presentation about the results of the NINR-funded study on POLST that drew clinicians, lawyers, and ethicists from the Indianapolis community. Based on the review of state laws (Hickman et al., 2008), it was clear that legislation was necessary in order to implement POLST in Indiana. Of specific concern were the Indiana OHDNR statutes, which were incompatible with the POLST Paradigm model because of the inclusion of narrow medical preconditions, a required witness signature, and a statutorily specified form that could not be modified to be compatible with POLST. Key legislators were approached and indicated they would be open to legislation if the group had grassroots support from across the community.

Indiana Physician Orders for Scope of Treatment (POST)
State Form 55317 (11-16)
Indiana State Department of Health – IC 16-36-6

INSTRUCTIONS: *This form is a physician's order for scope of treatment based on the patient's current medical condition and preferences. The POST should be reviewed whenever the patient's condition changes. A POST form is voluntary. A patient is not required to complete a POST form. A patient with capacity or their legal representative may void a POST form at any time by communicating that intent to the health care provider. Any section not completed does not invalidate the form and implies full treatment for that section. HIPAA permits disclosure to health care professionals as necessary for treatment. The original form is personal property of the patient. A facsimile, paper, or electronic copy of this form is a valid form.*

Patient Last Name	Patient First Name	Middle Initial
Birth Date (mm/dd/yyyy)	Medical Record Number:	Date Prepared (mm/dd/yyyy)

	DESIGNATION OF PATIENT'S PREFERENCES: The following sections (A through D) are the patient's current preferences for scope of treatment.
A *Check One*	**CARDIOPULMONARY RESUSCITATION (CPR):** Patient has no pulse AND is not breathing ☐ Attempt Resuscitation/CPR ☐ Do Not Attempt Resuscitation/DNR When not in cardiopulmonary arrest, follow orders in **B, C** and **D**
B *Check One*	**MEDICAL INTERVENTIONS:** If patient has pulse AND is breathing OR has pulse and is NOT breathing ☐ Comfort Measures (Allow Natural Death): Treatment Goal: Maximize comfort through symptom management. Relieve pain and suffering through the use of any medication by any route, positioning, wound care and other measures. Use oxygen, suction and manual treatment of airway obstruction as needed for comfort. Patient prefers no transfer to hospital for life-sustaining treatments. Transfer to hospital only if comfort needs cannot be met in current location. ☐ Limited Additional Interventions: Treatment Goal: Stabilization of medical condition. In addition to care described in Comfort Measures above, use medical treatment for stabilization, IV fluids (hydration) and cardiac monitor as indicated to stabilize medical condition. May use basic airway management techniques and non-invasive positive-airway pressure. Do not intubate. Transfer to hospital if indicated to manage medical needs or comfort. Avoid intensive care if possible. ☐ Full Intervention: Treatment Goal: Full interventions including life support measures in the intensive care unit. In addition to care described in Comfort Measures and Limited Additional Interventions above, use intubation, advanced airway interventions, and mechanical ventilation as indicated. Transfer to hospital and/or intensive care unit if indicated to meet medical needs.
C *Check One*	**ANTIBIOTICS:** ☐ Use antibiotics for infection only if comfort cannot be achieved fully through other means. ☐ Use antibiotics consistent with treatment goals.
D *Check One*	**ARTIFICIALLY ADMINISTERED NUTRITION:** Always offer food and fluid by mouth if feasible. ☐ No artificial nutrition. ☐ Defined trial period of artificial nutrition by tube. (Length of trial: _____ Goal: _____) ☐ Long-term artificial nutrition.
	OPTIONAL ADDITIONAL ORDERS:
	SIGNATURE PAGE: This form consists of two (2) pages. Both pages must be present. The following page includes signatures required for the POST form to be effective.

Page 1 of 2

FIGURE 17.1 Indiana physician orders for scope of treatment form (*continued*).

Source: Indiana State Department of Health (n.d.).

Patient Name: _____ Date of Birth: _____

	SIGNATURE OF PATIENT OR LEGALLY APPOINTED REPRESENTATIVE: In order for the POST form to be effective, the patient or legally appointed representative must sign and date the form below.
E	**SIGNATURE OF PATIENT OR LEGALLY APPOINTED REPRESENTATIVE** My signature below indicates that my physician or physician's designee discussed with me the above orders and the selected orders correctly represent my wishes.

Signature (*required by statute*)	Print Name (*required by statute*)	Date (*required by statute*)

F	**CONTACT INFORMATION FOR LEGALLY APPOINTED REPRESENTATIVE IN SECTION E (IF APPLICABLE):** If the signature above is other than patient's, add contact information for the representative.

Relationship of representative identified in Section E if patient does not have capacity (*required by statute*)	Address	Telephone Number

PHYSICIAN ORDER:

A POST form may be executed only by an individual's treating physician and only if:
  (1) the treating physician has determined that:
    (A) the individual is a qualified person; and
    (B) the medical orders contained in the individual's POST form are reasonable and medically appropriate for the individual; and
  (2) the qualified person or represent ative has signed and dated the POST form

A qualified person is an individual who has at least one (1) of the following:
  (1) An advanced chronic progressive illness.
  (2) An advanced chronic progressive frailty.
  (3) A condition caused by injury, disease, or illness from which, to a reasonable degree of medical certainty:
    (A) there can be no recovery; and
    (B) death will occur from the condition with in a short period without the provision of life prolonging procures.
  (4) A medical condition that, if the person were to suffer cardiac or pulmonary failure, resuscitation would be unsuccessful or within a short period the person would experience repeated cardiac or pulmonary failure resulting in death.

G	**DOCUMENTATION OF DISCUSSION: Orders discussed with (check one):** ☐ Patient (patient has capacity) ☐ Health Care Representative ☐ Legal Guardian ☐ Parent of Minor ☐ Health Care Power of Attorney
H	**SIGNATURE OF TREATING PHYSICIAN** My signature below indicates that I or my designee have discussed with the patient or patient's representative the patient's goals and treatment options available to the patient based on the patient's health. My signature below indicates to the best of my knowledge that these orders are consistent with the patient's current medical condition and preferences.

Signature of Treating Physician (*required by statute*)	Print Treating Physician Name (*required by statute*)	Date (*required by statute*)

Physician Office Telephone Number (*required by statute*)	Physician License Number (*required by statute*)	Health Care Professional preparing form if other than the physician

I	**APPOINTMENT OF HEALTH CARE REPRESENTATIVE:** As patient you have the option to appoint an individual to serve as your health care representative pursuant to IC 16-36-1-7. You are not required to designate a health care representative for this POST form to be effective. You are encouraged to consult with your attorney or other qualified individual about advance directives that are available to you. Forms and additional information about advance directives may be found on the ISDH web site at http://www.in.gov/isdh/25880.htm.

FIGURE 17.1 (*continued*)

In August 2010, the IPPC held its first formal meeting to develop a strategy for building support and creating draft legislation. Using a "snowball" method of recruitment, each new member was encouraged to identify and invite additional stakeholders. Membership was open to all, with a focus on recruiting individuals who could represent key stakeholder organizations and institutions—a strategy that helped ensure broad support and involvement. Quarterly meetings of the whole coalition were augmented with meetings of the smaller legislative committee. Through a process of regular and sometimes intense discussion, the diverse membership achieved consensus on several key issues.

First, the group decided that the Indiana program would be called the POST or Physician Orders for Scope of Treatment, reflecting the reality that the form represents a plan of care for the broader scope of treatment rather than orders specifically focused on life-sustaining therapies. Second, the group agreed that the POST form should require the signature of the patient or a legally authorized representative. Research suggests that most forms in use require a patient or surrogate signature (Hickman et al., 2010). Third, it was decided that the form itself should not be integrated into state statutes. Although the form contains required elements, the specific language is not specified by statute in order to permit future revisions if needed without requiring legislative action. Fourth, a subcommittee consisting primarily of clinicians worked together to review POLST form models from different states in order to develop the proposed Indiana version, a project that required significant discussion. Fifth, the group agreed that the form should be available for use with children. Sixth, it was agreed that it was unnecessary to require the signature of a witness. Finally, the group agreed conceptually that the POST legislation should build on the existing OHDNR statutes as much as possible. However, several issues remained that required extensive further discussion to identify differences of opinion, clarify misunderstandings, and achieve consensus.

Who Can Have a POST Form?

The existing Indiana OHDNR statutes contain a fairly narrow set of medical preconditions that are necessary in order for a patient to have an OHDNR. The patient must have either a terminal condition or a condition in which the patient is unlikely to benefit from CPR. Clinicians shared that they were uncomfortable using the label "terminal" with many of their patients and that the presence of this language on the form made the conversation about code status more difficult. Furthermore, these two categories omitted a large number of patients who might benefit from the POST form. Research describing the proposed trajectories of dying (Lunney, Lynn, Foley, Lipson, & Guralnik, 2003) and medical frailty (Fried et al., 2001) helped inform the discussion about potentially eligible patients, supporting a decision to expand the categories of patients who were eligible for POST to include patients with advanced chronic progressive illness or frailty.

Who Can Prepare a POST Form?

Research suggests that the POLST is often prepared by other members of the health care team, including nurses and social workers (Hickman et al., 2004). The group discussed the possibility of narrowly specifying who could prepare a POST form for review and signature by a physician, but it became apparent that it would be impossible to list everyone who might be appropriate in the various settings where the POST might be prepared and signed. Ultimately, the language was changed to permit preparation by a health care team member designated by the physician.

Who Can Sign and Activate a POST Form?

One of the more challenging discussions was focused on whether nurse practitioners or physician assistants could sign the POST form in order to activate the orders. Nurse practitioners play an important role in advance care planning conversations and have the authority to sign POLST forms in other states (Kim, Ersek, Bradway, & Hickman, 2015). However, only licensed physicians are allowed to sign an Indiana OHDNR order, so permitting nonphysicians to sign a POST form was viewed as an expansion in the scope of practice. Key stakeholders were unable to support the addition of physician extenders without endorsement by their members. This issue was therefore tabled for future discussion and the existing form restricted to physician signature only.

What If the Patient Lacks Decisional Capacity?

Indiana law permits legally appointed representatives to speak on behalf of patients who lack decisional capacity. If no one has been appointed, Indiana has default surrogate statutes that authorize family members to make decisions about life-sustaining treatments on behalf of patients without capacity. However, the list of default surrogates in statutes contains no hierarchy. Spouses, adult children, parents, and adult siblings are granted equal decision-making authority under the law, making it difficult to know who should serve as the surrogate in situations where there was no agreement about the best plan of care for the patient. The POST form was therefore restricted only to patients with decisional capacity or to the legally authorized representatives of patients without decisional capacity.

Ownership of the POST Form

A distinguishing feature of the POLST paradigm is that the form itself is designed to transfer with patients across settings. However, a few stakeholder organizations expressed concerns that they would be held liable if the form was inadvertently not transferred. There was strong resistance to including language on the form indicating it should be transferred with the patient. Therefore, the Indiana statute states that the POST form is the property of the patient and transferring remains a patient responsibility, despite concerns about whether a seriously ill patient could remember to bring a form in the middle of a medical crisis.

Religious and Faith-Based Considerations

From the very beginning, the group worked collaboratively with faith-based organizations and health care systems. In September 2011, the chair and co-chair were invited to present before three Indiana Catholic bishops during a meeting with Catholic health care leaders. These relationships proved to be critical given a growing national debate about whether the POLST Paradigm was consistent with Catholic values (Narin, 2013), and the legislation reflected this collaboration. Additions to the bill included a conscientious objector clause and clarification that the bill did not permit euthanasia or physician-assisted suicide.

The Legislative Path for POST

IPPC members with legislative expertise identified an ideal legislative sponsor in 2011: Representative Tim Brown, MD, a family physician who practiced in the emergency department and served as chair of the Indiana House Public Health Committee. This strong champion introduced House Bill 1114 in the 2012 Indiana General Assembly. Coalition members provided testimony about the research supporting the POLST model as well as professional and personal experiences illustrating the need for POLST. When the bill was tabled, stakeholders expressed concerns about a few issues that had not been resolved satisfactorily. After an additional year of discussion, House Bill 1182 was introduced with multiple bipartisan cosponsors. Similar to before, coalition members presented testimony about supporting research and the clinical case for POST. However, unlike before, all of the testimony was in favor of the legislation or neutral. A total of 28 stakeholder organizations and health systems expressed public support for the legislation, and no one testified in opposition. The bill passed in the Indiana House 99–0 and was introduced in the Senate with multiple bipartisan cosponsors, where it passed 48–1. The bill was signed into law by the Governor Michael R. Pence and the Indiana POST Act went into effect on July 1, 2013.

Translating Policy Into Practice

Translating research into policy is important, but represents just the first step along the way to changing practice. In order for the policy to take root, implementation requires significant effort and time as well as ongoing collaboration among multiple stakeholders. Following passage of the Indiana law, a top priority was to ensure that the POST form was available for use on July 1, 2013. The POST Act authorized the Indiana State Department of Health to develop and disseminate the POST form. The IPPC shared its draft POST form and met with leadership at the Indiana State Department of Health during the process of form development.

The IPPC continues to meet regularly, but the focus has shifted to discussions about implementation, outreach, and educational materials. To support this work, the group developed bylaws that outline membership criteria and a website to house resources (IPPC, 2016). Members developed model policies for hospitals, nursing homes, and hospices that were reviewed and approved by attorneys for stakeholder organizations prior to distribution. These policies can be readily adapted by organizations and put into practice. Partnerships have been leveraged to create resources, including an educational video for health care providers that includes a description of key research findings supporting use of the POLST paradigm (Indiana University Health, 2015).

The biggest educational outreach success to date in Indiana was garnering the support of the Emergency Medical Services Commission to require education for all newly certified and recertifying emergency medical responders in the state. A collaboration between the Indiana Department of Homeland Security, the Indiana Fire Chiefs Association Emergency Medical Services Section, and coalition members resulted in the development of an evidence-based training program for emergency medical responders (Indiana Department of Homeland Security, 2016). As a result, as of the end of 2015, a majority of emergency medical responders (85% or approximately 22,000/26,000) have received training about the Indiana POST. Success has been less uniform with other involved clinicians, including physicians, nurses, and social workers. Although there have been hundreds of presentations around the state reaching thousands of people, knowledge of the law and POST form is still highly inconsistent. A webinar for physicians is currently in development, as is a continuing nursing education article for nurses. Collaboration with key partners is ongoing. Recent discussion about the importance of advance care planning in preventing medical errors has resulted in the Indianapolis Coalition for Patient Safety identifying advance care planning as a safety focus. Similarly, the Indiana Cancer Consortium included advance care planning in the 2016–2020 Indiana Cancer Control Plan. Discussion is in progress about integrating advance care planning documents and POST into the health information exchange to facilitate accessibility across health systems, building upon work done at key hospitals to integrate POST into the electronic medical record.

POLICY AND RESEARCH IN INDIANA

The passage of the Indiana POST Act made it possible to launch two federally funded studies that address significant gaps in the POLST evidence base. Advance care planning and use of the POLST are key components of a Centers for Medicare and Medicaid demonstration program. Optimizing Patient Transfers, Impacting Medical Quality, and Improving Symptoms: Transforming Institutional Care (OPTIMISTIC) is designed to reduce potentially avoidable hospitalizations of long-stay nursing facility residents through enhanced geriatric care, a focus on transitions, and advance care planning in order to reduce costs and the negative effects that often result from unnecessary transfers of nursing home patients to the hospital (Unroe et al., 2015).

The funding announcement included a clear call for evidence-based interventions. POLST was included in the original proposal based on the strength of the NINR-funded multistate study finding that patients with POLST forms indicating comfort measures were 71% less likely to be hospitalized than patients with no POLST. These data suggested that it might be possible to further reduce avoidable hospitalizations by considering patient preferences in addition to clinical interventions. This notion represents a novel definition of avoidable hospitalizations. The intervention project began shortly before the Indiana POST statue went into effect in July 2013, placing the team and nurse interventionists on the forefront of implementation at all levels. Nurse interventionists are embedded in 19 Indianapolis nursing facilities with the support of a team of nurse practitioners. All enrolled patients are offered the opportunity to participate in conversations about goals of care using the structured, evidence-based Respecting Choices Last Steps® Facilitation model (www.gundersenhealth.org/respecting-choices), and POLST is being offered to all qualified patients.

In a preliminary analysis of data from 2,708 patients enrolled from August 2013 to December 2014, advance care planning conversations resulted in a change in orders 67% of the time. Most of these changes were recorded on a POLST form (Hickman, Unroe, Ersek, Buente, & Sachs, 2016). Future analyses will include an assessment of the effect of POLST on treatment outcomes and the relationship between use and cost savings yielded through averting hospitalizations. The project will also provide opportunities to evaluate patient and family experiences with POLST. Funding from the John A. Hartford Foundation for a planning grant is supporting further evaluation of the OPTIMISTIC model and dissemination opportunities. The OPTIMISTIC project was recently awarded an additional 4 years of funding by the Centers for Medicare and Medicaid Services to test a payment reform model that will be layered on top of the clinical intervention. A second group will be able to use the new codes to bill for providing care in the building, but will not be able to access the OPTIMISTIC clinical model (www.cms.gov). Findings have the potential to significantly impact policy decisions regarding reimbursement for nursing home care in a way that could dramatically shift the culture of care to prioritize patient preferences and goals.

A new study funded by NINR in 2015 (NR015255) was designed to address a significant unanswered question regarding how well POLST orders reflect patient and surrogate treatment preferences. Once POLST orders are signed by the treating clinician, the resulting orders direct care weeks and months into the future. It is unclear how well these orders represent patient preferences over time and how well patients and surrogates understand the orders documented on POLST. High decision quality is achieved when decisions reflect the values and preferences of informed patients (Winn, Ozanne, & Sepucha, 2015). This NINR-funded study will evaluate POLST decision quality, or how well existing POLST orders reflect current patient treatment preferences and how well the orders are understood. Interviews will be conducted with 320 randomly selected nursing home residents and surrogates in Indiana. In addition to data about the rate of POLST discordance, qualitative methods will be used to identify the reasons for discordance. Currently, the primary theory for discordance between advance care documentation and current preferences focuses on instability of preferences (Auriemma et al., 2014), but other reasons likely exist (Hickman, Hammes, Torke, Sudore, & Sachs, 2016). The potential state and federal policy implications of this NINR-funded study include the possibility that results will spur amendments to existing state POLST program legislation requiring period review, the implementation of mandatory POLST education programs tied to licensure or certification, and/or the identification of required conversation elements for reimbursement.

CONCLUSION

A growing body of evidence supports use of the POLST, fueled by research funding by NINR and private foundations. Research on the POLST has been used to drive change in health policy over the past 20 years at the local, regional, and state levels. An examination of the process of development in Indiana suggests that high-quality research is a requisite for creating a foundation on which to build sound health policy. Additional research is needed to address unanswered questions and provide direction to policy makers in the future.

REFERENCES

Auriemma, C. L., Nguyen, C. A., Bronheim, R., Kent, S., Nadiger, S., Pardo, D., & Halpern, S. D. (2014). Stability of end-of-life preferences: A systematic review of the evidence. *JAMA Internal Medicine, 174*(7), 1085–1092.

Beach, M. C., & Morrison, R. S. (2002). The effect of do-not-resuscitate orders on physician decision-making. *Journal of the American Geriatrics Society, 50*, 2057–2061.

Brinkman-Stoppelenburg, A., Rietjens, J. A. C., & van der Heider, A. (2014). The effects of advance care planning on end-of-life care: A systematic review. *Palliative Medicine, 28*, 1000–1025.

Christopher, M., & Bain, J. W. (Eds.). (2003). *Data-driven policymaking (an update): Using statistics to shape agendas and measure progress* (State Initiatives in End-of-Life Care, No. 18). Kansas City, MO: Midwest Bioethics Center.

Christopher, M., & Spann, J. (Eds.). (1999). *Implementing end-of-life treatment preferences across clinical settings* (State Initiatives in End-of-Life Care, No. 3). Kansas City, MO: Midwest Bioethics Center.

Dunn, P. M., Schmidt, T. A., Carley, M. M., Donius, M., Weinstein, M. A., & Dull, V. T. (1996). A method to communicate patient preferences about medically indicated life-sustaining treatment in the out-of-hospital setting. *Journal of the American Geriatrics Society, 44*(7), 785–791.

Fagerlin, A., & Schneider, C. E. (2004). Enough: The failure of the living will. *Hastings Center Report, 34*(2), 30–42.

Field, M. J., & Cassel, C. K. (1997). *Approaching death: Improving care at the end of life.* Washington, DC: National Academies Press.

Fried, L. P., Tangen, C. M., Walston, J., Newman, A. B., Hirsch, C., Gottdiener, J., . . . Cardiovascular Health Study Collaborative Research Group. (2001). Frailty in older adults: Evidence for a phenotype. *Journal of Gerontology, Series A: Biological Sciences and Medical Sciences, 56*, M146–M156.

Fromme, E. K., Zive, D., Schmidt, T. A., Cook, J. N., & Tolle, S. W. (2014). Association between physician orders for life-sustaining treatment for scope of treatment and in-hospital death in Oregon. *Journal of the American Geriatrics Society, 62*(7), 1246–1251.

Fromme, E. K., Zive, D., Schmidt, T. A., Olszewski, E., & Tolle, S. W. (2012). POLST registry do-not-resuscitate orders and other patient treatment preferences. *JAMA, 307*, 34–35.

Hammes, B. J., Rooney, B. L., & Gundrum, J. D. (2010). A comparative, retrospective, observational study of the prevalence, availability, and specificity of advance care plans in a county that implemented an advance care planning microsystem. *Journal of the American Geriatrics Society, 58*(7), 1249–1255.

Hammes, B. J., Rooney, B. L., Gundrum, J. D., Hickman, S. E., & Hager, N. (2012). The POLST program: A retrospective review of the demographics of use and outcomes in one community where advance directives are prevalent. *Journal of Palliative Medicine, 15*(1), 77–85.

Happ, M. B., Capezuti, E., Strumpf, N. E., Wagner, L., Cunningham, S., Evans, L., & Maislin, G. (2002). Advance care planning and end-of-life care for hospitalized nursing home residents. *Journal of the American Geriatrics Society, 50*(5), 829–835.

Hickman, S. E., Hammes, B. J., Moss, A. H., & Tolle, S. W. (2005). Hope for the future: Achieving the original intent of advance directives. *Hastings Center Report, Spec No.*, S26–S30.

Hickman, S. E., Hammes, B. J., Torke, A. M., Sudore, R., & Sachs, G. A. (2016). The quality of POLST (Physician Orders for Life-Sustaining Treatment) decisions: A pilot study. *Journal of Palliative Medicine*.

Hickman, S. E., Keevern, E., & Hammes, B. J. (2015). Use of the physician orders for life-sustaining treatment (POLST) in the clinical setting: A systematic review of the literature. *Journal of the American Geriatrics Society, 63*(2), 341–350. doi:10.1111/jgs.13248

Hickman, S. E., Nelson, C. A., Moss, A. H., Hammes, B. J., Terwilliger, A., Jackson, A., & Tolle, S. W. (2009). Use of the physician orders for life-sustaining treatment (POLST) paradigm program in the hospice setting. *Journal of Palliative Medicine, 12*(2), 133–141.

Hickman, S. E., Nelson, C. A., Moss, A. H., Tolle, S. W., Perrin, N. A., & Hammes, B. J. (2011). The consistency between treatments provided to nursing facility residents and orders on the physician orders for life-sustaining treatment form. *Journal of the American Geriatrics Society, 59*(11), 2091–2099.

Hickman, S. E., Nelson, C. A., Perrin, N. A., Moss, A. H., Hammes, B. J., & Tolle, S. W. (2010). A comparison of methods to communicate treatment preferences in nursing facilities: Traditional practices versus the physician orders for life-sustaining treatment program. *Journal of the American Geriatrics Society, 58*(7), 1241–1248.

Hickman, S. E., Nelson, C. A., Smith-Howell, E., & Hammes, B. J. (2014). Use of the physician orders for life-sustaining treatment program for patients being discharged from the hospital to the nursing facility. *Journal of Palliative Medicine, 17*(1), 43–49.

Hickman, S. E., Sabatino, C., Moss, A. H., & Nester Wehrle, J. (2008). The POLST (Physician Orders for Life-Sustaining Treatment) Paradigm to improve end-of-life care: Potential state legal barriers to implementation. *Journal of Law, Medicine, & Ethics, 36*(1), 119–140.

Hickman, S. E., Tolle, S. W., Brummel-Smith, K., & Carley, M. M. (2004). Use of the physician orders for life-sustaining treatment program in Oregon nursing facilities: Beyond resuscitation status. *Journal of the American Geriatrics Society, 52*(9), 1424–1429.

Hickman, S. E., Unroe, K. T., Ersek, M., Buente, B. B., & Sachs, G. A. (2016). An interim analysis of an advance care planning intervention in the nursing home setting. *Journal of the American Geriatrics Society, 64*, 2385–2392.

Holtzman, J., Pheley, A. M., & Lurie, N. (1994). Changes in orders limiting care and the use of less aggressive care in nursing home population. *Journal of the American Geriatrics Society, 42*, 275–279.

Indiana Department of Homeland Security. (2016). POST information. Retrieved from https://secure.in.gov/dhs/3818.htm

Indiana Patient Preferences Coalition. (2016). The Indiana POST (Physician Orders for Scope of Treatment) Program. Retrieved from http://www.indianapost.org

Indiana State Department of Health. (n.d.). Physicians Order for Scope of Treatment (POST) [PDF/Word]. Retrieved from http://www.in.gov/isdh/25880.htm

Institute of Medicine. (2014). *Dying in America: Improving quality and honoring individual preferences near the end of life.* Washington, DC: National Academies Press.

Indiana University Health. (2015). The Indiana POST form in action. Retrieved from www.indianapost.org

Kim, H., Ersek, M., Bradway, C., & Hickman, S. E. (2015). Physician orders for life-sustaining treatment for nursing home residents with dementia. *Journal of the American Association of Nurse Practitioners, 27,* 606–614.

Lee, M. A., Brummel-Smith, K., Meyer, J., Drew, N., & London, M. R. (2000). Physician orders for life-sustaining treatment (POLST): Outcomes in a PACE [Program of All-inclusive Care for the Elderly] program. *Journal of the American Geriatric Society, 48,* 1219–1225.

Lunney, J. R., Lynn, J., Foley, D. J., Lipson, S., & Guralnik, J. M. (2003). Patterns of functional decline at the end of life. *JAMA, 289,* 2387–2392.

Meyers, J. L., Moore, C., McGrory, A., Sparr, J., & Ahern, M. (2004). Physician orders for life-sustaining treatment form: Honoring end-of-life directives for nursing home residents. *Journal of Gerontological Nursing, 30*(9), 37–46.

Mirarchi, F. L., Cammarata, C., Zerkle, S. W., Cooney, T. E., Chenault, J., & Basnak, D. (2015). TRIAD VII: Do prehospital providers understand physician orders for life-sustaining treatment documents? *Journal of Patient Safety, 11,* 9–17.

Mirarchi, F. L., Doshi, A. A., Zerkle, S. W., & Cooney, T. E. (2015). TRIAD VI: How well do emergency physicians understand Physician Orders for Life-Sustaining Treatment (POLST) forms? *Journal of Patient Safety, 11,* 1–8.

Moore, K. A., Rubin, E. B., & Halpern, S. D. (2016). The problems with physician orders for life-sustaining treatment. *JAMA, 315,* 259–260.

Narin, T. (2013). The Catholic Medical Associations white paper, The POLST paradigm and form: Facts and analysis. *Health Care Ethics USA, 21*(3), 17–36.

Pedraza, S. L., Culp, S., Falkenstine, E. C., & Moss, A. H. (2016). POLST forms more than advance directives associated with out-of-hospital death: Insights from a state registry. *Journal of Pain and Symptom Management, 51,* 240–246.

Rahman, A. N., Bressette, M., Gassoumis, Z. D., & Enguidanos, S. (2015). Nursing home residents' preferences on physician orders for life sustaining treatment. *Gerontologist, 56*(4), 714–722.

Sabatino, C., & Karp, N. (2011). Improving advanced illness care: The evolution of state POLST programs. Retrieved from http://assets.aarp.org/rgcenter/ppi/cons-prot/POLST-Report-04-11.pdf

Schmidt, T. A., Hickman, S. E., Tolle, S. W., & Brooks, H. S. (2004). The physician orders for life-sustaining treatment program: Oregon emergency medical technicians' practical experiences and attitudes. *Journal of the American Geriatrics Society, 52*(9), 1430–1434.

Schmidt, T. A., Olszewski, E. A., Zive, D., Fromme, E. K., & Tolle, S. W. (2013). The Oregon physician orders for life-sustaining treatment registry: A preliminary study of emergency medical services utilization. *Journal of Emergency Medicine, 44*(4), 796–805.

Schmidt, T. A., Zive, D., Fromme, E. K., Cook, J. N. B., & Tolle, S. W. (2014). Physician orders for life-sustaining treatment (POLST): Lessons learned from analysis of the Oregon POLST registry. *Resuscitation, 85,* 480–485.

Silveira, M. J., Wiitala, W., & Piette, J. (2014). Advance directive completion by elderly Americans: A decade of change. *Journal of the American Geriatrics Society, 62*(4), 706–710.

Sugiyama, T., Zingmond, D., Lorenz, K. A., Diamant, A., O'Malley, K., Citko, J., & Wenger, N. S. (2013). Implementing physician orders for life-sustaining treatment in California hospitals: Factors associated with adoption. *Journal of the American Geriatrics Society, 61*(8), 1337–1344.

Tuck, K. K., Zive, D. M., Schmidt, T. A., Carter, J., Nutt, J., & Fromme, E. K. (2015). Life-sustaining treatment orders, location of death and co-morbid conditions in decedents with Parkinson's disease. *Parkinsonism and Related Disorders, 21,* 1205–1209.

Unroe, K., Nazir, A., Holtz, L. R., Maurer, H., Miller, E., Hickman, S. E., . . . Sachs, G. A. (2015). The OPTIMISTIC approach: Preliminary data of the implementation of a CMS nursing facility demonstration project. *Journal of the American Geriatrics Society, 63,* 165–169.

Vo, H., Pekmezaris, R., Guzik, H., Nouryan, C., Patel, C., Vij, B., . . . Wolf-Klein, G. (2011). Knowledge and attitudes of health care workers regarding MOLST (Medical Orders for Life-Sustaining Treatment) implementation in long-term care facilities. *Geriatric Nursing, 32,* 58–62.

Waldrop, D. P., Clemency, B., Maguin, E., & Lindstrom, H. (2014). Preparation for frontline end-of-life care: Exploring the perspectives of paramedics and emergency medicine technicians. *Journal of Palliative Medicine, 17,* 338–341.

Wilkinson, A., Wenger, N., & Shugarman, L. R. (2007). Literature review on advance directives. Retrieved from https://aspe.hhs.gov/sites/default/files/pdf/75141/advdirlr.pdf

Winn, K., Ozanne, E., & Sepucha, K. (2015). Measuring patient-centered care: An updated systematic review of how studies determine and report concordance between patient preferences and medical treatments. *Patient Education and Counseling, 98*(7), 811–821.

Zive, D. M., Fromme, E. K., Schmidt, T. A., Cook, J. N. B., & Tolle, S. W. (2015). Timing of POLST form completion by cause of death. *Journal of Pain and Symptom Management, 50,* 650–658.

Zweig, S. C., Kruse, R. L., Binder, E. F., Szafara, K. L., & Mehr, D. R. (2004). Effect of do-not-resuscitate orders on hospitalization of nursing home residents evaluated for lower respiratory infections. *Journal of the American Geriatrics Society, 52*(1), 51–58.

18

Nursing Research and Health Policy Through the Lens of Pediatric Palliative, Hospice, and End-of-Life Care

Kim Mooney-Doyle, Lisa C. Lindley, and Pamela S. Hinds

Tragically, 28,000 infants and nearly 25,000 children between the ages of 1 and 19 years die each year in America (Field & Behrman, 2003; www.cdc.gov/nchs/fastats/adolescent-health.htm). Their dying and death can place their family members at high health risk. Parents are significantly more likely to experience depression and anxiety, experience a first psychiatric hospitalization, be unable to meet the emotional or developmental needs of their surviving children, have low levels of social functioning, experience high rates of accidents, leave the workforce because of health-related issues, and die earlier than parents who do not experience the death of a child (Boyden, Kavanaugh, Issel, Eldeirawi, & Meert, 2014; Goodenough, Drew, Higgins, & Trethewie, 2004; Harper, O'Connor, & O'Carroll, 2014; Hendrickson, 2009; Hinds, Schum, Baker, & Wolfe, 2006; Kreicbergs, Valdimarsdóttir, Onelöv, Henter, & Steineck, 2004; Kreicbergs, Valdimarsdóttir, Steineck, & Henter, 2004; Lannen, Wolfe, Prigerson, Onelöv, & Kreicbergs, 2008; Li, Laursen, Precht, Olsen, & Mortensen, 2005; Li, Precht, Mortensen, & Olsen, 2003; McCarthy et al., 2010; Rosenberg, Baker, Sryjala, & Wolfe, 2012; Valdimarsdóttir et al., 2007). This research also describes how the child's death can threaten the health and functional status of parents and families—an impact that can continue for generations of a family and a community. Because of this, pediatric palliative and end-of-life care is a pressing public health issue. In particular, such care is urgently needed to prevent or reduce the negative effects on the health of family members—thus a primary prevention focus—even as a child is dying and after a child family member dies.

This chapter addresses the interface of nursing science and policy in pediatric palliative and end-of-life research and care. The levels of policy to be addressed include local institution, state, professional association, and national initiatives.

Exemplar policies and programs exist at the level of nations, but we limit our focus here to the United States because context (including political, social, and financial) uniquely shapes the interface of nursing science and policy.

CONTENT CONCEPTUAL FRAMEWORK

The content conceptual framework created for this chapter has two sources: the five recommendations from the 2014 Institute of Medicine (IOM) report, *Dying in America: Improving Quality and Honoring Individual Preferences Near the End of Life*, and the three pillars of public health policy advocated by the Institute for Healthcare Improvement (IHI): care quality, cost, and care access (Table 18.1). By combining these two sources, the very recently released, evidence-based recommendations from the IOM and the public health policy pillars from the IHI, we were able to identify the extent to which evidence exists in each pillar for each of the five IOM palliative and end-of-life recommendations and to interpret the extent of evidence contributed from nursing science. The combined framework also helped in discerning the actual and possible impact of nursing science on health policy related to pediatric palliative and end-of-life care in the United States, including the impact on preventing serious health consequences for families who have experienced the death of a child family member. A brief description of these two foundations of the conceptual framework follows.

RECOMMENDATIONS FROM THE 2014 INSTITUTE OF MEDICINE REPORT, *DYING IN AMERICA*

The IOM convened a group of palliative and end-of-life care experts to review all available evidence and develop recommendations that could contribute to improved care for persons of all ages with a serious illness who are likely approaching death. The first IOM recommendation was:

> Government health insurers and care delivery programs as well as private health insurers should cover the provision of comprehensive care for individuals with advanced serious illness who are nearing the end of life. (IOM, p. S-8)

This recommendation addressed the need for readily available, seamless, patient- and family-focused palliative and end-of-life care at all times and to have that care delivered by competent professionals who have the requisite training and skill. An interdisciplinary health care team was specifically recommended to provide this level of care. Quite importantly, the care provided is to be fully consistent with the values and goals of those receiving the care, and care recipients are to have been well-informed about options and been able to express their care preferences.

(*text continues on page 324*)

TABLE 18.1 *Evidence Matrix of Pediatric Palliative Care, Hospice, and End-of-Life Care Research Positioned With IOM Recommendations to IHI Triple Aim*

	Cost	Quality	Access

IOM 1.
Government health insurers and care delivery programs should cover the provision of comprehensive care for individuals nearing the end of life.
	• Federal
	• State
	  a. California (Gans et al., 2012; Lindley & Lyon, 2013)
	  b. Florida (Knapp, Thompson, Vogel, Madden, & Shenkman, 2009)
	What is known: Care for children at end of life is costly; early evidence shows that state PPC programs reduce costs.
	What is unknown: Long-term effects of programs on costs, age differences in cost reductions, federal policies' impact on costs, lack of baseline cost data.
	Bottom line: Cost of end-of-life care policies is unknown.
	
	Recommendations: Need national data to assess cost of federal policies, nurse researchers with training in economics and costs analysis. Need baseline cost data at national and state levels. Need to translate cost findings for nurses to use in practice.
		• Federal policies: ACA 2302 (Lindley, 2011; Miller, LaRagione, Kang, & Feudtner, 2012)
		• State policies
		  a. California (Gans et al., 2012)
		What is known: Conflicting early evidence about whether initial implementation of policies (state or federal) actually reduces or improves quality, but long-term gains expected.
		What is unknown: No standard measures of quality, no reports on impact of state or federal policies on quality.
		Bottom line: Quality of end-of-life care policies is unknown
		
		Recommendations: Standard measures of pediatric end-of-life quality and industry acceptance and implementation of measures to aid nursing research. Need to translate quality findings for nurses to use in practice.
			• Federal policies: ACA 2302 (Lindley, 2011; Lindley, Edwards, & Bruce, 2014; Keim-Malpass, Hart, & Miller, 2013)
			• State policies
			  a. Overall (Keim-Malpass et al., 2013)
			  b. Tennessee (Lindley & Edwards, 2015)
			  c. California (Dabbs, Butterworth, & Hall, 2007)
			  d. Florida (Knapp et al., 2008, 2009)
			  e. Massachusetts (Bona, Bates, & Wolfe, 2011)
			What is known: States led the way at improving access to care through policies; access issues remain in states with certificate of need rules; federal policy not uniformly implemented, which affects access.
			What is unknown: The effect of federal policy on access; how state policies can be expanded beyond their initial target county areas.
			Bottom line: State policies have positively impacted access, but federal policy impact is unknown.
			
			Recommendations: Need national data to assess federal policies. Need to translate access findings for nurses to use in practice. Need approaches to engage nurses to advocate for improving access to care.

(continued)

315

TABLE 18.1 *Evidence Matrix of Pediatric Palliative Care, Hospice, and End-of-Life Care Research Positioned With IOM Recommendations to IHI Triple Aim (continued)*

	Cost	Quality	Access
IOM 2: **Professional groups should develop standards for clinician–patient communication and ACP that are measurable, actionable, and evidence-based.**	• What is known: Health systems have a cost and quality incentive to integrate palliative care into care of AYA with life-threatening illnesses (Weiner, Weaver, Bell, & Sansom-Daly, 2015); enrollment in PPC program associated with reduced hospitalization, length of stay, and lower cost of care for children without cancer (Postier, Chrastek, Nugent, Osenga, & Friedrichsdorf, 2014); integration is associated with lower inpatient care and intensive care utilization and lower financial burden for families (Weiner et al., 2015).	• What is known: Professional groups promote quality in clinician–family interactions (e.g., NANN position statement by Catlin, Brandon, Woole, & Mendes, 2015; HPNA position statement, 2015a). Highlights heterogeneity within subspecialty groups and contextual concerns (perinatal needs versus neonatal needs; within NICU versus during transport).	• What is known: The number of pediatric palliative and hospice clinicians is small, which means that palliative care needs must be met through other clinicians in primary or subspecialty care. Thus, the need to provide generalist training in conversations about goals of care and advanced care planning is crucial.
	• Costs incurred by upfront investment needed for training staff and curriculum development; states that have implemented PPC programs described the initial costs as low relative to the long-term savings and advantages of having the programs in place; the costs of programs that provide this training to clinicians range from none (in-house training) to several hundred for continued education training, such as ELNEC or EPEC, to several thousand for education within the context of degree-granting programs (AACN, 2016a).	• In neuro-oncology, intervention development and testing of delivery of early palliative and end-of-life communication with families of children with aggressive brain tumors (Hendricks-Ferguson et al., 2015); focused on nurses and physicians working collaboratively with families and incorporating bereaved parents as teachers; concerns expressed about scheduling and the impact on the bereaved parents who served as teachers.	• Nurses broadly endorsed the significance of palliative care goals and the presence of problems, but differed on the importance of these PPHIC goals and problems; the hospital unit was the most significant predictor of how nurses collaborated with the PPC team (Tubbs-Cooley et al., 2011). Thus, there may be differences across a single institution by unit or individual clinician, which may affect the quality of PPC provided in the institution or sought for the child and family in the community.
	• Disparity in U.S. because of differences in program availability across states (Weiner et al., 2015).	• Interdisciplinary training (within one institution): nursing research has been influential in interdisciplinary communication training (Hendricks-Ferguson et al., 2015; Meyer et al., 2009) across disciplines (although mostly nurses and physicians) and across experience levels; unit-based initiatives to improve quality; challenges in implementation of palliative care in acute care (Docherty, Miles, & Brandon, 2007), yet efforts in stem cell transplant (LaFond, Kelly, Hinds, Sill, & Michael, 2015) were welcomed, feasible, and families reported satisfaction with this intervention.	• Implementation of a NICU-based palliative care program provides access for children and families who would not otherwise receive care and did not experience increases in withdrawal of life support; this improved communication with families and improved symptom management (Younge et al., 2015).

(continued)

316

Cost	Quality	Access
• Unit and institutional level costs of implementing programs: addition of PPHC teams potentially improves job retention and satisfaction by decreasing moral distress in the NICU (Younge et al., 2015) and other pediatric settings (Petteys et al., 2015); decreases costs of losing and retraining clinicians who leave due to moral distress and diminished job satisfaction.	• Communication in PPHC is emphasized through formal education programs at graduate (DNP: Hendricks-Ferguson et al., 2015) and undergraduate levels and undergraduate (O'Shea et al., 2015) palliative care education; elements of high-quality PPHC, especially those around communication and advanced care planning, should be integrated from generalist education. Gaps also identified (Shea, Grossman, Wallace, & Lange, 2010).	• What is unknown: What are the ideal ways to initiate a discussion and elicit preferences, especially for training across the board for nonpalliative care specialists? How best to integrate this training into curriculum? Finally, is access to high-quality palliative care communication and ACP limited by limited scope of practice laws (especially those that pertain to nurses)?
• What is unknown: Feasibility of federal or more comprehensive oversight of standards, funding, access, education, and research, as has been demonstrated in other nations; cost of training needed to have sustained impact on children and families.	• What is unknown: Despite different avenues of clinician education and training, longitudinal outcomes have rarely been assessed; how palliative care conversations will be evaluated and graded; how to account for variation across state lines because of institutional and state differences in APN scope of practice laws; improvement in care delivered by DNP-prepared APNs in palliative care.	
• Potential first steps: Track the impact of ELNEC (or any other training) past clinician-reported ratings of comfort with having conversations or implementing knowledge to linking the care provided by PPHC-educated nurses to patient and family outcomes; assessing the most meaningful, cost-effective, and impactful ways to train primary and subspecialty care professionals in PPHC for further integration.	• Potential next steps: Assess the impact on child/family outcomes and the impact over time; how to grade these communication efforts; gap in the delivery of palliative/end-of-life care during cancer clinical trials; this may be an avenue for nursing to explore—are there trigger points in a clinical trial that should prompt discussions about ACP and goals of care? (Levine et al., 2015, and others); assess quality of interventions holistically assessed by ascertaining family perspective.	

(continued)

	Cost	Quality	Access
IOM 3: Educational institutions, credentialing bodies, etc. should establish the appropriate training, certification, and licensure requirements to strengthen palliative care knowledge and skills of all clinicians who care for individuals who are nearing end of life.	What is known: The AACN has formalized recommendations for undergraduate palliative care curricula, including the competencies needed at that level of nursing (http://www.aacn.nche.edu/news/articles/2016/elnec; Zolot, 2016). The primary certification body for pediatric and perinatal hospice and palliative nursing care is the Hospice & Palliative Credentialing Center. Seven types of nursing certification are offered by this center, which is the official credentialing arm of the HPNA. The Centers for Medicare and Medicaid Services has recognized the Hospice and Palliative Certification Board at the advanced practice level as a national certifying body (http://www.aacn.nche.edu/elnec/New-Palliative-Care-Competencies.pdf). The costs of taking the certification exam are generally assumed by the individual nurse or (totally or partially) by the employer of the nurse. Standards for palliative care, including those for PPC nurses, have been established for communication and other skills by the National Consensus Project and applied to nursing (Goldsmith, Ferrell, Wittenberg-Lyles, & Ragan, 2013), but these are not reflected in licensure requirements. Standards for hospitals and certification criteria for palliative care have been established by The Joint Commission and have direct care and policy level implications for nursing (www.jointcommision.org/certification/palliative_care.aspx).	What is known: Using a questionnaire developed for this survey study, Kehl documented in the responses of 1,434 (51% response rate) HPNA members that certified nurses were more likely to report tailoring their care based on the ill patient's education, diagnosis, and prognosis than were the noncertified nurses. However, few other differences between the two groups of nurses were detected (Kehl, 2014). What is unknown: It is too early to determine the uptake and the outcomes of the new AACN palliative care standards for undergraduate nursing curricula, but both could be assessed over the next few years. The difference in patient and family care outcomes related to symptom management, emotional and spiritual suffering when receiving care from a team that includes certified nurses compared to a team that does not include certified nurses is unknown. The actual time and resources needed to implement PPC standards related to training and certification needs in academic programs, specialty offerings, and employer-offered education and to obtain the desired level of palliative care skill achievement are unknown.	What is known: Access to certified PPC nurses is limited by the number of certifying bodies (HPNA) and the number of nurses who view themselves to be a part of that specialty group. Because the new AACN recommendations for undergraduate nursing palliative care competencies and standards have recently been issued, we can anticipate that nurses graduating in the next several years will have primary palliative care skills. What is unknown: Assess the palliative care skill achievement longitudinally and care outcomes to determine the impact of primary palliative care being required at the undergraduate level.

(continued)

TABLE 18.1 *Evidence Matrix of Pediatric Palliative Care, Hospice, and End-of-Life Care Research Positioned With IOM Recommendations to IHI Triple Aim (continued)*

Cost	Quality	Access
Federally funded curricula have been implemented in pediatric nursing, including nurse-specific offerings (i.e., ELNEC) and interdisciplinary offerings (EPEC-Pediatrics; Ferrell, Malloy, & Virani, 2015; Ferrell, Virani, Paice, Coyle, & Coyne, 2010; O'Shea et al., 2015; Widger et al., 2016). Curricula delivered in workshop, seminar, and online formats have been determined to be feasible and satisfying for a majority of nurse and other discipline participants (Ferrell et al., 2010; Jacobs, Ferrell, Virani, & Malloy, 2009; O'Shea et al., 2015). Curricula with bereaved parents as instructors have also been implemented; in a small sample, 9 bereaved parents who served as instructors reported meaning-making secondary to participating in this role and 11 health care professionals reported increased mutual understanding and learning and the likelihood of openness having been limited to some extent by the parents' presence (Adams, Green, Towe, & Huett, 2013).	Recommendations: Palliative care skill standards should be consistently implemented by all academic and employers of nurses at all levels of care (primary and secondary palliative care skills) and used to evaluate nurse skill achievements and care outcomes for patients and families.	
Integrating the perinatal and pediatric ELNEC curricula into the nursing curricula of one private university and one public university was evaluated in one study and integration was determined to be feasible and to increase knowledge related to palliative care (O'Shea et al., 2015). What is unknown: The actual cost of embedding palliative care content or offerings into curricula at the undergraduate, graduate, or employer level has not been determined (Goldsmith et al., 2013), nor has the sustainability of such an effort been assessed.		

(continued)

TABLE 18.1 *Evidence Matrix of Pediatric Palliative Care, Hospice, and End-of-Life Care Research Positioned With IOM Recommendations to IHI Triple Aim (continued)*

Cost	Quality	Access
Costs of curricula offered via diverse formats have not yet been evaluated.		

Cost/benefit ratio for impact of palliative care education and certification on direct patient and family care delivered and the outcomes of that care has not been determined.

Costs for hospitals to achieve the palliative care certification offered by The Joint Commission have not been reported.

Recommendations:

The costs of creating interdisciplinary PPC learning experiences should be documented and shared across the participating schools or divisions and the costs and outcomes of such interdisciplinary curricular approaches should be compared with those that are discipline-specific.

Do a formal assessment of the cost/benefit ratio of a purposefully coordinated approach to implementing palliative care content in academic nursing programs and reflecting this content in licensing and certifying requirements and metrics as well as with orientation and in-service programs offered by employers of nurses. The outcomes of such a coordinated effort should also be evaluated.

The costs to maintain individual nurse and institution competencies in palliative care should be documented and the association with care outcomes should be assessed.

(continued)

	Cost	Quality	Access
IOM 4: **Care delivery programs should integrate the financing of medical and social services to support care that is consistent with the values, goals, and informed preferences of people nearing the end of life.**	• Quality and cost are interrelated. High-quality care may diminish costs because it provides care that is aligned with child/family preferences, is rooted in open and honest communication that allows parents to make decisions with the best available information, and avoids costly measures that may provide little benefit or are not desired. • What is known: Nurses have an instrumental hand in developing PPC programs that span both inpatient/outpatient/home environments; patient- and family centered, nurse-driven program cut down on emergency department visits for symptom management ($250–$3000) with home-based symptom management (average cost = $172), as well as subsequent admissions; continuity of care provided by the palliative care teams allowed for consistent support and a more open environment for end-of-life discussions, which led to a decrease in admissions for end-of-life care and diminished use of life-sustaining interventions (Mastro, Johnson, McElvery, & Preuster, 2015); philanthropic funding has been vital in starting and maintaining PPC programs, as well as billing for physician services (Duncan, Spengler, & Wolfe, 2007).	• What is known: Provision of high-quality palliative care is an extension of nursing's social contract. Growing recognition of the needs of family caregivers (most notably parents). There is also work on unearthing how to best support family caregivers. • High-quality delivery programs are patient- and family-centered (Baird, Davies, Hinds, Baggott, & Rehm, 2015; Davies, Baird, & Gundsmunsdottir, 2013), yet competing perceptions and goals among parents and clinicians may impede this. Parents face significant barriers to full participation in their ill child's care in the critical care setting (Baird et al., 2015). High-quality engagement with parents may help parents achieve or reframe their definition of being a good parent; interventions to promote this are feasible and may help parents emotionally survive the death of their child (Hinds et al., 2001, JPM); implications for the care of the ill child's healthy siblings (Mooney-Doyle & Deatrick, 2016); child's chart may not fully capture family's needs, preferences, or competing priorities, and therefore clinicians may not provide care consistent with child and family needs and values. • What is unknown: How best to broaden the impact of this research and move it from institutional or unit level policy to broader, regional, state, or federal level policy. How to fully incorporate child and family voice into broader policy.	• What is known: High-quality, cost-effective palliative and hospice care is made accessible in two ways: through generalists trained in basic provision of palliative care and initiation of conversations around goals of care and specialist palliative and hospice care that is provided by certified individuals or as part of a palliative care team. How do we train clinicians to provide palliative, hospice, and end-of-life care that is consistent with the wishes and needs of children and their families? • Research done by Lindley (2013) demonstrates increased access to core palliative care services (as defined by CMS) from 2002 to 2008 for children in California; the rates of access to noncore or other hospice services, such as skilled therapists, did not change in the study period. This is concerning since the rates of children with complex chronic conditions whose quality of life would be enhanced with the use of skilled therapist services as part of their care increased 26%; physician services were the least common core service available in pediatric hospice, which may potentially hamper care for children with increased complexity and symptom severity. Policy implication of this work: important baseline data to assess the impact of the concurrent care provision on the availability of hospice care for children.

(continued)

TABLE 18.1 *Evidence Matrix of Pediatric Palliative Care, Hospice, and End-of-Life Care Research Positioned With IOM Recommendations to IHI Triple Aim (continued)*

Cost	Quality	Access
• Program use by children and families: Medicaid eligibility and private insurance are each related to hospice use in children (Lindley & Shaw, 2014). Profit status of a hospice may predict if children are enrolled for care; nonprofit hospices are more likely to have a specialized pediatric program and have more experience caring for children (Lindley, Mixer, & Mack, 2012). Enrollment in home-based PPC service was associated with decreased emergency room and hospital length of stay and total hospital charges versus the time prior to enrollment for children without a cancer diagnosis (Postier et al., 2014). • What is unknown: How to achieve more equitable distribution of PPC programs and hospices equipped to care for them.		• Lindley, Mixer, and Cozad (2014) describes the children who are utilizing hospice; mid–late adolescents were more likely to receive hospice services, as were those with certain diagnoses (such as neuromuscular diseases and cancer). Any child was more likely to be enrolled in hospice if one was located within the family's community; infants requiring hospice care may have less access to community-based hospices because of the lack of pediatric knowledge in many community hospices (Lindley et al., 2012); nonprofit hospices may be more likely to care for highly complex patients. Thus, there may be a significant subset of children for whom hospice care is not available or accessible. Children with certain diseases, of particular ages, or residing in certain communities may not be referred to hospice by their clinicians or may not have access even if they are referred. • Access can also be adjusted through an institution. Doorenbos et al. (2013) found that automatic referrals across intensive care settings for children receiving ECMO can increase access for children and families. • What is unknown: How to make distribution of resources more equitable across populations and regions. How to increase scale of training initiatives and best practices.

(continued)

TABLE 18.1 *Evidence Matrix of Pediatric Palliative Care, Hospice, and End-of-Life Care Research Positioned With IOM Recommendations to IHI Triple Aim (continued)*

	Cost	Quality	Access
IOM 5: All organizations should engage their constituents and provide fact-based information about care of people nearing end of life to encourage ACP and informed choices.		What is known: Emerging evidence that pediatric ACP may be emotionally relieving and facilitate communication and decision making. What is unknown: Effect of communications/ACP on quality of end-of-life care (NQF measures)	What is known: Many national health care organizations are providing information about accessing pediatric end-of-life care and ACP (including POLST) to constituents; these include NINR (conversations matter; science of compassion), HPNA (position statements), NHPCO/ChiPPs (toolkits, protocols), and ONS (podcasts). Local and regional organizations are also active, such as Pediatric Palliative Care Coalition, Greater Illinois Pediatric Palliative Care Coalition, Children's Hospice and Palliative Care Coalition. Scholars have examined the process of accessing (provision and use) among adolescents. Clinicians still have issues with conducting these conversations with family and children. What is unknown: Little is known about access to information and ACP for younger children, especially infants and their families. Also little is known about the best timing of these conversations/information. Recommendation: Need conversations with families in the NICU and prenatally if necessary. Continued professional education.

The second IOM recommendation was:

Professional societies and organizations that establish quality standards should develop standards for clinician–patient communication and advance care planning that are measurable, actionable, and evidence based. These standards should change as needed to reflect the evolving population and health system needs and be consistent with emerging evidence, methods, and technologies. Payers and health care delivery organizations should adopt these standards and their supporting processes, and integrate them into assessments, care plans, and the reporting of health care quality. (IOM, p. S-10)

These quality standards were viewed as so essential by the IOM working committee that they recommended payers tie reimbursements to the successful achievement of such standards and that professional associations embed quality standards into their credentialing processes. The recommendation also reflected that children be allowed, as desired, to have a voice in their care decision making and that their voice be sought over time and changing circumstances as preferences and values can change.

The third IOM recommendation was:

Educational institutions, credentialing bodies, accrediting boards, state regulatory agencies, and health care delivery organizations should establish the appropriate training, certification, and/or licensure requirements to strengthen the palliative care knowledge and skills of all clinicians who care for individuals with advanced serious illness who are nearing the end of life. (IOM, p. S-11)

This recommendation more directly addressed the need for all clinicians, regardless of discipline or specialty, to be prepared to provide primary or basic palliative care. Quite preferably, this education would begin at the first level of training for professionals and would continue throughout careers. Just as educational institutions need to provide this kind of training, accrediting organizations should require this content in reviewed programs, and certifying bodies should require this knowledge in their criteria for competency in pediatric palliative and end-of-life care. Relatedly, the same expectations apply for the specialty level (expert) of pediatric palliative and end-of-life care across institutions, organizations, and professional associations. Of concern to the IOM committee members was the tradition of separate educational preparation for disciplines in terms of primary and specialty palliative and end-of-life care, the absence of curriculum content related to palliative and hospice care, and insufficient attention given to talking directly to children and others with advanced disease who cannot survive their illness.

The fourth recommendation was:

Federal, state and private insurance and health care delivery programs should integrate the financing of medical and social services to support the provision of quality care consistent with the values, goals and informed preferences of people with advanced serious illness nearing the end of life. To the extent that additional legislation is necessary to implement this recommendation, the administration should seek and Congress should enact such legislation. In addition, the federal government should require public reporting on quality measures, outcomes, and costs regarding care near the end of life (e.g., in the last year of life) for programs that it funds or administers (e.g., Medicare, Medicaid, the Department of Veterans Affairs). The federal government should encourage all other payment and health care delivery systems to do the same. (IOM, p. S-13)

The recommendation specifically urged financial incentives for well-coordinated care across types of settings and clinicians and improved decision making about care, including advanced care planning, to minimize the use of unnecessary treatment interventions and care services. The language supporting the recommendation also urged the use of interoperable electronic health records such that the care recipient's care preferences and advance care planning were readily available across time, settings, and clinicians.

The fifth and final IOM recommendation was:

Civic leaders, public health and other governmental agencies, community-based organizations, faith-based organizations, consumer groups, health care delivery organizations, payers, employers, and professional societies should engage their constituents and provide fact-based information about care of people with advanced serious illness to encourage advance care planning and informed choice based on the needs and values of individuals. (IOM, p. S-15)

The additional supportive language for this recommendation indicated the need for media forms (e.g., billboards, pamphlets, flyers, blogs) to effectively and appropriately reach groups regarding care options, decision making, the value of dialogue among involved individuals (including family, clinicians, and others) regarding preferences, values, and care goals related to serious illness and further, to purposefully undo false information regarding care and care systems connected to end of life.

THE IHI'S TRIPLE AIM FRAMEWORK

The second part of the conceptual framework is the three pillars of public health policy advocated by the IHI and referred to as the Triple Aim Framework; the three pillars are care quality, cost, and care access and all three are population-focused. These pillars were developed to focus national attention on improving the experience of patient care in the United States and improving the health of all its citizens at a reasonable cost (www.ihi.org/sites/search/pages/results.aspx?K=triple+aim+framework). This framework aligns well with assessing policy impact on population health, such as the impact of nursing science on public policy to prevent or minimize the harmful consequences that can occur to a family following the death of a child family member. Importantly, both the Triple Aim Framework and the IOM 2014 recommendations support the quest for high-quality, individualized care for the dying in America and at a reasonable cost. In summary, this content conceptual framework represents the current evidence contributed from the discipline of nursing that is now guiding pediatric palliative, hospice, and end-of-life care and facilitates the analysis of the impact of this evidence in terms of care quality, cost, and care access.

NURSING SCIENCE AND HEALTH POLICY IMPACT IN PEDIATRIC PALLIATIVE AND END-OF-LIFE CARE AND SCIENCE

The following sections describe the nursing research that has informed various levels of health policy in pediatric palliative and end-of-life research and care. For each of the IOM recommendations and across each IHI Triple Aim pillar, we highlight the contributions of nursing science and nurse researchers to understanding the quality, cost, and care access to high-quality pediatric palliative and end-of-life care.

IOM I

Government, health insurers, and care delivery programs should cover the provision of comprehensive care for individuals nearing the end of life.

Cost of Care

The IOM report recommends that government, health insurers, and care delivery programs cover the provision of comprehensive care for children nearing the end of life, but at what cost? The expense to the health care system for children with life-limiting conditions is staggering. These children are often in the top 10% of health care expenditures for government and private health insurers, with an average annual cost of $82,000 per child (Buescher, Whitmire, Brunssen, & Kluttz-Hile, 2006; Lindley & Lyon, 2013). To manage the high cost of care, several states have implemented palliative care programs through their Medicaid plans. In 2005, the United States Department of Health and Human Services assisted states in waiving hospice eligibility by supporting PPC policies in Florida, Massachusetts, Washington, Colorado, Illinois, and California (Bona et al., 2011; Knapp et al., 2008). Early evidence from non-nursing researchers in California, Massachusetts, and Florida is sparse. California's palliative care policy resulted in a cost savings of $1,677 per child per month on average or an 11% reduction in spending monthly (Gans et al., 2012). The Massachusetts palliative care program had costs that ranged from $1,520 to $7,421 per child, while the Florida palliative care program had average annual predicted costs for infants and children of $149,071 per child per year for inpatient care and $2,784 per child per year for hospice care (Table 18.1; Bona et al., 2011;

Knapp et al., 2009). Thus, state programs designed to reduce costs have shown moderate cost saving for children enrolled in palliative care programs.

At the federal level, passage of the "Concurrent Care for Children" provision of the Affordable Care Act (ACA 2302) allows children to receive hospice care along with curative treatments, which might influence cost of care (Lindley, 2011). Although researchers have engaged in state-level studies of costs, research on the federal level has been limited. One possible explanation is the timing of the "Concurrent Care for Children" provision. ACA 2302 was passed in 2010; however, by 2012 more than 30% of states had not implemented this requirement (Lindley, Edwards, & Bruce, 2014). Thus, data are only now becoming available to conduct these studies. Nurse researchers might benefit from partnering with health care economists to explore the cost-effectiveness and cost benefit of policies and programs aimed at improving costs for children at end of life. Collaborations with political scientists might encourage the use of alternative methods such as natural experiment designs to investigate the effect of policy changes on costs. Therefore, nursing research examining the cost implications of pediatric state and federal policies has the potential to expand and provide a significant contribution to our understanding of how policies can influence the cost of care for children at end of life.

Quality of Care

Although end-of-life care quality measures have emerged recently through the Hospice Item Set (Centers for Medicare and Medicaid Services, 2013), "Measuring What Matters" in palliative care (Dy et al., 2015), National Quality Forum Palliative and End-of-Life Quality Measures (National Quality Forum [NQF], 2016), and clinical practice guidelines for quality palliative care (National Consensus Project for Quality Palliative Care, 2013), there are limited standard quality measures for providing end-of-life care specifically for children and their families.

The *Standards of Practice for Pediatric Palliative Care and Hospice* issued by the National Hospice and Palliative Care Organization (NHPCO) is one of the few sources that includes quality measures for pediatric end-of-life care (NHPCO, 2009). As an example, end-of-life care should be patient- and family-centered. Nurse researchers have found that families and children are generally satisfied with the patient- and family-centered care delivered by pediatrics hospices and palliative care (Contro, Larson, Scofield, Sourkes, & Cohen, 2002; Davies et al., 2005; Gans et al., 2012). In addition, pediatric end-of-life care should be congruent with the individual and family preferences, values, and cultural beliefs. Emerging evidence suggests that pediatric hospices generally deliver culturally competent end-of-life care, with the majority of hospices providing translation services (74.9%) and interpreter services (87.1%) for children and families (Lindley et al., 2016). Finally, all aspects of care should be sensitive to the needs of the child and family. Gans et al. (2012), in a study of 33 families, found the California palliative care program improved family quality of life, as demonstrated by reports of less difficulty sleeping, less feelings of nervousness, tension, or worry about their child. The families also reported that care coordination, family education, massage therapy, child life therapy, and the 24/7 nurse line offered through the policy were helpful in reducing stress and worry at end of life. Thus, children and families may be receiving quality care at end of life.

Overall, the limited evidence suggests that providing quality end-of-life care for children and families is a critical component for the well-being of the child and family, but that the lack of standard quality measures specific to this population has limited the advancement of pediatric end-of-life science. Nurse researchers have a leadership opportunity to engage the pediatric end-of-life clinical and scholarly communities in identifying and developing quality measures specific to pediatrics. Creating measures that are meaningful for clinicians and appropriate for research will promote and enable the translation of findings to improve care for children and their families.

Access to Care

The IOM report also suggests that government, health insurers, and care delivery programs should provide access to care for children at the end of life. However, nursing studies have found that provision of end-of-life care for children is not common and the availability of pediatric providers is declining. In a longitudinal study of 311 California hospice providers, Lindley and colleagues reported that the percentage of hospices providing care for children declined from 40% in 2002 to 28% in 2008 (Lindley, Mark, et al., 2013). However, the care offered by pediatric providers varied significantly. In a 7-year time period (2002–2008), the proportion of California pediatric hospices offering nursing care, physician, social, counseling, medication, inpatient, transportation, imaging and laboratory, outpatient, and chemotherapy services increased, while home health aide and homemaker services, equipment and supplies services, and therapy services declined in that same time period (Lindley, 2013). Thus, nursing research suggests that access to pediatric care may be concentrating in a few providers, but that no standard services are offered to children and families.

Consequently, the provision of pediatric end-of-life care may not match the need for care. Using innovative geographic information system techniques, a recent nursing study examined the geographic distribution of pediatric hospice need and supply and identified areas lacking pediatric hospice care in Tennessee over a 3-year time period (Lindley & Edwards, 2015). The study showed a consistent need for care among children with cancer across the state. Most urban areas were supplied by pediatric hospices, except the Knoxville area. The authors identified that while the supply of pediatric hospice care declined, the need for hospice care was unchanging. Therefore, nursing research has begun to identify that access to care, particularly hospice care, which is a continual problem for children and their families.

Research from nurse researchers have found that states lead the way at improving access to care at the end of life for children. Although state Medicaid fee-for-service programs provide comprehensive services for children with life-limiting conditions (Lindley & Lyon, 2013), state PPC policies have sought to improve access to supportive services at diagnosis that are concurrent with treatments and therapies

(Keim-Malpass, Hart, & Miller, 2013). For example, the palliative care policy in California did not have any effect on hospice enrollment; however, the policy was positively associated with increasing days in hospice care (Lindley, 2016). The rate of hospice length of stay increased by a factor of 5.61 for children in palliative care counties, compared to children unaffected by the policy. At the federal level, while we expect that the "Concurrent Care for Children" will improve access to care for children at end of life nationally (Lindley, 2011; Keim-Malpass et al., 2013), no empirical studies were identified that explored the impact of the law on access to care. Future research is needed to examine broadly the impact of state policies on access, while developing studies to explore the influence of federal policy. Therefore, based on past contributions, nurse researchers are poised to continue contributing to the evidence on access to pediatric end-of-life care. See Table 18.1 for a display of the current evidence.

There are critical implications for nurse researchers investigating government, health insurers, and care delivery programs' provision of comprehensive care for children nearing the end of life. First, research questions about costs of pediatric end-of-life care provide an opportunity for nurses to partner with health care economists or gain additional economic training to further their analytic skills. Second, nurses need to bring their clinical knowledge to the quality discussions within the hospice and palliative care research community. For example, nurse expertise in symptom assessment/management, along with child and family communication, is a valuable contribution to ensuring that quality of pediatric end-of-life care is accurately and appropriately measured. Finally, nurse researchers must continue advocating for their programs of research in the provision of comprehensive care for children and their families at end of life. As new legislation is implemented at the state and federal level and policies are enacted within organizations, nurses need to continue to ask questions about the effectiveness of these policies on the care for children and their families.

IOM 2

Professional societies and other organizations that establish quality standards should develop standards for clinician–patient communication and advance care planning that are measurable, actionable, and evidence based. These standards should change as needed to reflect the evolving population and health system needs and be consistent with emerging evidence, methods, and technologies. Payers and health care delivery organizations should adopt these standards and their supporting processes, and integrate them into assessments, care plans, and the reporting of health care quality.

Cost of Care

Research with adolescents and young adults (AYA) is an avenue through which to examine advanced care planning in pediatrics. Nurses have been involved in research to promote AYA advanced care planning in life-threatening illness and its integration across subspecialties (Weaver et al., 2015, 2016). Researchers report that the cost of advanced care planning is minimal when compared to the long-term benefit to patients, families, institutions, and health care systems. Costs are incurred for training health care clinicians in advanced care planning, in initiating and facilitating conversations to uncover patient and family hopes and priorities, and in discussions about reframing goals of care (Wiener et al., 2015).

Health systems have a cost and quality incentive to integrate palliative care into care of children with life-threatening and life-limiting illnesses. For example, the value in the integration of palliative care with care of AYA is associated with lower inpatient care, intensive care utilization, and lower financial burden for families While costs are incurred to make the upfront investment needed for adequately trained staff and curriculum development, states that have implemented PPC programs described the initial costs as low relative to the long-term savings and advantages of having the programs in place. The disparity in the United States, however, exists because of differences in program availability across states (Wiener et al., 2015). The integration of palliative care, high-quality communication and advanced care planning into neonatal transport is another example of how upfront institutional investment can diminish disparities faced by newborns and their parents and provide care consistent with family goals. In this case, increased costs may be incurred if the parents and ill infant are transported to the receiving institution together, but this intervention maintains high-quality, family-centered palliative care (Dulkerian, Douglas, & Taylor, 2011). Nurse researchers must share their voices in advocacy to raise awareness to prompt research and policy discussions.

Another consideration is costs incurred by institutions that lose staff because of burnout, moral distress, or feelings of disempowerment. Such feelings are perpetuated when staff do not have adequate palliative care training or access to palliative care services. One interdisciplinary team of neonatal researchers (Younge et al., 2015) found lower moral distress and less desire to leave a job within 6 months of implementation of the quality-of-life (QOL) team in the neonatal intensive care unit (NICU). This could impact costs of losing nursing and physician staff and training new staff. Such findings allow us to reframe the addition of PPHC teams as a measure to impact retention and job satisfaction and prevent moral distress among clinicians (Petteys, Goebel, Wallace, & Singh-Carlson, 2015). Considering these interventions not only in terms of patient and family satisfaction, but also in terms of employee job satisfaction, enhancing employee desire to stay in their current position may be an important cost consideration. Therefore, policies must be enacted at the unit, institutional, and governmental levels to promote an (a) interdisciplinary collaboration; (b) support interdisciplinary clinician training; and (c) reimbursement for palliative and end-of-life conversations to promote equitable and high-quality pediatric palliative and end-of-life care for children. These policy measures may also promote clinician health in the workplace so that an experienced, resilient workforce is maintained.

What remains unknown, in the context of the United States, is the feasibility of federal or more comprehensive oversight of standards, funding, access, education, and research. How feasible is it to have comprehensive oversight of standards that foster the provision of adequate funding for services and research, equitable access to care, interdisciplinary education and training, and research, when many broad pediatric palliative and end-of-life care efforts are emphasized at the state level? Children and families may experience inequities in care while living a mile apart but across a state line. How will the call for linking the broader communication competencies be filled across disciplines? Will advanced practice nurses (APNs) be able to bill and be reimbursed for initiating and conducting discussions around advanced care planning and assessing goals of care? What are nurses called to do when these standards conflict with the culture of the institution in which they practice? Will nurses and APNs be allowed to practice to their full scope? We need nurse researchers to partner with nurse clinicians at all levels to understand the limitations imposed upon their care that are not consistent with standards promoted by professional organizations (Hospice and Palliative Nurses Association [HPNA]) or national-level organizations focused on health care policy (IOM, Robert Wood Johnson Foundation [RWJF]). In addition, nurse researchers must share this information as part of their dissemination plan beyond peer-reviewed journals, by sharing research findings and professional concerns with policy makers at institutional, local, state, and federal levels.

Quality of Care

Professional groups promote quality in clinician–family interactions through their evidence-based position statements. One example is the National Association of Neonatal Nurses (NANN) position statement (Catlin, Brandon, Woole, & Mendes, 2015), in which the authors provided an updated and broader perspective on delivering palliative care and conducting conversations around goals of care during the perinatal period. Also highlighted was the importance of communication between parents and the transport team around end-of-life choices if the infant is at risk for dying during transport, indicating that infants and families have palliative care needs that cross settings and that there is heterogeneity within the subset of perinatal palliative care. The HPNA also affirms nursing's role in communication and advanced care planning in its position statement for both generalist and advanced practice nurses (HPNA, 2013b, 2015a). Position statements such as those create a vision for the membership and outline new developments in the field or responses to current events in the field in order to keep the membership abreast of changes. Interestingly, while the HPNA position statements are geared to those members in clinical practice, it does not emphasize the role of the nurse scientist or researcher in palliative care leadership (HPNA, 2015b). For leadership to be truly transformational and nursing research in communication and advanced care planning to be meaningfully adopted and affect health policy, emphasis on nurses leading research and creating knowledge beyond following and applying the research is warranted.

Nursing research has been influential in creating communication training (Hendricks-Ferguson et al., 2015; Meyer et al., 2009) across disciplines (although including primarily nurses and physicians) and across experience levels. Meyer et al. (2009) examined 5-month outcomes on self-ascribed feelings and competencies and found that interdisciplinary clinicians felt more confident and prepared for difficult conversations and less anxious. This demonstrated that the one-day intervention conducted in the study was rooted in relational abilities and communication skills meaningful to participating clinicians, useful in the clinical setting, and feasible. To improve palliative care communication in the neuro-oncology setting, Hendricks-Ferguson et al. (2015) developed an intervention to test delivery of early palliative and end-of-life communication with families of children with aggressive brain tumors. The intervention dually focused on nurses and physicians working collaboratively with families and incorporated bereaved parents as teachers. Clinicians found it to be helpful overall, but faced challenges regarding scheduling and were concerned about the impact on bereaved parents who served as teachers. Learning which interventions are difficult to implement or burdensome for clinicians is instructive for the development of future interventions. These efforts demonstrate how nurses and nursing research have been foundational to disentangling the challenges of this sensitive communication and for designing feasible and effective interventions to promote high-quality communication and advanced care planning.

The findings of this research can inform policy makers at the institutional level by prompting them to ensure that clinicians have adequate time to conduct these discussions in the outpatient setting and that APNs are allowed to practice to the full scope allowed by their state practice acts and reimbursement policy. For example, an institution prohibits an APN from initiating an advanced care planning discussion, yet he or she may be allowed to do so through the state practice act and be eligible to receive compensation for the advanced care planning discussions. At the state level, policy makers must ensure that mechanisms exist for children and adolescents/young adults to receive comprehensive pediatric palliative and end-of-life care that includes reimbursement for advanced care planning discussions. Several states have implemented comprehensive programs, yet the clear expectation that advanced care planning discussions will take place and include children as they are able is missing (NHPCO, 2012). Finally, comprehensive federal policy to expand the provision of palliative care to those children who would benefit while living with life-limiting and life-threatening diseases is necessary. This would eliminate geographic disparities that afflict children and their families. Nursing research, as outlined here, can inform actions reimbursed through policy. In addition, nurse researchers can partner with policy makers to construct policy that is inclusive and that takes down barriers to care for children and families that is informed by current evidence.

An important way to assess quality of communication and advanced care planning is through dialogue with children and families living with life-threatening illnesses. While Docherty, Miles, and Brandon (2007) outlined the challenges of implementing palliative care in acute care, other nurse researchers have demonstrated a potential path forward. In stem cell transplant, LaFond et al. (2015) found that nurse-led palliative care consultations in the context of hematopoietic stem cell transplant (HSCT) were welcomed and feasible, and families reported satisfaction with this intervention. Similarly, Akard et al.'s (2015) use of digital storytelling represents a mode of quality palliative and end-of-life care delivery that remains with the family after the child has died. These studies stand out as examples in which quality can be more holistically assessed because family perspective is ascertained and provide evidence of outcomes and the return on investment of family-focused interventions that prompt policy makers to create family-focused health and social policy.

The second IOM recommendation also calls for evaluation of palliative care conversations, especially those including advanced care planning and those elucidating goals of care. What also remains to be documented, however, is how these conversations will be evaluated. National efforts at evaluation may be limited because of state variation in PPC coverage and reimbursement and variation in institutional rules and state laws that dictate APN scope of practice. A next step in evaluating palliative care conversations should include assessment of child/family outcomes over time resulting from palliative care conversations and the creation of an evaluation tool of these desired communication efforts. Nurse researchers can assist this process and engage with policy makers to create evidence-based evaluation standards and criteria to guide assessment of conversations, as well as implement such standards and criteria into the educational setting for clinicians and students. Levine et al. (2015), along with oncology nurse researchers, highlighted a gap in the delivery of palliative and end-of-life care during cancer clinical trials; this may be an avenue for future nursing research: Are there trigger points in a clinical trial that should prompt discussions about advance care planning and goals of care? Finally, as the authors note, communication needs cross many pediatric life-threatening illnesses and thus require the same level of attention. A potential policy action rooted in this evidence is that all children enrolled in federally funded or industry-sponsored clinical trials to treat a life-threatening condition or alleviate symptoms of such a condition receive screening for these trigger points while enrolled in research. Nurse researchers could work with funding agencies, parent/family advocacy groups, industry sponsors, and policy makers to design protocols of when to assess for goals of care and how to conduct these conversations in the context of clinical trials.

Access to Care

The number of pediatric palliative and hospice clinicians is small, which means that palliative care needs must be met through other clinicians in primary or subspecialty care. Thus, the need to provide training to generalists in holding conversations about goals of care and advanced care planning is crucial. Tubbs-Cooley et al. (2011) described nurses' perceptions of pediatric palliative and hospice care (PPHC) across subspecialty units at a large, tertiary children's hospital with a palliative care consultative service. While the nurses broadly endorsed the significance of palliative care goals and the presence of problems, they differed on the importance of these PPHC goals and problems. Interestingly, the hospital unit was the most significant predictor of how nurses collaborated with the PPC team. Thus, there may be differences across a single institution by unit or individual clinician that may affect the quality of PPC provided in the institution or sought for the child and family in the community. Younge et al. (2015) described the initiation of a NICU-based palliative care program that was found to improve communication with families and provide more aggressive symptom management near end of life, as evidenced through more family meetings and sedative use. Few infants who die in the NICU receive PPC (Brandon, Docherty, & Thorpe, 2007; Feudtner et al., 2011). For example, implementation of a NICU-based palliative care program provided access for children and families who would not otherwise receive care and did not experience increases in withdrawal of life support (Younge et al., 2015); this implementation was associated with increased parental satisfaction (Petteys et al., 2015). Table 18.1 displays the current evidence.

Communication and advanced care planning are foundational and important aspects of pediatric palliative and end-of-life care, yet require skill, sensitivity, and meaningful representation of all clinicians. Nursing research has contributed to efforts to improve these essential skills across disciplines and to provide a pathway for a multitude of voices to be heard. Among the most important of these voices, which our research must continue to include, is that of all children affected by life-threatening illness, both ill children and their healthy siblings. Our research, and the interventions or practice changes that arise from such research endeavors, should be rooted in the developmental state of the children and should incorporate measures that tap into children's innate creativity and meet their developmental, contextual needs. In order to better understand and elucidate these needs, we may need to utilize innovative research methods to dive deeper into the experiences of children affected by life-threatening illness. Such efforts take training, time, solid mentorship, and adequate funding. These efforts also require collaborative and cooperative research groups that are not afraid of the sampling challenges of pediatric palliative and end-of-life care research, the complexity of research with families, and the nuanced skills that are needed to elicit the perspectives of children. To move the science forward, these urgent needs must be met.

IOM 3

Educational institutions, credentialing bodies, accrediting boards, state regulatory agencies, and health care delivery organizations should establish the appropriate training, certification, and/or licensure requirements to strengthen the palliative care knowledge and skills of all clinicians who care for individuals with advanced serious illness who are nearing the end of life.

Costs of Care

Standards for palliative care, including pediatrics, have been put forward by specialty groups and certifying bodies at the level of individual skill achievement, curricula for nursing at the undergraduate and graduate levels, and for employers of nurses. The early efforts to promote standards were most noteworthy in federally funded or foundation-funded curricula, with the exemplar in this category being the End-of-Life Nursing Education Consortium (ELNEC) that has now been offered in all 50 states and the District of Columbia. The exact costs associated with implementing and sustaining this curriculum have not been reported, though positive participant reports mentioning increased palliative care knowledge and continued enrollments have been noteworthy (Ferrell, Malloy, & Virani, 2015; Goldsmith et al., 2013; Jacobs et al., 2009; O'Shea et al., 2015). This educational curriculum has been offered as a freestanding workshop, online (certain modules), and (in a recent demonstration project) embedded into an undergraduate nursing curriculum (Jacobs et al., 2009; O'Shea et al., 2015; Wittenberg-Lyles, Goldsmith, Ferrell, & Burchett, 2014). Two interdisciplinary PPC curricula, one now concluded (the Initiative for Pediatric Palliative Care) and one ongoing (Education in Palliative and End-of-Life Care for Pediatrics [EPEC-Pediatrics]) also had nurse faculty and nurse participants (Solomon, Browning, Dokken, Merriman, & Rushton, 2010; Widger et al., 2016). Costs for implementation or sustainment have also not been reported for these two initiatives, but cost information would be quite helpful to estimate dollars needed to expand the scale and reach of this type of educational initiative and to calculate the cost/benefit ratio in terms of program costs linked to improved patient and family care outcomes.

In 2016, the American Association of Colleges of Nursing (AACN) issued new recommendations for palliative care content for undergraduate nursing curricula (AACN, 2016b). Specific new competencies are included in the recommendations. These recommendations expand the practice expectation for baccalaureate nursing graduates stated in the AACN (2008) document, *The Essentials of Baccalaureate Education for Professional Nursing Practice*, related to symptom management, support of rituals, and respect for patient and family preferences during palliative and end-of-life care. Together, these two documents have the strong likelihood of influencing the undergraduate curriculum such that in a few short years, the nursing graduates of baccalaureate programs can be assumed to have had exposure to primary palliative care. Evaluating the costs of uptake of the recommendations (speed of uptake, extent of uptake, methods used for the uptake) is needed and will be quite informative, as will information on the undergraduate nurses' knowledge, confidence, and application of the learned skills. Eventually, the new knowledge infused into the undergraduate nursing curricula will be reflected in the nursing licensure exam, an achievement that will give further emphasis to primary palliative care being a part of nursing practice at the generalist level.

Certification for nurses in pediatric and perinatal palliative care is provided by the Hospice & Palliative Credentialing Center, which is the certifying arm of the HPNA. As of 2014, only 160 nurses in America were certified through this credentialing center in hospice and palliative nursing (IOM, 2014, 4–17), indicating an alarmingly low number given the annual number of infants, children, and adolescents who die in America and the number of children being treated for a complex chronic condition each year. This discrepancy from need to access to specialty palliative care nurses conveys the frank need for programs that formally prepare nurses to provide this level of care.

Palliative care certification from The Joint Commission is also available in the United States. The criteria for this certification have direct effects on nursing, including the role composition of the palliative care service and the skill and education of the members of that service. The costs for hospitals to achieve and maintain this certification have not been reported.

Several gaps in our understanding of nursing palliative care certification and licensure remain, such as (a) determining the most effective methods for nursing skill achievement and confidence in addressing palliative care needs of children and their families, (b) determining how pilot projects of embedding primary palliative care in undergraduate and graduate nursing curricula can be brought to scale across nursing programs and the costs of such uptake, and (c) assessing the costs of linking and extending palliative care content from nursing academic programs to education offerings by their employers. In summary, the costs of providing primary or specialty palliative care education to nurses through academic, degree-granting programs, professional associations, or employers have not been assessed in a standardized approach and have not been reported publicly. It does not appear that recommended content related to palliative care nursing, including pediatrics, has been implemented in undergraduate curricula to a uniform degree such that content can be assumed for the nursing licensure exam or for certification requirements. Nurse researchers are well-positioned to elucidate the key measures and methods to assess the cost/benefit ratio of palliative care educational endeavors and the formal content linkage between academic programs, licensing bodies, and certification groups.

Quality of Care

The link between standards of PPC and nursing care and the important link to patient and family care outcomes have not been measured to date. This is the central set of relationships that must be measured. Perhaps, because the care standards from national organizations such as the NQF or The Joint Commission have not been universally adopted and the 2016 AACN recommendations for palliative care content or the AACN baccalaureate curriculum standards have not been implemented in a standardized manner, measurement has been limited to small-scale reports of single-site or single-program implementation. The absence of data for this central set of relationships in PPC nursing is alarming.

Access to Care

As soon as the 2016 recommendations from the AACN are fully actualized, the number of nurses exposed to primary palliative care nursing skills will be exponentially greater. How those nurses apply the skills will merit careful documentation as a form of feedback about the strength of the AACN recommendations when translated into actual curricula. Similarly, with only 160 PPC-certified nurses in America (IOM, 2014), their accessibility to seriously ill children and their families is quite limited. Determining their direct impact on care will be difficult on a large-scale basis, so impact may have to be narrowly defined initially for measurement purposes—but it must be addressed and established. *Nurses certified in pediatric and perinatal palliative care are uniquely positioned to address the need for their skills within and beyond their own institutions of care and own communities. In this way, this small group of well-prepared nurses can influence public health policy.*

IOM 4

Federal, state, and private insurance and health care delivery programs should integrate the financing of medical and social services to support the provision of quality care consistent with the values, goals, and informed preferences of people with advanced serious illness nearing the end of life. To the extent that additional legislation is necessary to implement this recommendation, the administration should seek and Congress should enact such legislation. In addition, the federal government should require public reporting on quality measures, outcomes, and costs regarding care near the end of life (e.g., in the last year of life) for programs it funds or administers (e.g., Medicare, Medicaid, the Department of Veterans Affairs). The federal government should encourage all other payment and health care delivery systems to do the same.

Cost of Care

The fourth recommendation of the IOM encourages health care payers and systems to integrate financing health and social services in order to provide care that is consistent with patient and family values, goals, and preferences. This recommendation reminds clinicians of the need to elicit values, goals, and preferences of children, AYA, and their families. It also reminds all palliative care professionals of the need to engage in and lead public discourse around palliative and end-of-life care, while understanding the options available for care at this phase of life, hallmarks of high-quality care, and the meaning and significance of advanced care planning discussions.

Quality and cost are interrelated. High-quality care in this domain may be costly initially, but it may diminish costs because it provides care that is aligned with child/family preferences, is rooted in open and honest communication that allows parents to make decisions with the best available information, and avoids costly measures that may provide little benefit or are not truly desired.

Nurses have an instrumental hand in developing PPC programs that span both inpatient/outpatient/home environments. One study led by a nurse executive noted that the development of their patient- and family-centered, nurse-driven program cut down on emergency department visits for symptom management ($250–$3,000) due to home-based symptom management (average cost = $172) and subsequent admissions. The continuity of care provided by the pediatric palliative care team allowed for consistent support and a more open environment for end-of-life discussions, which led to a decrease in admissions for end-of-life care and diminished use of life-sustaining interventions (Mastro, Johnson, McElvery, & Preuster, 2015). Duncan, Spengler, and Wolfe (2007) demonstrated how philanthropic funding has been vital in starting and maintaining PPC programs, as well as billing for physician services.

In terms of program use by children and families, Medicaid eligibility and private insurance are both related to hospice use by children (Lindley & Shaw, 2014). Profit status of a particular hospice may also predict if children are enrolled for care; nonprofit hospices are more likely to have a specialized pediatric program and have more experience caring for children (Lindley et al., 2012). Enrollment in home-based PPC service was associated with decreased emergency room and hospital length of stay and total hospital charges versus the time prior to enrollment for children without a cancer diagnosis (Postier et al., 2014).

A gap that nursing research can fill is related to nursing's social contract: How can we achieve more equitable distribution of PPC services and hospices equipped to render them?

Quality of Care

Provision of high-quality palliative care is an extension of nursing's social contract. Nursing research, thus far, has done a remarkable job elucidating what is important to families, clinicians, and to a lesser extent, children. Thus, nursing research has been another avenue through which nurses can uphold the social contract with some of the most vulnerable members of our society and their families.

High-quality delivery programs are patient- and family-centered (Baird et al., 2015; Davies, Baird, & Gundsmunsdottir, 2013), yet competing perceptions and goals among parents and clinicians may impede this. In a study of nursing care provided in a pediatric intensive care unit, parents reported facing significant barriers to full participation in their ill child's care in the critical care setting (Baird et al., 2015). A concept that helps clinicians and researchers understand parents' experiences when their child is ill stems from nursing research (Hinds et al., 2009). This concept, "being a good parent to my seriously ill child," emerged from the words of parents themselves and describes their "perceived obligation to make beneficial health care decisions and remain at the child's side despite difficult circumstances" (Hinds et al., 2009, p. 5982). High-quality engagement with parents may be rooted in helping parents achieve or reframe their definition of being a good parent in the care of their child with life-threatening illness. As reported by Hinds and colleagues, interventions to promote this are feasible and may help parents emotionally survive the death of their child (Hinds et al., 2012). This may also have implications for the care of the ill child's healthy siblings (Mooney-Doyle & Deatrick, 2016). Documentation in a child's chart may not fully capture family's needs, preferences, or competing priorities; therefore, clinicians may not provide care consistent with child and family needs and values. Research reporting the feasibility of responding to family care needs can inform and support clinical practice. These studies provide data to be translated to policy makers documenting the need for supportive care.

Because the intersection of health and social care is at the heart of nursing's social contract, nursing research is poised to elucidate the best ways to broaden the impact of this research and move it from institutional- or unit-level policy to broader, regional, state, or federal level policy. How should the voices of children and families be incorporated into broader health and social policy? High-quality care is rooted in research that elicits and disseminates child and family preferences (Hinds, Drew, et al., 2005) and, as demonstrated in the IOM report, there is a growing recognition of the needs of family caregivers (most notably parents). There is also work in unearthing how best to support family caregivers, such as illuminating key factors in caring for dying children and families (Hinds, Schum, et al., 2006), assessing parental goals and priorities (Hill et al., 2015; Hinds et al., 2009), and developing guidelines and interventions in supportive communication with children and families (Hinds et al., 2001, 2012; Hinds & Kelly, 2010). The data from the program of research of Hinds and colleagues have been used with the Food and Drug Administration (FDA) to begin the dialogue of incorporating the child's voice and perspective into reporting adverse events of new therapies to inform the FDA, including the feasibility and acceptability of asking and documenting the child's self-report on symptoms, function, and treatment toxicities during treatment for life-threatening illness.

Access to Care

High-quality, cost-effective palliative and hospice care is made accessible in two ways: (a) through generalists trained in basic provision of palliative care and initiation of conversations around goals of care; and (b) specialist palliative and hospice care that is provided by certified individuals or as part of a palliative care team. How do we train clinicians to provide palliative, hospice, and end-of-life care that is consistent with the wishes and needs of children and their families so that access is equitable?

Lindley and Shaw (2014) described the children who are utilizing hospice. They found that mid–late adolescents were more likely to receive hospice services, as were those with certain diagnoses (such as neuromuscular diseases and cancer). A child was more likely to be enrolled in hospice if one was located within the family's community. Similarly, Lindley et al. (2012) found that infants requiring hospice care may have less access because of the lack of pediatric knowledge in many community hospices. In addition, nonprofit hospices may be more likely to care for highly complex patients. Thus, there may be a significant subset of children for whom hospice care is not available or accessible. Children with certain diseases, of particular ages, or residing in certain communities may not be referred to hospice by their clinicians or may not have access even if they are referred.

Access can also be adjusted through an institution. Doorenbos et al. (2013) found that automatic referrals across intensive care settings for children receiving extracorporeal membrane oxygenation (ECMO) can increase access for children and families. Additionally, Tubbs-Cooley et al. (2011) found that the hospital unit was the most significant predictor of how nurses collaborated with the PPC team, even controlling for individual differences. This highlights the specific needs that acute care, inpatient nurses have concerning provision of PPHC, which affects the access to and quality of palliative care provided in the hospital setting. Table 18.1 provides a display of the current evidence.

The IOM report calls for health care delivery programs to support integration of medical and social services for children affected by life-threatening illness and their families. A gap in this call, however, is the gravity or consequences for families affected by a pediatric life-threatening illness. What is key to recognize in our research and policy work is this: life-threatening illness is disruptive to family life and this disruption causes ripples during diagnosis; treatment (sometimes for years), as families live each day with the ups and downs of illness and try to meet their various duties; and with the death of the ill child. Families wrestle with decisions that are nearly unfathomable for many of us and are painful. Nursing research has illuminated how this very context can be both painful and joyful, yet we may have missed a single important question: What do families need to survive this experience as intact as possible? Additionally, we need further research and policy leadership on how to make distribution of palliative care resources more equitable across populations and regions and how to increase the scale of training initiatives and best practices so that children and families across the United States have access to high-quality palliative and end-of-life care and that this survival is possible for all families caring for an ill child.

IOM 5

All organizations should engage their constituents and provide fact-based information about care of people nearing end of life to encourage advance care planning (ACP) and informed choices.

Cost of Public Education and Engagement

The cost of providing fact-based information about care of children with advanced serious illnesses by health care delivery organizations, government agencies, payers, and health care professional societies is relatively unknown. There is a lack of cost information on advance care planning and informed choices that is based on the needs and values of the child and family. Although reports from the adult end-of-life literature have found that patient and family education and engagement in advance care planning affects costs (Dixon, Matosevic, & Knapp, 2015; Khandelwal, Benkeser, Coe, & Curtis, 2016; Klinger, in de Schmitten, & Marckmann, 2016; Korfage et al., 2015), there is no similar evidence in pediatrics. One possible explanation is that cost data on advance care planning is often unavailable. Many health care delivery systems and payers do not collect data on specific services such as advance care planning. The costs may be considered part of a palliative care consultation or physician/nurse practitioner visit. Identifying the direct costs contributed to advance care planning may not be feasible. Alternatively, there are significant methodological challenges to conducting cost analysis studies of advance care planning.

The cost of care at end of life for children often involves a variety of services, programs, and clinicians. Modeling whether advance care planning influences costs is complicated because many confounding factors, such as geographic location, diagnosis, and payer type, may impact costs. However, these confounding factors must be included in the model or results will potentially be biased. In addition, there is a concern of reverse causality or endogeneity in cost studies that must be controlled. For example, does the delivery of advance care planning influence costs, or do costs influence the delivery of advance care planning? Arguments could be made in both directions. Cost researchers must be knowledgeable of sophisticated analytics including instrumental variables and variable time lagging to address this concern. Thus, nurse researchers interested in contributing knowledge to this important gap in our understanding of advance care planning would benefit from advanced education in quantitative methods and statistics. Partnering with health care economists might also provide insight into the analytic techniques needed to investigate research questions involving advance care planning and costs.

Quality of Public Education and Engagement

Newly emerging evidence by nurse researchers is showing that public education and engagement in advance care planning is benefiting teens and families. A randomized controlled trial found that participating in advance care planning does not unduly distress adolescents with serious illness (Lyon, Garvie, Briggs, et al., 2010). When advance care planning is conducted with trained facilitators, there is increased congruence in adolescent/parent preferences for end-of-life care, decreased decisional conflict, and enhanced communication quality (Lyon, Garvie, McCarter, et al., 2009). Adolescents demonstrated low depressive symptoms and high quality of life, compared to adolescents who did not participate in advance care planning (Lyon, Jacobs, Briggs, Cheng, & Wang, 2014). Families generally rated the advance care planning discussion as worthwhile (Lyon et al., 2014); however, timing of such discussions is dependent on the receptivity of the parents (Erby, Rushton, & Geller, 2006). One challenge for nurse researchers remains exploring questions of quality among families of young children and infants. For families with seriously ill infants and young children, conversations about advance care planning may be viewed as taking away hope for a cure or that death is imminent (Hill et al., 2015). These are special challenges that nurse researchers, who provide care for these children and families, are uniquely positioned to explore. Another challenge is navigating this research space with no defined measures of pediatric end-of-life care, as already discussed.

Access to Public Education and Engagement

There are encouraging examples of nurse involvement and leadership in ensuring access to advance care planning for children and their families. Nursing-focused government agencies such as the National Institute of Nursing Research (NINR) have provided information on pediatric advanced care planning with their

"Conversations Matter" initiative (https://www.ninr.nih.gov/newsandinforma tion/conversationsmatter/conversations-matter-newportal). Nursing health care professional societies have also been actively involved in the development and dissemination of information about pediatric advance care planning. The HPNA has issued position statements in support of advance care planning for all ages to its membership of nurses (HPNA, 2013b), and the Oncology Nursing Society offers podcasts on the topic that are publicly available. The NHPCO offers toolkits and protocols for practitioners directly involved in pediatric advance care planning (NHPCO, 2015). Pediatric end-of-life coalitions such as the Pediatric Palliative Care Coalition, Greater Illinois Pediatric Palliative Care Coalition, and Children's Hospice and Palliative Care Coalition advocate for and engage in meaningful dialogue about pediatric advance care planning among their members and the community at large. Given this broad and comprehensive approach to providing constituents with information about advance care planning, there is still a lack of knowledge about whether these efforts are reaching children and families, especially in underserved populations. Recent studies have investigated advance care planning for teens with cancer and HIV (Lyon, Garvie, McCarter, et al., 2009; Lyon, Jacobs, Briggs, Cheng, & Wang, 2013), but little is known about whether racial/ethnic disparities exist in accessing pediatric advance care planning. This area of inquiry provides opportunities for future nursing research. Table 18.1 provides a display of the current evidence.

There are several implications for nurse researchers in the area of organization engagement with constituents to provide information about nearing end of life for children and families. The first implication is that nurse researchers might benefit from additional training in the advanced statistical methods needed to conduct sophisticated cost studies, which would be a significant contribution to the literature. Another implication is that as the science of advance care planning develops, nurse researchers are poised to expand the evidence to seriously ill infants and young children. Our experience in the NICUs and pediatric intensive care units enables nurses to build trust and confidence among families to participate in studies examining difficult conversations about end of life. A third implication is that nurse researchers have a leadership opportunity to expand our knowledge on racial and ethnic disparities in access to pediatric advance care planning. The current lack of knowledge in this area suggests that nurse researchers might add valuable insight into the social dynamics of end-of-life care for children and their families.

CONCLUSION

In conclusion, nurses have actively engaged in research examining pediatric palliative and end-of-life care, though the short- and longer-term impacts on health policy are not fully established. However, challenges still remain.

Challenge 1. Nurse researchers often struggle with obtaining access to data for national studies of children at end of life. Due to small sample sizes and the specialty nature of pediatric end-of-life care, many national databases such as Fair Health cannot provide a study cohort. In addition, the Medicaid pediatric end-of-life sample size is increasingly becoming smaller as states move children from fee-for-service to managed care, a payment structure not currently captured in the Medicaid data files by the Centers for Medicare and Medicaid Services (2013). Nurse researchers have found that state data sources can provide pediatric end-of-life data, but at the cost of generalizability. Researchers need access to national data.

Challenge 2. Not enough nurse researchers are engaged in the hospice and palliative care research community. Nurse researchers are well prepared to address issues related to measurement and data, including those about measuring quality and developing data repositories. Pediatric nurses are well-positioned to participate and lend their voices to the challenges of measurement and data within pediatrics.

Challenge 3. Nurse researchers are challenged with securing extramural funding for pediatric end-of-life studies. Although pediatric end-of-life research has funding champions in the NINR and National Cancer Institute, funding for pediatric policy research is very restricted. In the current tight funding environment, policy studies are often limited to private organizations such as the RWJF. Pediatric end of life is often considered too narrow a topic or too specialized a field for many funding agencies. Therefore, nurse policy researchers must advocate for a pediatric program of research among data owners, end-of-life research groups, and funding agencies.

Challenge 4. Nurse educators and nurse researchers in partnership could determine the education methods and curricula that effectively prepare all nurses to have primary palliative care skills, including those for use in pediatrics. Further, this partnership could then examine the application of these methods and curricula through the actual delivery of nursing primary palliative care and the patient care outcomes of that care. Examining the effects of these skills on nurse morale and longevity in the pediatric palliative and end-of-life care specialty and on the rate of PPC certification would also be a priority consideration.

Challenge 5. Translation of pediatric end-of-life policy research must improve. Whether the research is directly related to policy or has policy implications, nursing research is typically not disseminated to policy makers or advocates. In the case of Concurrent Care for Children in the 2010 Affordable Care Act, there was no formal or anecdotal evidence cited in the development of this policy. Nurse researchers might benefit from developing a dissemination plan for their research beyond peer-reviewed journal and conference presentations, to include local, state, and federal policy makers. In addition, identifying policy advocate groups that can use research to advance pediatric end-of-life legislation might improve policy dissemination (Feetham, 2011; Feetham & Doering, 2015; Sullivan-Bolyai & Feetham, 2013). Simply creating a list of policy makers or advocates contacts/e-mails to send study findings may facilitate nurse researchers' engagement in the political conversation about improving costs, quality, and access to end-of-life care for children. Nurses have an opportunity to provide critical policy leadership on issues of pediatric end of life, while navigating the challenges of conducting and translating policy research.

REFERENCES

Adams, G., Green, A., Towe, S., & Huett, A. (2013). Bereaved caregivers as educators in pediatric palliative care: Their experiences and impact. *Journal of Palliative Medicine, 16*(6), 609–615. doi:10.1089/jpm.2012.0475

Akard, T. F., Dietrich, M. S., Friedman, D. L., Hinds, P. S., Given, B., Wray, S., & Gilmer, M. J. (2015). Digital storytelling: An innovative legacy-making intervention for children with cancer. *Pediatric Blood and Cancer, 62*(4), 658–665.

American Association of Colleges of Nursing. (2008). The essentials of baccalaureate education for professional nursing practice. Washington, DC: Author. Retrieved from http://www .aacn.nche.edu/education-resources/BaccEssentials08.pdf

American Association of Colleges of Nursing. (2016a). ELNEC fact sheet. Retrieved from http:// www.aacn.nche.edu/elnec/about/fact-sheet

American Association of Colleges of Nursing. (2016b). CARES: Competencies and recommendations for educating nursing students: Preparing nurses to care for the seriously ill and their families. Retrieved from http://www.aacn.org/wd/practice/content/palliative-and-end -of-life-care.pcms?menu=practice

Baird, J., Davies, B., Hinds, P. S., Baggott, C., & Rehm, R. S. (2015). What impact do hospital and unit-based rules have upon patient- and family-centered care in the pediatric intensive care unit? *Journal of Pediatric Nursing, 30*(1), 133–142.

Bona, K., Bates, J., & Wolfe, J. (2011). Massachusetts' pediatric palliative care network: Successful implementation of a novel state-funded pediatric palliative care program. *Journal of Palliative Medicine, 14*(11), 1217–1223.

Boyden, J. Y., Kavanaugh, K., Issel, L. M., Eldeirawi, K., & Meert, K. L. (2014). Experiences of African American parents following perinatal or pediatric death: A literature review. *Death Studies, 38*(6), 374–380.

Brandon, D., Docherty, S. L., & Thorpe, J. (2007). Infant and child deaths in acute care settings: Implications for palliative care. *Journal of Palliative Medicine, 10*(4), 910–918.

Buescher, P. A., Whitmire, J. T., Brunssen, S., & Kluttz-Hile, C. E. (2006). Children who are medically fragile in North Carolina: Using Medicaid data to estimate prevalence and medical care costs in 2004. *Maternal Child Health Journal, 10*(5), 461–466.

Catlin, A., Brandon, D., Woole, C., & Mendes, J. (2015). NANN position statement: Palliative and end-of-life care for newborns and infants. *Advances in Neonatal Care, 15*(4), 239–240.

Centers for Medicare and Medicaid Services. (2013). Medicare program; FY2014 hospice wage index and payment rate update; hospice quality reporting requirements; and updates in payment reform; final rule. *Federal Register, 78*(152), 48233–48281.

Contro, N., Larson, J., Scofield, S., Sourkes, B., & Cohen, H. (2002). Family perspectives on the quality of pediatric palliative care. *Archives of Pediatrics & Adolescent Medicine, 156*(1), 14–19.

Dabbs, D., Butterworth, L., & Hall, E. (2007). Tender mercies: Increasing access to hospice services for children with life-threatening conditions. *MCN: The American Journal of Maternal/ Child Nursing, 32*(5), 311–319.

Davies, B., Baird, J., & Gudmundsdottir, M. (2013). Moving family-centered care forward: Bereaved fathers' perspectives. *Journal of Hospice and Palliative Nursing: JHPN, 15*(3).

Davies, B., Collins, J. B., Steele, R., Cook, K., Brenner, A., & Smith, S. (2005). Children's perspectives of a pediatric hospice program. *Journal of Palliative Care, 21*(4), 252–261.

Dixon, J., Matosevic, T., & Knapp, M. (2015). The economic evidence for advance care planning: Systematic review of evidence. *Palliative Medicine, 29*(10), 869–884.

Docherty, S. L., Miles, M. S., & Brandon, D. (2007). Searching for the "dying point": Providers' experiences with palliative care in pediatric acute care. *Pediatric Nursing, 33*(4), 335–341.

Doorenbos, A. Z., Starks, H., Bourget, E., McMullan, D. M., Lewis-Newby, M., Rue, T. C., . . . Wilfond, B. S. (2013). Examining palliative care team involvement in automatic consultations for children on extracorporeal life support in the pediatric intensive care unit. *Journal of Palliative Medicine, 16*(5), 492–495.

Dulkerian, S. J., Douglas, W. P., & Taylor, R. M. (2011). Redirecting treatment during neonatal transport. *The Journal of Perinatal & Neonatal Nursing, 25*(2), 111–114.

Duncan, J., Spengler, E., & Wolfe, J. (2007). Providing pediatric palliative care: PACT in action. *MCN: The American Journal of Maternal/Child Nursing, 32*(5), 279–287.

Dy, S. M., Kiley, K. B., Ast, K., Lupu, D., Norton, S. A., McMillan, S. C., . . . Casarett, D. J. (2015). Measuring what matters: Top-ranked quality indicators for hospice and palliative care from the American Academy of Hospice and Palliative Medicine and Hospice and Palliative Nurses Association. *Journal of Pain and Symptom Management, 49*(4), 773–781.

Erby, L. H., Rushton, C., & Geller, G. (2006). "My son is still walking": Stages of receptivity to discussions of advanced care planning among parents of sons with Duchenne muscular dystrophy. *Seminars in Pediatric Neurology, 13*(2), 132–140.

Feetham, S. (2011). The role of science policy in programs of research and scholarship. In A. S. Hinshaw & P. A. Grady (Eds.), *Shaping health policy through nursing research* (pp. 53–71). New York, NY: Springer Publishing.

Feetham, S., & Doering, J. J. (2015). Career cartography: A conceptualization of career development to advance health and policy. *Journal of Nursing Scholarship, 47*(1), 70–71. doi:10.1111/jnu.12103

Ferrell, B., Malloy, P., & Virani, R. (2015). The End-of-Life Nursing Education Nursing Consortium project. *Annals of Palliative Medicine, 4*(2), 61–69.

Ferrell, B., Virani, R., Paice, J. A., Coyle, N., & Coyne, P. (2010). Evaluation of palliative care nursing education seminars. *European Journal of Oncology Nursing, 14*(1), 74–79.

Feudtner, C., Kang, T. I., Hexem, K. R., Friedrichsdorf, S. J., Osenga, K., Siden, H., . . . Wolfe, J. (2011). Pediatric palliative care patients: A prospective multicenter cohort study. *Pediatrics, 127*, 1094–1101.

Field, M. J., & Behrman, R. E. (2003). *When children die: Improving palliative and end-of-life care for children and their families.* Washington, DC: National Academies Press.

Gans, D., Kominski, G. F., Roby, D. H., Diamant, A. L., Chen, X., Lin, W., & Hohe, N. (2012). Better outcomes, lower costs: Palliative care program reduces stress, costs of care for children with life-threatening conditions. *UCLA Center for Health Policy Research: Health Policy Brief,* (PB2012-3), 1–8.

Goldsmith, J., Ferrell, B., Wittenberg-Lyles, E., & Ragan, S. L. (2013). Palliative care communication in oncology nursing. *Clinical Journal of Oncology Nursing, 17*(2), 163–167. doi:10.1188/13.cjon.163-167

Goodenough, B., Drew, D., Higgins, S., & Trethewie, S. (2004). Bereavement outcomes for parents who lose a child to cancer: Are place of death and sex of parent associated with differences in psychological functioning? *Psycho-Oncology, 13*(11), 779–791.

Harper, M., O'Connor, R. C., & O'Carroll, R. E. (2014). Factors associated with grief and depression following the loss of a child: A multivariate analysis. *Psychology, Health & Medicine, 19*(3), 247–252.

Hendricks-Ferguson, V. L., Kane, J. R., Pradhan, K. R., Shih, C. S., Gauvain, K. M., Baker, J. N., & Haase, J. E. (2015). Evaluation of physician and nurse dyad training procedures to deliver a palliative and end-of-life communication intervention to parents of children with a brain tumor. *Journal of Pediatric Oncology Nursing, 32*(5), 337–347.

Hendrickson, K. C. (2009). Morbidity, mortality, and parental grief: A review of the literature on the relationship between the death of a child and the subsequent health of parents. *Palliative and Supportive Care, 7*(01), 109–119.

Hill, D. L., Miller, V. A., Hexem, K. R., Carroll, K. W., Faerber, J. A., Kang, T., & Feudtner, C. (2015). Problems and hopes perceived by mothers, fathers, and physicians of children receiving palliative care. *Health Expectations, 18*(5), 1052–1065.

Hinds, P. S., Drew, D., Oakes, L. L., Fouladi, M., Spunt, S. L., Church, C., & Furman, W. L. (2005). End-of-life care preferences of pediatric patients with cancer. *Journal of Clinical Oncology, 23*(36), 9146–9154.

Hinds, P. S., & Kelly, K. P. (2010). Helping parents make and survive end of life decisions for their seriously ill child. *Nursing Clinics of North America, 45*(3), 465–474.

Hinds, P. S., Oakes, L., Furman, W., Quargnenti, A., Olson, M. S., Foppiano, P., & Srivastava, D. K. (2001). End-of-life decision making by adolescents, parents, and healthcare providers in pediatric oncology: Research to evidence-based practice guidelines. *Cancer Nursing, 24*(2), 122–134.

Hinds, P. S., Oakes, L. L., Hicks, J., Powell, B., Srivastava, D. K., Baker, J. N., . . . Furman, W. L. (2012). Parent-clinician communication intervention during end-of-life decision making for children with incurable cancer. *Journal of Palliative Medicine, 15*(8), 916–922.

Hinds, P. S., Oakes, L. L., Hicks, J., Powell, B., Srivastava, D. K., Spunt, S. L., . . . Furman, W. L. (2009). "Trying to be a good parent" as defined by interviews with parents who made phase I, terminal care, and resuscitation decisions for their children. *Journal of Clinical Oncology, 27*(35), 5979–5985.

Hinds, P. S., Schum, L., Baker, J. N., & Wolfe, J. (2006). Key factors affecting dying children and their families. *Journal of Palliative Medicine, 8*(Suppl. 1), s70–s78.

Hospice and Palliative Nurses Association. (2013a). HPNA position statement: Assuring high-quality palliative nursing. Retrieved from http://hpna.advancingexpertcare.org/wp-content/uploads/2015/08/Assuring-High-Quality-in-Palliative-Care.pdf

Hospice and Palliative Nurses Association. (2013b). HPNA position statement: The nurse's role in advance care planning. Retrieved from https://www.hpna.org/filemaintenance_view.aspx?ID=23

Hospice and Palliative Nurses Association. (2015a). HPNA position statement: Value of the advanced practice nurse in palliative care. Retrieved from http://hpna.advancingexpertcare.org/wp-content/uploads/2015/08/Value-of-the-Advanced-Practice-Registered-Nurse-in-Palliative-Care.pdf

Hospice and Palliative Nurses Association. (2015b). HPNA position statement: Palliative nursing leadership. Retrieved from http://advancingexpertcare.org/wp-content/uploads/2016/05/Palliative-Nursing-Leadership.pdf

Institute of Medicine. (2014). *Dying in America: Improving quality and honoring individual preferences near the end of life.* Washington, DC: National Academies Press.

Jacobs, H. H., Ferrell, B., Virani, R., & Malloy, P. (2009). Appraisal of the pediatric end-of-life Nursing Education Consortium training program. *Journal of Pediatric Nursing, 24*(3), 216–221.

Kehl, K. A. (2014). The relationship of patient population and nurses certification status on nurses' practices in preparing families for the end of life. *Journal of Hospice and Palliative Nursing, 16*(8), 503–513. doi:10.1097/njh.0000000000000108

Keim-Malpass, J., Hart, T. G., & Miller, J. R. (2013). Coverage of palliative and hospice care for pediatric patients with life-limiting illness: A policy brief. *Journal of Pediatric Health Care, 27*, 511–516.

Khandelwal, N., Benkeser, D. C., Coe, N. B., & Curtis, J. R. (2016). Potential influence of advance care planning and palliative consultation on ICU costs for patients with chronic and serious illness. *Critical Care Medicine, 44*(8), 1474–1481.

Klinger, C., in der Schmitten, J., & Marckmann, G. (2016). Does facilitated advance care planning reduce the costs of care near the end of life? Systematic review and ethical considerations. *Palliative Medicine, 30*(5), 423–433.

Knapp, C. A., Madden, V. L., Curtis, C. M., Sloyer, P. J., Huang, I. C., Thompson, L. A., & Shenkman, E. A. (2008). Partners in care: Together for kids: Florida's model of pediatric palliative care. *Journal of Palliative Medicine, 11*(9), 1212–1220.

Knapp, C. A., Shenkman, E. A., Marcu, M. I., Madden, V. L., & Terza, J. V. (2009). Pediatric palliative care: Describing hospice users and identifying factors that affect hospice expenditures. *Journal of Palliative Medicine, 12*(3), 223–229.

Korfage, I. J., Rietjens, J. A., Overbeek, A., Jabbarian, L. J., Billekens, P., Hammes, B. J., . . . van der Heide, A. (2015). A cluster randomized controlled trial on the effects and costs of advance care planning in elderly care: Study protocol. *BMC Geriatrics, 15*, 87.

Kreicbergs, U., Valdimarsdóttir, U., Onelöv, E., Henter, J. I., & Steineck, G. (2004). Anxiety and depression in parents 4–9 years after the loss of a child owing to a malignancy: A population-based follow-up. *Psychological Medicine, 34*(08), 1431–1441.

Kreicbergs, U., Valdimarsdóttir, U., Steineck, G., & Henter, J. I. (2004). A population-based nationwide study of parents' perceptions of a questionnaire on their child's death due to cancer. *The Lancet, 364*(9436), 787–789.

Lafond, D. A., Kelly, K. P., Hinds, P. S., Sill, A., & Michael, M. (2015). Establishing feasibility of early palliative care consultation in pediatric hematopoietic stem cell transplantation. *Journal of Pediatric Oncology Nursing, 32*(5), 265–277.

Lannen, P. K., Wolfe, J., Prigerson, H. G., Onelöv, E., & Kreicbergs, U. C. (2008). Unresolved grief in a national sample of bereaved parents: Impaired mental and physical health 4 to 9 years later. *Journal of Clinical Oncology, 26*(36), 5870–5876.

Levine, D. R., Johnson, L. M., Mandrell, B. N., Yang, J., West, N. K., Hinds, P. S., & Baker, J. N. (2015). Does phase 1 trial enrollment preclude quality end-of-life care? Phase 1 trial enrollment and end-of-life care characteristics in children with cancer. *Cancer, 121*(9), 1508–1512.

Li, J., Laursen, T. M., Precht, D. H., Olsen, J., & Mortensen, P. B. (2005). Hospitalization for mental illness among parents after the death of a child. *New England Journal of Medicine, 352*(12), 1190–1196.

Li, J., Precht, D. H., Mortensen, P. B., & Olsen, J. (2003). Mortality in parents after death of a child in Denmark: A nationwide follow-up study. *The Lancet, 361*(9355), 363–367.

Lindley, L. C. (2011). Health care reform and concurrent curative care for terminally ill children: A policy analysis. *Journal of Hospice and Palliative Nursing, 13*(2), 81–88.

Lindley, L. C. (2013). Trends in services among pediatric hospice providers during 2002 to 2008. *American Journal of Hospice and Palliative Medicine, 30*(1), 68–74.

Lindley, L. C. (2016). The effect of pediatric palliative care policy on hospice utilization among California Medicaid beneficiaries. *Journal of Pain and Symptom Management, 52*(5), 688–694.

Lindley, L. C., & Edwards, S. L. (2015). Geographic access to hospice care for children with cancer in Tennessee, 2009 to 2011. *American Journal of Hospice and Palliative Medicine, 32*(8), 849–854.

Lindley, L. C., Edwards, S. L., & Bruce, D. J. (2014). Factors influencing the implementation of healthcare reform: An examination of the concurrent care for children provision. *American Journal of Hospice and Palliative Medicine, 31*(5), 527–533.

Lindley, L. C., Held, M. L., Henley, K. M., Miller, K. A., Pedziwol, K. E., & Rumley, L. E. (2016). Nursing unit environment associated with provision of language services in pediatric hospices. *Journal of Racial and Ethnic Health Disparities, 1–7.* doi:10.1007/s40615-016-0224-1

Lindley, L. C., & Lyon, M. E. (2013). A profile of children with complex chronic conditions at end of life among Medicaid beneficiaries: Implications for healthcare reform. *Journal of Palliative Medicine, 16*(11), 1388–1393.

Lindley, L. C., Mark, B. A., Lee, S.-Y., Domino, M., Song, M., & Jacobson-Vann, J. (2013). Factors associated with the provision of pediatric hospice care. *Journal of Pain and Symptom Management, 45*(4), 701–711.

Lindley, L. C., Mixer, S., & Mack, J. (2012). Profit status and delivery of hospice care for infants: The mediating role of pediatric knowledge. *Journal of Palliative Medicine, 15*(2), 1369–1373.

Lindley, L. C., Mixer, S. J., & Cozad, M. J. (2014). The effect of pediatric knowledge on hospice care costs. *American Journal of Hospice and Palliative Medicine, 31*(3), 269–274.

Lindley, L. C., & Shaw, S. L. (2014). Who are the children using hospice care? *Journal for Specialists in Pediatric Nursing, 19*(4), 308–315.

Lyon, M. E., Garvie, P. A., Briggs, L., He, J., Malow, R., D'Angelo, L. J., & McCarter, R. (2010). Is it safe? Talking to teens with HIV/AIDS about death and dying: A 3-month evaluation of Family Centered Advance Care (FACE) planning—anxiety, depression, quality of life. *HIV AIDS (Auckl), 2,* 27–37.

Lyon, M. E., Garvie, P. A., McCarter, R., Briggs, L., He, J., & D'Angelo, L. J. (2009). Who will speak for me? Improving end-of-life decision-making for adolescents with HIV and their families. *Pediatrics, 123*(2), e199–e206.

Lyon, M. E., Jacobs, S., Briggs, L., Cheng, Y. I., & Wang, J. (2013). Family-centered advance care planning for teens with cancer. *JAMA Pediatrics, 167*(5), 460–467.

Lyon, M. E., Jacobs, S., Briggs, L., Cheng, Y. I., & Wang, J. (2014). A longitudinal, randomized, controlled trial of advanced care planning for teens with cancer: Anxiety, depression, quality of life, advanced directives, spirituality. *Journal of Adolescent Health, 54*(6), 710–717.

Mastro, K. A., Johnson, J. E., McElvery, N., & Preuster, C. (2015). The benefits of a nurse-driven, patient- and family-centered pediatric palliative care program. *Journal of Nursing Administration, 45*(9), 423–428.

McCarthy, M. C., Clarke, N. E., Ting, C. L., Conroy, R., Anderson, V. A., & Heath, J. A. (2010). Prevalence and predictors of parental grief and depression after the death of a child from cancer. *Journal of Palliative Medicine, 13*(11), 1321–1326.

Meyer, E. C., Sellers, D. E., Browning, D. M., McGuffie, K., Solomon, M. Z., & Truog, R. D. (2009). Difficult conversations: Improving communication skills and relational abilities in health care. *Pediatric Critical Care Medicine, 10*(3), 352–359.

Miller, E. G., LaRagione, G., Kang, T. I., & Feudtner, C. (2012). Concurrent care for the medically complex child: Lessons of implementation. *Journal of Palliative Medicine, 15*(11), 1281–1283.

Mooney-Doyle, K., & Deatrick, J. A. (2016). Parenting in the face of childhood life-threatening conditions: The ordinary in the context of the extraordinary. *Palliative and Supportive Care, 14*(03), 187–198.

National Consensus Project for Quality Palliative Care. (2013). Clinical practice guidelines for quality palliative care. Retrieved from https://www.hpna.org/multimedia/NCP_Clinical_Practice_Guidelines_3rd_Edition.pdf

National Hospice and Palliative Care Organization. (2009). Standards of practice for pediatric palliative care and hospice. Retrieved from http://www.nhpco.org/sites/default/files/public/quality/Peds-Standards_article_NL-0209.pdf

National Hospice and Palliative Care Organization. (2012). Pediatric palliative care. Alexandria, VA. Retrieved from http://www.nhpco.org/sites/default/files/public/ChiPPS/Continuum_Briefing.pdf

National Hospice and Palliative Care Organization, Children's Project on Palliative/Hospice Services. (2015). Advance planning in pediatric hospice/palliative care. Retrieved from http://www.nhpco.org/sites/default/files/public/ChiPPS/ChiPPS_ejournal_Issue-39.pdf

National Quality Forum. (2016). Palliative and end-of-life care project 2015–2016. Retrieved from http://www.qualityforum.org/Palliative_and_End-of-Life_Care_Project_2015-2016.aspx

O'Shea, E. R., Campbell, S. H., Engler, A. J., Beauregard, R., Chamberlin, E. C., & Currie, L. M. (2015). Effectiveness of a perinatal and pediatric End-of-Life Nursing Education Consortium (ELNEC) curricula integration. *Nurse Educator Today, 35*(6), 765–770.

Petteys, A. R., Goebel, J. R., Wallace, J. D., & Singh-Carlson, S. (2015). Palliative care in neonatal intensive care effects on parent stress and satisfaction: A feasibility study. *American Journal of Hospice and Palliative Medicine, 32*(8), 869–875.

Postier, A., Chrastek, J., Nugent, S., Osenga, K., & Friedrichsdorf, S. J. (2014). Exposure to home-based pediatric palliative and hospice care and its impact on hospital and emergency care charges at a single institution. *Journal of Palliative Medicine, 17*(2), 183–188.

Rosenberg, A. R., Baker, K. S., Syrjala, K., & Wolfe, J. (2012). Systematic review of psychosocial morbidities among bereaved parents of children with cancer. *Pediatric Blood & Cancer, 58*(4), 503–512.

Shea, J., Grossman, S., Wallace, M., & Lange, J. (2010). Assessment of advanced practice palliative care nursing competencies in nurse practitioner students: Implications for the integration of ELNEC curricular modules. *Journal of Nursing Education, 49*(4), 183–189.

Solomon, M. Z., Browning, D. M., Dokken, D. L., Merriman, M. P., & Rushton, C. H. (2010). Learning that leads to action: Impact and characteristics of a professional education approach to improve the care of critically ill children and their families. *Archives of Pediatrics & Adolescent Medicine, 164*(4), 315–322.

Sullivan-Bolyai, S. L., & Feetham, S. (2013). History lesson: How a little girl and her family moved mountains to change care and policy to help children with special health care needs go home. *Journal of Family Nursing, 19*(2), 278–280.

Tubbs-Cooley, H. L., Santucci, G., Kang, T. I., Feinstein, J. A., Hexem, K. R., & Feudtner, C. (2011). Pediatric nurses' individual and group assessments of palliative, end-of-life, and bereavement care. *Journal of Palliative Medicine, 14*(5), 631–637.

Valdimarsdóttir, U., Kreicbergs, U., Hauksdóttir, A., Hunt, H., Onelöv, E., Henter, J. I., & Steineck, G. (2007). Parents' intellectual and emotional awareness of their child's impending death to cancer: A population-based long-term follow-up study. *The Lancet: Oncology, 8*(8), 706–714.

Weaver, M. S., Heinze, K. E., Bell, C. J., Wiener, L., Garee, A. M., Kelly, K. P., . . . Hinds, P. S. (2016). Establishing psychosocial palliative care standards for children and adolescents with cancer and their families: An integrative review. *Palliative Medicine, 30*(3), 212–223.

Weaver, M. S., Heinze, K. E., Kelly, K. P., Wiener, L., Casey, R. L., Bell, C. J., . . . Hinds, P. S. (2015). Palliative care as a standard of care in pediatric oncology. *Pediatric Blood & Cancer, 62*(Suppl. 5), S829–S833.

Widger, K., Friedrichsdorf, S., Wolfe, J., Liben, S., Pole, J. D., Bouffet, E., . . . Rapoport, A. (2016). Protocol: Evaluating the impact of a nation-wide train-the-trainer educational initiative to enhance the quality of palliative care for children with cancer. *BMC Palliative Care, 15*(1), 1.

Wiener, L., Weaver, M. S., Bell, C. J., & Sansom-Daly, U. M. (2015). Threading the cloak: Palliative care education for care providers of adolescents and young adults with cancer. *Clinical Oncology in Adolescents and Young Adults, 9*(5), 1–18.

Wittenberg-Lyles, E., Goldsmith, J., Ferrell, B., & Burchett, M. (2014). Assessment of an interprofessional online curriculum for palliative care communication training. *Journal of Palliative Medicine, 17*(4), 400–406.

Younge, N., Smith, P. B., Goldberg, R. N., Brandon, D. H., Simmons, C., Cotten, C. M., & Bidegain, M. (2015). Impact of a palliative care program on end-of-life care in a neonatal intensive care unit. *Journal of Perinatology, 35*(3), 218–222.

Zolot, J. (2016). The AACN recommends increased palliative care training in undergraduate nursing education. *American Journal of Nursing, 116*(5), 16.

19

Palliative and End-of-Life Care Issues: Policy Perspective

Jeri L. Miller

A FRAMEWORK FOR SCIENCE POLICY IN PALLIATIVE AND END-OF-LIFE CARE

Better care is possible now, but we also need better data and scientific knowledge to guide efforts to deliver more effective care, educate professionals to provide such care, and design supportive public policies. (Field & Behrman, 2002, p. 3)

Since the publication of *Shaping Health Policy Through Nursing Research* (Grady & Hinshaw, 2011), a significant number of evidence-informed health policies have been implemented that affect the care of individuals approaching the end of life. Nursing science has played a critical role in shaping the evidence base of many of these new efforts through the establishment of a compelling and informative research literature. The impact made on health care policy by the field of end-of-life and palliative care science is evident in many renewed discussions of what it means to experience a serious, advanced illness in today's health care environment. End-of-life and palliative care science has also strengthened the public consciousness of the important role of nursing science to substantiate the evidence within many health care initiatives that place value on high-quality, effective, and meaningful care. End-of-life and palliative care science, both in the past and in the present, has elevated and strengthened national recognition that the care of those at the end of life is a significant issue and a public health care priority (Morhaim & Pollack, 2013). New, informative, and persuasive data from a growing body of studies have demonstrated the significance of research in shaping policy efforts and influencing thought leaders, and many new research findings from the nursing science community have stimulated national media attention on the need for and continued support of end-of-life care. Evidence-informed conversations about end-of-life care

are now being underscored by scientific data that serve as the underpinning for polices designed around the central premise of an individual's preferences, goals, and values for end-of-life care.

Research evidence remains a mainstay of many of issues found in today's public discourse surrounding end-of-life care and subsequent efforts in new health care policy development. Data-driven information continues to inform difficult policy discussions on issues such as pain management and opioid misuse, use or lack of use of advance directives, and withdrawal from life-sustaining treatments. New research findings continue to draw attention to the identification and treatment of advanced symptoms and the need for quality standards of clinical practice. A growing research literature has substantiated new legislative and regulatory policies that affect the provision of hospice and palliative care (Lorenz, Shugarman, & Lynn, 2006, p. 731). In addition, data from numerous studies have reinforced palliative care as a mainstay of health care with demonstrated value in improving health outcomes and health care utilization (Kamal et al., 2015).

Because of nursing science, the evidence base has significantly contributed to an increasing national awareness of end of life as a public health issue in terms of suffering and illness burden. For nurse scientists, health policy issues in end-of-life and palliative care extend into numerous areas that are well known in the community, from equitable access to comprehensive quality care, practice metrics and outcomes, reimbursement, and workforce needs, among others (Dubois & Reed, 2014; Paice et al., 2006). Nurse scientists identify and develop the new evidence-based improvements to end-of-life care, which are adopted into clinical practice through policy change across the entire health care system (Institute of Medicine [IOM], 2011, p. 222). In the complex and ever-changing area of palliative and end-of-life care, today's scientists must be policy-savvy and ever cognizant of the many health, social, and political implications of translating and implementing new evidence in a manner that is shared effectively with health policy communities (AcademyHealth, 2015a).

Recognizing the importance of end-of-life and palliative care science in health policy requires an awareness of the complexity of the policy world and an understanding of assumptions underlying divergent processes of policy framing, agenda building, and consensus building (Prewitt, Schwandt, & Straf, 2012, p. 6). This chapter provides an overview of the interaction between science and policy in end-of-life and palliative care and the fundamental components of how this science has evolved to shape and inform a number of new and emerging health care initiatives. The chapter begins with an historical overview of the early contributions of the scientific community toward creating an infrastructure for research that provided a rich evidence base to generate data that has influenced health policy programs. Portraits of nursing science that have informed both policy and practice are highlighted along with resources that can strengthen the scientist's understanding of health policy in end-of-life and palliative care. The chapter focuses on how nursing science has played a key role in informing end-of-life health care, and concludes with a discussion of strategic areas that future researchers may consider in ensuring that their work remains relevant to policy makers and public stakeholders.

BUILDING THE SCIENCE: AN INFRASTRUCTURE FOR POLICY CHANGE

Science contributes to knowledge, which serves as a critical component in shaping policy making and influencing emerging political decisions (van den Hove, 2007). The IOM 1997 report, *Approaching Death: Improving Care at the End of Life*, called for the collective efforts of policy makers, consumer groups, and health systems to work with researchers to increase knowledge and improve the quality of the experiences of individuals at the end of life. This landmark report was incentivized by a series of public and private initiatives to improve the care of dying patients and to respond to a growing awareness of deficiencies in end-of-life care that was emerging from a new body of compelling scientific data (Field & Cassel, 1997, p. 32). The 1995 *Study to Understand Prognoses and Preferences for Outcomes and Risks of Treatment* (SUPPORT; The Writing Group for the SUPPORT Investigators, 1995) served as a trigger point in singularly escalating the national discourse and raising the political awareness of the numerous shortfalls in the care provided to those at the end of life. Amid the subsequent public and political outcry to address the gaps in and dissatisfaction with the experiences of end-of-life care identified by the study, SUPPORT also served as an affirmation of the significant contribution that scientific research provides to inform and to guide quality health care services throughout the entire spectrum of living with and dying from an advanced illness (NINR, 2013).

The 1997 IOM report, the SUPPORT study, and subsequent IOM initiatives (e.g., Field & Behrman, 2002) helped to amass the existing data into informative messages that shaped national reconsideration of health policies in end-of-life care. The 1997 IOM report's inclusion of research data substantiated the enormity of the issues that needed to be understood. The data also served as talking points in a collaborative "call to action" by national leaders, policy makers, and the broader scientific establishment to develop new and evidence-informed care for those at the end of life. As a result, numerous research funding opportunities were created by both the public and the private sectors to build a stronger research base in end-of-life science (NINR, 2013). In 1997, the National Institute of Nursing Research (NINR, 2015) at the National Institutes of Health (NIH) held the first federally cosponsored workshop on symptoms of terminal illness, in an effort to bring together leading experts in the field to evaluate the breadth of current research and to define the scope of future scientific inquiry. The workshop laid the foundation for a standing program in end-of-life science at NIH and NINR's designation by the director of the NIH to serve as the lead institute on research in end-of-life care. NINR followed with a program announcement soliciting research on the *Management of Symptoms at the End of Life* and in 1999, a second request for applications targeted continued development of evidence in end-of-life care. These NINR efforts were the basis for subsequent directed funding by NIH and other federal agencies to define the scientific focus for end-of-life care and to identify areas for future research investment and health care policy development. NINR, along with the Office of Medical Applications of Research (OMAR), sponsored the *NIH State-of-the-Science Conference, Improving*

End-of-Life Care (Grady, 2005), which resulted in consensus of priorities for building research networks, funding research training and career development, and collaboration across interinstitute, interagency, and public–private programs (Grady, 2005; Lorenz et al., 2006).

Other U.S. Department of Health and Human Services (HHS) agencies responded to the *State-of-the-Science* recommendations with a number of initiatives focused on increasing research translation and informing the public. The Agency for Healthcare Research and Quality (AHRQ) developed several evidence-based reports, including a critical analysis of the existing literature's impact on quality improvement strategies for transforming health care quality (Dy et al., 2012). The National Center for Health Statistics (NCHS) actively engaged in the development of critical data briefs (Bercovitz, Sengupta, Jones, & Harris-Kojetin, 2011) and the HHS Office of the Assistant Secretary for Planning and Evaluation (ASPE) produced a *Report to Congress on Advance Directives and Advance Care Planning* that emphasized a national need for continued attention to these issues (U.S. Department of HHS, 2008).

The accumulating data became part of federal policy language. For example, research data were important in shaping several bipartisan efforts in the U.S. Congress pertaining to legislation to promote research, professional training, and public awareness around palliative and end-of-life care (e.g., the Personalize Your Care Act of 2013, H.R. 1173; the Care Planning Act of 2015, S. 1549). Bills included language on advance care planning (e.g., the *Physician Orders for Life-Sustaining Treatment* [POLST]) whose relevance to health care was based on research evidence (Hickman, Keevern, & Hammes, 2015). Support for provider–patient advance care planning discussions, through tools such as the POLST paradigm, became part of proposed legislation to reduce health care costs through Medicare reimbursement under the Patient Protection and Affordable Care Act (ACA, 2010) which, when first introduced, resulted in significant public and political debate over the influence of so-called "death panels" on decisions to avoid medical care. Though first defeated as part of the introduction of the ACA legislation, the issue was revisited and in 2015, the Centers for Medicare and Medicaid Services (CMS) released final payment rules for advance care planning reimbursement—an effort that rose out of a wide range of stakeholder support, professional input, research evidence, and bipartisan congressional recommendations (CMS, 2015).

Other new legislative efforts were shaped by a growing awareness of new data focused on individual and family caregiver education and support, professional training, workforce development, payment reform, and the need to increase palliative and end-of-life care research. The Advance Planning and Compassionate Care Act (S. 1150, H.R. 2911) and the Critical Care Assessment and Improvement Act (H.R. 2651) called for an NIH central coordinating entity for end-of-life and palliative care research—an initiative that NINR had independently and proactively pursued in 2013 through the establishment of the NINR Office of End-of-Life and Palliative Care Research (OEPCR), whose mandate includes the support of research to inform health policy. The importance of research in shaping health policy reached full circle in the 2014 IOM report, *Dying in America: Improving Quality and Honoring Individual Preferences Near the End of Life*, which noted the progress of the research community to build a substantial body of evidence to support broad improvements to end-of-life care. At a subsequent NINR-hosted briefing of the IOM Committee at the NIH in 2015, members of the IOM Report Committee reemphasized the continued need for such research development and for science to further advance evidence-based models of seamless, high-quality, integrated, and culturally appropriate palliative and end-of-life care.

These examples provide a broad overview of the important influence that the palliative and end-of-life research institution has played in building an infrastructure that continues to generate science that informs health policy. Since the early SUPPORT trial, the efforts of the research community have resulted in numerous publications and initiatives that have exemplified the important underpinning of "best" evidence to ensure that quality care is a priority for advanced illness. The significance of end-of-life and palliative care science—from building strong integrative research programs that provide the evidentiary impetus for change to the dissemination of results into meaningful health care policies and practices—remains unparalleled in its capacity to demonstrate the necessity for high-quality end-of-life care. Today, there is a new and evolving landscape associated with recent health care reform (Kamal et al., 2015). Palliative care has grown rapidly in the United States (Meier, Casarett, von Gunten, Smith, & Porter Storey, 2010) and is now recognized as a subspecialty certification in both nursing (Hospice and Palliative Credentialing Center, 2016) and medicine (American Board of Medical Specialties, 2016). Leaders in the field have created the National Consensus Project for Quality Palliative Care (2013) as a process to define quality care, and the National Quality Forum (NQF, 2006) has been created to generate preferred practice frameworks for providers. End of life is now a consistent contemporary issue in the popular press, such as *Being Mortal: Medicine and What Matters in the End* (Gawande, 2014), and the social media continue to inundate the public with informative and compelling information from numerous studies that draw attention to end-of-life care.

In summarizing both the past and the present progress on building science not only to improve the care of those approaching death, but also to create an impetus for change, it is clear that research remains a key proponent in shaping health care policy, and that nursing science continues to play a critical role in advancing this agenda. Going forward, it is an important time for science in end-of-life and palliative care and a "new era" for research as a critical component in shaping future policy. An important task for forthcoming health policy will be to continue to substantiate needs and solutions through an evolving and pragmatic evidence base (Taylor, Bhavsar, Harker, & Kassner, 2015) and to reframe scientific thinking to encompass a cognizance of how decision makers look to research results to improve the processes of policy making (Prewitt et al., 2012). The next section describes how science, and in particular nursing science, can be shaped to influence health policy decisions and how researchers should conceptualize their science to support tangible changes in palliative and end of-life care.

BRIDGING THE GAP

For those in end-of-life and palliative care science, the nature of the topic area and its highly political and public profile require adeptness at bridging the gap between scientific information and policy implementation. The processes that connect this gap, however, may not be linear. Science can both influence and be influenced by politics and policy and in many ways have different purposes:

> Scientific knowledge often raises more questions than it answers. Policy formation, on the other hand, is inherently inductive and aimed at concrete solutions. This difference in purposes often leaves policymakers frustrated with the inability of science to provide clear answers to political questions. (Neal, Smith, & McCormick, 2008, p. 13)

Thus, bridging the gap between science and policy is a responsibility of the research community that produces the data and those who use it (AcademyHealth, 2015a).

Historically, health policy in end-of-life care emerged from a number of sources, including research, clinical practice, the community, and changing political influences and high-profile issues. Today, ever-changing political contexts require scientists to continuously consider how research may be formulated to play a role in health policy discussions and how research may be interpreted and used by various political or social entities (World Health Organization, 2007). At the onset of research formulation, investigators must consider how their science may contribute to policy processes such as problem identification, formulation of new strategies or new options for health care, the creation of new standards for care, or opportunities for program evaluation (Norse & Tschirley, 2000). A number of policy reviews specific to palliative and end-of-life care highlight how scientific data can be formulated to play an important role in bridging policy concerns such as advance care planning, metrics, outcomes, payment reform, workforce, and training issues (e.g., Morhaim & Pollack, 2013; Reb, 2003; Tilden & Thompson, 2009; Wiener & Tilly, 2003). Professional organizations such as the American Nurses Association (2016), the Hospice and Palliative Nursing Association (2016), and the Oncology Nursing Society (2014), among others, provide position statements, policy briefs, and advocacy resources on a number of advanced care concerns. These associations feature profiles of political candidates or pending legislation that can inform nurse scientists about the viewpoints of those within policy circles and activities in policy development or implementation. Other resources that help connect science to policy include the Center to Advance Palliative Care (CAPC), leading health policy journals (e.g., *Health Affairs*) or popular blogs (e.g., *GeriPal* or *PalliMed*), all of which routinely discuss palliative care matters that help one form perspectives on how policy pundits view evidence gaps or social issues. In addition, attendance at national conferences often features regulatory or advocacy updates on palliative or hospice care—and the proceedings and the press releases from these events often are informational resources for policy makers (e.g., the *National Hospice & Palliative Care Organization Public Policy Committee Legislative Agendas for Congress*). Emerging nurse scientists can also obtain policy training through various academic programs or private foundations (e.g., the Robert Wood Johnson Foundation). These, and other opportunities, allow scientific engagement by the research community on health care issues that are impacting palliative and hospice care (IOM, 2011), and help to create an awareness in the research community of processes to consider in designing research that has the potential to shape future health policy. These include issue framing, agenda setting, and context messaging which are described in the following sections.

Issue Framing

The eventual fate of a policy proposal is also a function of how it is formulated in the first place—how it defines the problems to be attacked and what it offers in the way of policy solutions. (Porter, 1995, p. 15)

The way an issue may be shaped or "framed" will influence the solutions that may be proposed. For end-of-life and palliative care scientists, understanding the framing of a research topic is a necessary step in creating evidence to inform health policy. In their *Health Policy Checklist* (Wiener & Johns Hopkins University, 2005), a critical first step is to consider how to clearly define the policy implications of a research topic by addressing the scope and magnitude of the issue. For example: What is the problem or need? Who is affected? What is the impact of the problem if a solution is or is not achieved? Thinking through a topic from a policy perspective challenges researchers to focus beyond whether their research was used in a policy to instead examine *how* it was used in shaping the policy (Lavis, Ross, McLeod, & Gildiner, 2003, p. 165).

In issue framing, researchers are aware that different policy stakeholders may perceive the same issue and its solutions from different perspectives. Evidence may serve to inform policy rather than create or change it; as Lombrozo (2016) noted, "Science can (and should) inform most policy decisions, but science, on its own, won't settle policy." Scientists should, when applicable, consider the political, social, and economic contexts in which policy makers might connect with and use evidence. The Pew–MacArthur Results Initiative (2014, p. 2) described the process of issue framing as using the best available research and information to highlight gaps, identify what works, and create a framework that allows for informed choices, better outcomes, and accountability of results. Policy makers may look at evidence as a way to identify if a program is working, if the benefits of solutions outweigh the costs, and how information addresses the impact of one particular program compared to an alternate solution (p. 8). AcademyHealth has also created a series of "evidence road maps" intended to help policy analysts and research users better understand whether a perceived research gap represents an actual lack of evidence or a failure of existing evidence to reach the policy arena (AcademyHealth, 2015b). One such road map report focuses on research related to Medicare's role in providing and paying for services during the last part of beneficiaries' lives, including the Medicare hospice benefit (AcademyHealth, 2015b). Another helpful resource for issue framing is the Coalition to Transform Advanced Care (C-TAC) *Policy Review*, which provides information to help policy makers understand gaps in advanced care delivery (Sabatino & Schoeberl, 2015). Other organizations, such as RAND Health, have produced white papers on end-of-life care that synthesize research evidence to frame health policy issues and needs in areas such as demographic and cost components, gaps in the current health care system, reform measures, and adoption of new health care systems (Lynn & Adamson, 2003). The 2015 Pew Charitable Trust initiative, *Improving End-of-Life Care*, focuses on efforts to advance policies to assist individuals in making decisions about treatment preferences, improving the documentation of these preferences, and holding health care providers accountable. Within the publically available documents from this initiative are descriptions of policy needs that intersect with research communities, such as the development of quality metrics and the evaluation and dissemination of promising care delivery models—two areas in which nursing science has contributed and continues to contribute significant research data (see Box 19.1 as an example).

Without an awareness of the political, social, and other contexts that may influence how research is interpreted and used, research may not fit the needs of the policy community. The Health Policy Checklist (Wiener & Johns Hopkins University, 2005) provides several helpful considerations to make the science–policy connection work. First, policy analysts look for clear and understandable descriptions of background literature, any existing or new data that support the scope of a policy or social problem, its relevance to a target population, and clear, substantiated research that is topical and clearly addresses a policy need (Hawkins & Parkhurst, 2015). Second, analysts may look for best practices or benchmarks within the research literature, particularly if the best practices involve stakeholder interests (Wiener & Johns Hopkins University, 2005). Policy choices may then occur due to a number of reasons: political considerations, value preferences, the accuracy and persuasiveness of the research analysis, data reliability, the level of certainty on the causal inferences

---

BOX 19.1   *Framing Research Gaps to Impact Policy*

The National Institute of Nursing Research (NINR) Office of End-of-Life and Palliative Care Research (now OEPCR) facilitated the development of an informational resource that highlighted many past and ongoing contributions of science and provided a framework for understanding gap areas and needs that were useful in several policy discussions, such as the 2014 Institute of Medicine report, *Dying in America*. The NINR initiative, *Building Momentum: The Science of End-of-Life and Palliative Care: A Review of Research Trends and Funding, 1997–2010*, was framed to present useful data and information to public (and policy) stakeholders detailing the nature and extent of published end-of-life and palliative care research—from what diseases and conditions were being studied, what populations, and what settings. A link from data to policy issues was created by providing information on federal research awards and the public and private stakeholders who fund this science. On a policy level, the report provided examples as to how the research establishment has demonstrated leadership in bringing stakeholders together for workshops, symposia, and conferences that have created consensus on current knowledge and future research needs. Many of the recommendations from the report have been incorporated into white papers, federal reports, press releases, and policy pieces (www.ninr.nih.gov/eolspotlight).

linking an intervention to a desired outcome, the potential of evidence to address issues or pending issues, or whether the evidence addresses concerns, social values, or political interests (Prewitt et al., 2012, p. 15). Scientists should thus look at data relevancy through a policy lens: How will the data impact a broader range of constituents? What are the costs and benefits of this change to these entities? What ramifications to a policy would the data create? In framing a topic, researchers should consider many of these policy-relevant issues, using agenda setting as discussed in the next section.

AGENDA SETTING IN POLICY-RELEVANT ISSUES

One reason policy development has failed in the past is because it has been developed without a strong evidence base of strategies and models that have proven to be successful. (Sabatino & Schoeberl, 2015, p. 105)

Agenda setting focuses on actually getting an issue on a formal policy agenda to be addressed by policy makers in an engaged process. To increase uptake of research into policy agendas, one must understand effective policy relationships (Brownson & Jones, 2009, p. 313). Often a policy agenda exists within a time-restricted window of opportunity and is poised to quickly address an issue of national importance. The point when scientific information may be of value to policy makers may be brief and unpredictable, and thus the time between evidence translation and policy implementation may not be similar (Clancy, Glied, & Lurie, 2012, p. 342). In early end-of-life health care policies, public sentiment and controversial court rulings drove an awareness of the need for end-of-life evidence to support health care change. But recently, media attention on controversial issues in end-of-life care has been driven by factors and voices that may not include the scientific community but have reached the attention of decision makers because an issue resonates with private interest groups or various policy circles. Nurse scientists face challenging topics such as palliative sedation, withdrawal of life-sustaining treatments, aggressive end-of-life care, or physician-assisted suicide (e.g., the case of Brittany Maynard; Brittany Maynard Fund, 2016). In many instances, researchers find that the process of policy development in end-of-life care exists in evolutionary contexts much different than more familiar processes of research (Sabatino & Schoeberl, 2015). The timing challenge between science and policy is underscored by national survey data noting that only 14% of research findings in medicine are translated into clinical practice at an average of 17 years before being incorporated into care (Tierney et al., 2007). For research to be useful for policy agendas and the national debate, it has to be timely and accessible. Contemporary palliative and end-of-life care research must thus be formulated with an awareness of important problems in the field, how those problems are being discussed, and the time frames within which new policies might occur (Clancy et al., 2012, p. 343).

The current landscape of end-of-life care requires scientists to recognize that the policy environment is complex, involving multiple individuals, multiple motivations, and a multifaceted interplay between the two. A National Research Council (2012) report on evidence-based policy making noted how a research framework may be formulated to align science in health policy: "Science, when it has something to offer, should be at the policy table. But it shares that table with an array of nonscientific reasons for making a policy choice" (Prewitt et al., 2012, p. 3).

Data from research may be only a part of a larger number of variables that influence policy decisions (Stoker, 2010, p. 53). The evidence is often viewed in terms of relevance to a political issue, resource needs, or acceptability to public need. It is important to reflect on the impact of data on an organization, the time and resources needed to implement change, and the complexity required to make all this happen (IOM, 2014, p. 22). Within interdisciplinary publications of all kinds, scientists can convey the relevance of study results: How will findings create change and impact palliative and end-of-life care? How is this knowledge useful? An advanced agenda for policy development ensures that data is supported across a diverse population and that there are valid methods in which to measure the quality of care throughout the entire advanced illness trajectory. An important effort in this area was the creation of quality and performance metrics for palliative and supportive care (e.g., the *National Consensus Project Clinical Practice Guidelines for Quality Palliative Care* by the National Quality Forum). Box 19.2 provides an example of how relevant research was able to address relevant policy issues of the importance of early, concurrent palliative care.

Engaging in end-of-life care science requires one to take an active role in being current with ever-changing public issues, emerging policy needs, and advocacy interests, and to remain diligent as how evidence may contribute to informing the dialogue. Nimbleness in responding to issues requires being up to date on changing

---

BOX 19.2   *Policy-Relevant Issues. Innovative Models of Care*

Dr. Marie Bakitas is a palliative care nurse scientist whose work has reverberated across evidence-based models of care, advance care planning, and the implementation of interventions based on individual- and family-centered goals and preferences for care. Bakitas has spearheaded initiatives in pain and symptom management through quality improvement, research, and policy change projects. Through her membership in the Oncology Nursing Society, she made significant and sustained contributions to advancing innovations in pain relief, beginning in 1991 as a participant in the "Pain State of the Science" conference that in part stimulated the Joint Commission to adopt pain as the "Fifth Vital Sign." In the late 1990s, the Robert Wood Johnson Foundation funded demonstration projects to test approaches to improve end-of-life care, including ENABLE (Educate, Nurture, Advise, Before Life Ends), the first nurse-led early concurrent palliative care model for rural persons with newly diagnosed advanced cancer and their caregivers. Bakitas demonstrated the effectiveness of ENABLE in improving quality of life, mood, and survival for patients with advanced cancer, and by doing this, reduced burden in their family caregivers. Today, she is building the policy relevance of this trial by implementing the ENABLE model in the rural Deep South to reduce disparities in access to palliative care for minority, underserved, and veteran populations.

Source: Bakitas et al. (2015).

public and policy needs and continuously reviewing information related to gaps, barriers, or emerging issues that will impact end-of-life and palliative practice. In end-of-life science, there is a cautionary and historical challenge concerning how data may be used or misused in highly public, controversial issues about end of life. In discussing the relevance of science in creation of a policy agenda, researchers can assist in policy formulation by providing concise discussions of the pros and cons of their current research and its gaps (Norse & Tschirley, 2000). Many palliative care conferences and symposia offer opportunities for researchers and policy makers to discuss agendas through sharing knowledge, identifying gaps, and advising on important research findings. The National Hospice and Palliative Care Organization/Hospice Action Network regularly hosts a policy symposium to bring together policy makers, thought leaders, and experts to engage in in-depth discussions of issues important to hospice and palliative care. The American Society of Clinical Oncology's Government Relations Committee establishes and shares policy priorities on an annual basis. The Coalition for Compassionate Care holds various state meetings focused on best practices and policy, and C-TAC hosts summits that congregate national leaders from policy, practice, research, and the public to address issues of significance in advanced illness. These, and many other opportunities, can assist researchers to become informed of health-policy-relevant issues that may become policy agendas.

MESSAGING: CREATING SHARED DIALOGUE

Content may be king, but context is the king's prime minister. Content increasingly needs to be considered through a lens of context, framed and associated with relation to the issues of the day by effective messengers. (AcademyHealth, 2015a, p. 9)

The 2009 "Death Panel" debate served as a learning opportunity in how to communicate the impact of science in ways that are meaningful to the public and policy needs (Taylor et al., 2015, p. 9). Dissemination of research findings in a policy-literate manner is not a simple task, due in part to the fact that palliative care is not well understood. The CAPC conducted a public opinion poll, which identified that only 3% of the respondents indicated they were "knowledgeable" about palliative care. After considering evidence from the point of its relevancy, data must then be shared across a cadre of stakeholders, including the public, health professionals, health care organizations, consumers, and policy makers (Pearson, Jordan, & Munn, 2012). And although "[t]he right messenger is critical to dissemination," the "right messenger is not always the researcher or research organization that produced the study" (AcademyHealth, 2015a, p. 3). Thus, researchers need to consider how to articulate data from findings that will infuse a greater understanding surrounding the meaning and the value of palliative care (see Box 19.3 as an example). New texts (e.g., Wittenberg et al., 2015) provide guidance on contemporary ways to communicate

---

BOX 19.3   *Messaging: Creating a Shared Dialogue*

While many researchers, policy makers, and patient advocates cite the numerous benefits of hospice care in providing appropriate end-of-life care to Medicare patients, questions have been raised about the growth in for-profit hospice agencies and differences in the average care needs of the patients they serve compared with those served by nonprofit agencies. The NINR-supported researcher Dr. Melissa Aldridge (Carlson) described the implications of expanding eligibility for the Medicare hospice benefit for the structure and delivery of hospice and palliative care and the costs to the Medicare program. Her research led to the first cross-sectional study of hospice utilization and underscored the complexity of the hospice population and the resource requirements of serving patients with higher comorbidity burden (Aldridge et al., 2014). Publication of these data generated widespread commentaries in the media and critical citations in Centers for Medicare and Medicaid Services reviews of the hospice benefit (Hunt et al., 2014).

---

skillful messages that reflect cultural communication, sensitivity to barriers, and approaches to discussing palliative care with specific patient populations, and best messaging in research data on pain, life support, advance care planning, and quality of life. The AHRQ Health Literacy and Palliative Care Workshop at the Institute of Medicine provides examples of challenges and solutions in health literacy. The National Cancer Institute's *Making Data Talk: A Workbook* (2011) offers key information, practical suggestions, and examples on how to effectively communicate health-related scientific data to the public, policy makers, and the media. Suggestions include use of "plain language" writing styles in sharing research and creating compelling narratives, blog discussions, or infographics of descriptive and quantitative statistics as tools to simplify often complex data.

While there is a need for both public education and engagement, there is a distinction between the two (Meghani & Hinds, 2015, p. S7). A fundamental process of policy development is to identify and debate issues, exchange perspectives, find common ground, and reach consensus. Researchers can actively engage in this dialogue by using a range of media to disseminate important research messages that can add to an informed debate and information sharing. This may mean publishing outside of discipline-specific journals and participating in social media blogs, Twitter "chats," or presenting at professional conferences about the important policy implications of one's work. Well-constructed "sound bites" of new findings will help disseminate and engage conversations on key issues (Meghani & Hinds, 2015), and researchers can actively participate in systematic reviews of research findings to help shape important messages that can easily be understood and assimilated by different audiences (Grimshaw, Eccles, Lavis, Hill, & Squires, 2012, p. 1). Position papers by the various professional organizations can be used to construct critical language that may speak to issues of interest to decision makers. For example, AARP (2016) provides a policy booklet that describes in plain language several key policy areas, including the need for continued research support by policy makers and the importance of growing the evidence base of information to improve the quality of end-of-life care. These and other resources are important to ensure that researchers become active in translating the meaning and implications of their findings to the public and to policy makers (Collins & Coates, 2000, p. 1390).

CONCLUSION

Science is essential to develop the evidence base for enhancement of clinical care delivery and distinguishing the spectrum of challenges in advanced illness care. As the field moves forward, it will be important to determine what level of evidence is "good enough" to clarify new issues, support emerging policy agendas, and increase the leverage of evidence to shape meaningful changes to end-of-life care (Taylor et al., 2015). The research community will need to give thought to what information will be useful to policy communities in emerging topical areas such as quality standards, metrics, and outcomes (C-TAC, 2013; Pew Charitable Trusts, 2014). Those formulating new health policies will need to look to the strength of the evidence to support new models of comprehensive and integrated palliative care that are responsive to a shortage of skilled palliative care providers and refined reimbursement policies. Much still must be done to determine if new and emerging policies related to end-of-life and palliative care truly demonstrate an impact on the quality, access, and provision of care to all individuals and their families (Goodridge, 2010). Data will be needed to substantiate processes that will incentivize engagement in conversations about advance care planning based on goals, values, and preferences. Nurse scientists will need to ensure that the data are representative of diverse populations, health care settings, age groups, and changing national demographics. An ongoing dialogue about critical policy and research issues will remain part of efforts to continue to accelerate and to sustain current progress in advanced illness care (IOM, 2014) and, for nursing science, to develop the kinds of evidence that are meaningful to clinical practice, public health, and policy needs. Looking to the future of shaping policies through nursing research, Kamal et al. (2015, p. 243) provide a conceptual challenge for future end-of-life and palliative care research communities to think of scientific contributions to health policy as not "here is what we do," but rather, "this is how well we do it" and "let's see how we can do it better." It is incumbent on nursing science in end-of-life and palliative care to lead these efforts.

REFERENCES

AARP Office of Policy Integration. (2016). *Priorities book: Building a better future 2015–2016.* Retrieved from http://www.aarp.org/policybook

AcademyHealth. (2015a). *Moving health services research into policy and practice: Lessons from inside and outside the health sector* (Report from an AcademyHealth Workshop, April 28–29, 2014). Washington, DC: Author.

AcademyHealth. (2015b). *Evidence roadmap: End-of-life care and Medicare's hospice benefit.* Washington, DC: Author.

Advance Planning and Compassionate Care Act of 2014. S.3009, 113th Congress.

Aldridge, M. S., Schlesinger, M., Barry, C. L., Morrison, R. S., McCorkle, R., Huzeler, R., & Bradley, E. H. (2014). National Hospice Survey results: For-profit status, community engagement, and service. *JAMA Internal Medicine, 174*(4), 500–506.

American Board of Medical Specialties Certification. (2016). Certification for hospice and palliative medicine specialists. Retrieved from http://aahpm.org/career/certification

American Nurses Association. (2016). *Position statement: Registered nurses' roles and responsibilities in providing expert care and counseling at the end of life.* Retrieved from http://www.nursing world.org

Bakitas, M. A., Tosteson, T. D., Li, Z., Lyons, K. D., Hull, J. G., Li, Z., . . . Ahles, T. A. (2015). Early versus delayed initiation of concurrent palliative oncology care: Patient outcomes in the ENABLE III randomized controlled trial. *Journal of Clinical Oncology, 33*(13), 1438–1445.

Bercovitz, A., Sengupta, M., Jones, A., & Harris-Kojetin, L. D. (2011). Complementary and alternative therapies in hospice: The National Home and Hospice Care Survey: United States, 2007. *National Health Statistics Report, 33*(1), 1–20.

Brittany Maynard Fund. (2016). Retrieved from http://thebrittanyfund.org

Brownson, R. C., & Jones, E. (2009). Bridging the gap: Translating research into policy and practice. *Preventive Medicine, 49*, 313–315.

Care Planning Act of 2015. (2015–2016). S.1549, 114th Congress.

Centers for Medicare and Medicaid Services. (2015, July 8). 42 C.F.R. pts. 405, 410, 411, 414, 425, 495. Retrieved from https://s3.amazonaws.com/public-inspection.federalregister.gov/2015 -16875.pdf

Clancy, C. M., Glied, S. A., & Lurie, N. (2012). From research to health policy impact. *HSR: Health Services Research, 47*(1), 337–343.

Coalition to Transform Advanced Care. (2013). Advanced illness policy review: The landscape for improving advanced illness care in America. Retrieved from http://www.thectac.org/ wp-content/uploads/2015/04/Advanced-Illness-Policy-Review-Landscape-for-Improving -Advanced-Illness-Care-in-America.pdf

Collins, C., & Coates, T. J. (2000). Science and health policy: Can they cohabit or should they divorce? *American Journal of Public Health, 90*(9), 1389–1390.

Critical Care Assessment and Improvement Act. (20132014). H. R. 2651, 113th Cong.

DuBois, J. C., & Reed, P. G. (2014). The nurse practitioner and policy in end-of-life care. *Nursing Science Quarterly, 27*(1), 70–76.

Dy, S. M., Aslakson, R., Wilson R. F., Fawole, O. A., Lau, B. D., Martinez, K. A., . . . Bass, E. B. (2012). *Improving health care and palliative care for advanced and serious illness. Closing the quality gap: Revisiting the state of the science* (Evidence Report No. 208). Rockville, MD: Agency for Healthcare Research and Quality.

Field, M. J., & Behrman, R. E. (Eds.), for Institute of Medicine Committee on Palliative and End-of-Life Care for Children and Their Families. (2002). *When children die.* Washington, DC: National Academies Press.

Field, M. J., & Cassel, C. K. (Eds.). (1997). *Approaching death: Improving care at the end of life.* Washington, DC: National Academies Press.

Gawande, A. (2014). *Being mortal: Medicine and what matters in the end.* New York, NY: Henry Holt.

Goodridge, D. (2010). End of life care policies: Do they make a difference in practice? *Social Science and Medicine, 70*, 1166–1170.

Grady, P. A. (2005). Introduction: Papers from the National Institutes of Health state-of-the-science conference on improving end-of-life care. *Journal of Palliative Medicine, 8*, (Supp. 1), S1–S3.

Grady, P. A., & Hinshaw, A. S. (Eds). (2011). *Shaping health policy through nursing research.* New York, NY: Springer Publishing.

Grimshaw, J. M., Eccles, M. P., Lavis, J. N., Hill, S. J., & Squires, J. E. (2012). Knowledge translation of research findings. *Implementation Science, 7*(50), 1–17.

Hawkins, B., & Parkhurst, J. (2015). The "good governance" of evidence in health policy. *Evidence and Policy*, 1–18.

Hickman, S. E., Keevern, E., & Hammes, B. J. (2015). Use of Physician Orders for Life-Sustaining Treatment (POLST) in the clinical setting: A systematic review of the literature. *Journal of the American Geriatrics Society, 63*(2), 341–350.

Hospice & Palliative Nurses Association. (2016). Joint position statements. Retrieved from http://www.advancingexpertcaer.org/educaiton/positoin-statements

Hospice and Palliative Credentialing Center. (2016). Retrieved from http://hpcc.advancing expertcare.org

Hunt, M., Rezaee, M. E., Luallen, J., Pozniak, A., Gerteis, J., Edwards, A., . . . Plotzke, M. (2014). *Medicare Hospice Payment Reform: A review of the literature* (HHSM-500-2005-00191, May 1, 2014). *Medicare and Medicaid Research Review, 4*(2).

Institute of Medicine. (2011). *The future of nursing: Leading change, advancing health.* Washington, DC: National Academies Press.

Institute of Medicine. (2014). *Dying in America: Improving quality and honoring individual preferences near the end of life.* Washington, DC: National Academies Press.

Kamal, A. H., Hanson, L. C., Casarett, D. J., Dy, S. M., Pantilat, S. Z., Lupu, D., & Abernethy, A. P. (2015). The quality imperative for palliative care. *Journal of Pain and Symptom Management, 49*(2), 243–253.

Lavis, J., Ross, S., McLeod, C., & Gildiner, A. (2003). Measuring the impact of health research. *Journal of Health Services Research & Policy, 8*(3), 165–170.

Lombrozo, T. (2016, January 25). Science can quantify risks, but it can't settle policy. National Public Radio (NPR Blog). Retrieved from http://www.npr.org

Lorenz, K. A., Shugarman, L. R., & Lynn, J. A. (2006). Health care policy issues in end-of-life care. *Journal of Palliative Medicine, 9*(3), 731–749.

Lynn, J., & Adamson, D. M. (2003). *Living well at the end of life: Adapting health care to serious chronic illness in old age.* Santa Monica, CA: RAND.

Meghani, S. H., & Hinds, P. S. (2015). Policy brief: The Institute of Medicine report *Dying in America*: Improving quality and honoring individual preferences near the end of life. *Nursing Outlook, 63*, 51–59.

Meier, D. E., Casarett, D. J., von Gunten, C. F., Smith, W. J., & Porter Storey, Jr., C. (2010). Palliative medicine: Politics and policy. *Journal of Palliative Medicine, 13*(2), 1–6.

Morhaim, D. K., & Pollack, K. M. (2013). End-of-life care issues: A personal, economic, public policy, and public health crisis. *American Journal of Public Health, 103*(6), e8–e10.

National Cancer Institute. (2011). Making data talk: A workbook. Retrieved from https://www.cancer.gov/publications/health-communication/making-data-talk.pdf

National Consensus Project for Quality Palliative Care. (2013). *Clinical practice guidelines for quality palliative care* (3rd ed.). Pittsburgh, PA: National Consensus Project.

National Institute of Nursing Research. (2013). *Building momentum: The science of end-of-life and palliative care. A review of research trends and funding, 1997–2010.* Bethesda, MD: Author.

National Institute of Nursing Research. (2015). Special briefing on IOM report—*Dying in America*. Retrieved from http://www.ninr.nih.gov

National Quality Forum. (2006). A national framework and preferred practices for palliative and hospice care quality. Retrieved from http://www.qualityforum.org

Neal, H. A., Smith, T., & McCormick, J. (2008). *Beyond Sputnik: U.S. science policy in the twenty-first century.* Ann Arbor: University of Michigan Press.

Norse, D., & Tschirley, J. B. (2000). Links between science and policy making. *Agriculture Ecosystems & Environment, 82*, 15–26.

Oncology Nursing Society. (2014). Palliative care for people with cancer. Retrieved from https://www.ons.org/advocacy-policy/positions/practice/palliative-care

Paice, J. A., Ferrell, B. R., Virani, R., Grant, M., Malloy, P., & Rhome, A. (2006). Appraisal of the graduate end-of-life nursing education consortium training program. *Journal of Palliative Medicine, 9*(2), 353–360.

Patient Protection and Affordable Care Act. Pub. L. No. 111-148, Sec. 3026. (2010).

Pearson, A., Jordan, Z., & Munn, Z. (2012). Translational science and evidence-based healthcare: A clarification and reconceptualization of how knowledge is generated and used in healthcare. *Nursing Research and Practice, 12*, 1–6.

Personalize Your Care Act of 2013. H.R. 1173, 113th Cong.

Pew Charitable Trusts. (2014). Evidence-based policymaking. A guide for effective government. Retrieved from http://www.pewtrusts.org/en/research-and-analysis/reports/2014/11/evidence-based-policymaking-a-guide-for-effective-government

Pew Charitable Trusts. (2015). *Improving end-of-life care.* Washington, DC: Author. Retrieved from http://www.pewtrusts.org/en/projects/improving-end-of-life-care

Pew–MacArthur Results Initiative. (2014). Retrieved from http://www.pewtrusts.org/en/research-and-analysis/fact-sheets/2015/07/the-pew-macarthur-results-first-initiative

Porter, R W. (1995). *Knowledge utilization and the process of policy formation: Toward a framework for Africa.* Washington, DC: Academy for Educational Development.

Prewitt, K., Schwandt, T. A., & Straf, M. L. (Eds.), for the National Research Council Division of Behavioral and Social Sciences and Education. (2012). *Using science as evidence in public policy: Committee on use of social science knowledge in public policy.* Washington, DC: National Academies Press.

Reb, A. M. (2003). Palliative and end-of-life care: Policy analysis. *Oncology Nursing Forum, 30*(1), 35–50.

Sabatino, C., & Schoeberl, M. (2015). The role of policy and advocacy. In B. Novelli, T. Koutsoumpas, & B. Workman (Eds.). *A roadmap for success. Transforming advanced illness care in America.* Washington, DC: American Hospital Association and AARP.

Stoker, G. (2010). Translating experiments into policy. *Annals of the American Academy of Political and Social Science, 628*(1), 47–58.

Taylor, D., Bhavsar, N., Harker, M., & Kassner, C. (2015). Evaluating a new era in Medicare hospice and end-of-life policy. Retrieved from http://healthaffairs.org/blog/2015/12/22s

Tierney, W. M., Oppenheimer, C. C., Hudson, B. L., Benz, J., Finn, A., Hickner, J. M., . . . Gaylin, D. S. (2007). A national survey of primary care practice-based research networks. *Annals of Family Medicine, 5*(3), 242–250.

Tilden, V. P., & Thompson, S. (2009). Policy issues in end-of-life care. *Journal of Professional Nursing, 25*, 363–368.

U.S. Department of Health and Human Services, Office of the Assistant Secretary for Planning and Evaluation. (2008). *Advance directives and advance care planning: Report to Congress.* Washington, DC: Author. Retrieved from http://aspe.hhs.gov/_/office_specific/daltcp.cfm

van den Hove, S. (2007). A rationale for science-policy interfaces. *Futures, 39*(7), 807–826.

Wiener, J., & The Johns Hopkins University. (2005). *Health policy analysis checklist* (Johns Hopkins Bloomberg School of Public Health). Retrieved from http://ocw.jhsph.edu/courses/Intro HealthPolicy/PDFs/Bardach_Outline_IHP_7b.pdf

Wiener, J. M., & Tilly, J. (2003). End-of-life care in the United States: Policy issues and model programs of integrated care. *International Journal of Integrated Care, 3*(7), 1568–4156.

Wittenberg, E., Ferrell, B., Goldsmith, J., Smith, T., Glajchen, M., Handzo, G., & Ragan, S. L. (Eds.). (2015). *Textbook of palliative care communication.* Oxford, UK: Oxford University Press.

World Health Organization. (2007). *People-centered health care: A policy framework.* Geneva, Switzerland: WHO Press.

The Writing Group for the SUPPORT Investigators. (1995). A controlled trial to improve care for seriously ill hospitalized patients: The Study to Understand Prognoses and Preferences for Outcomes and Risks of Treatments (SUPPORT). *JAMA, 274*, 1591–1598.

20

Expanding Health Care Policy: The Ties That Bind

Ada Sue Hinshaw and Patricia A. Grady

This book explores the process of using nursing research to shape health policy. There is no single best approach to accomplish this, but there are a number of ties that bind research to health policy. Some of these are actual, some are implied, and others have the potential to be realized in the future. This text focuses on all three of these in the overview, the contexts that are provided, and the examples that are given. In this chapter, several areas are highlighted: the concepts used by the researchers, innovative clinical patterns that have emerged, lessons learned from the illustrative examples provided in the chapters, and finally the policy directives shaped by the examples provided.

INNOVATIVE CLINICAL PATTERNS

The first section of this text deals with innovative clinical patterns that are influencing nursing science and health policy, including expanding areas of clinical and basic science, team science, data science, and implementation science.

Expanding Areas of Clinical and Basic Science

Over time, there has been a shift in the type of research nurse scientists are engaging in, although the focus remains primarily clinical. As pointed out by Cashion and Austin, nurses are incorporating more biological measures and themes into their research. With the expansion of genetics into genomics and the surge of other areas of "omics," additional knowledge is required to conduct cutting-edge research that will improve patient care. Symptom science, the core of nursing, has evolved over time. Still focusing on the patient, it now incorporates the explosion of new information, adapting it in ways that support the nursing research agenda. A good example of this approach is the National Institutes of Health Symptom Science Model (NIH-SSM; Cashion & Grady, 2015). This model integrates biological, psychological, and sociological components. It identifies a symptom, develops the related phenotype, and uses omics methodologies to identify biomarkers that will lead to development of clinical interventions for individuals. A good example of the clinical and basic science interface, examined by Williams in Chapter 4, is the work of Starkweather et al. (2016) in phenotyping and management of low back pain. This study was designed in a manner that would facilitate translation into policy.

This confluence of clinical and basic science that is emerging is particularly relevant to nursing science, as nurses have a strong clinical focus and are better able to recognize appropriate opportunities and tie them to the basic science knowledge in ways that may be more challenging for other disciplines.

Team Science

Team science, once considered a new idea, is now becoming essential as the level of complexity of science continues to grow. There are numerous examples of team science in the chapters contained in this book. Naylor, in Chapter 5, makes the point that team science is necessary because the concept of health itself is very complex. She identifies key points related to team science in the area of health that are necessary for successful knowledge development and translation. She characterizes the successes of the Transitional Care Model (TCM) developed and implemented by her team, and describes activity based on that success. Her chapter also identifies the important contributions that nurses make to interdisciplinary teams: nurses contribute unique knowledge and skills to share with other disciplines, and their collaboration with other disciplines is essential for safe and effective health care; nurse leadership of interdisciplinary teams is associated with improved safety and higher quality outcomes; and nurse team leadership is associated with greater team interdependence, fosters greater respect among members, and positively contributes to organizational culture of interprofessional learning.

Interdisciplinary team approaches are key in most of the examples contained in this text. Team science is most often understood in terms of clinical studies, but due to the growing complexity of science, it is increasingly seen in the basic sciences as well. Dorsey's work is a good example to illustrate this. Although her work is framed in the clinical health problem of neuropathic pain, she is currently carrying out primarily basic science studies. Within that context, to help her carry out those studies, she has created an interdisciplinary team of experts that include geneticists, clinicians, pain experts, and neuroscientists, to name a few.

The expertise of members who constitute an effective team can cover a broad span, as demonstrated by the chapters in this book. Increasingly, patients and community members are becoming a formal part of teams. Hill has shown the important role of the community in achieving successful outcomes working with African American males with hypertension; Hickman, using the Physician Orders for Life-Sustaining Treatment (POLST) tool, has formally incorporated the patient in ways that are essential in facilitating the achievement of their health care preferences toward the end of life; Hinds has developed strategies to include families in a more practical and essential way to improve outcomes for their dying children. Her approach has positive outcomes that span the period of bereavement of surviving parents.

Szanton's work with homebound older adults helps to redefine the potential range of expertise that can constitute a successful team, including handymen, social workers, and occupational therapists. Hickman's team has included the clergy, lawyers, and legislators in order to create and implement the POLST method of incorporating patient care wishes. Rantz has included engineers, architects, university administrators, and city planners on the team she created to develop TigerPlace, Missouri's first Aging in Place site.

Data Science

The area of data science is considered one of the most rapidly expanding areas of science. Clinical nurses and nurse scientists have long been generating enormous amounts of data, through patient histories, health records, and observations. The challenge moving forward is how to collect such large amounts of data in meaningful ways and how best to store, analyze, and share it so that the most can be extracted from all the information that is collected. This is also an area primed for and in need of health policy formation, given the issues related to privacy, data sharing, and resource allocation and utilization. The National Consortium on Data Science has released a relevant white paper covering these issues (Ahalt et al., 2014); the NIH has formulated a Big Data to Knowledge (BD2K) Initiative, which will provide an NIH Data Commons and a toolkit for research (NIH, 2016); and the International Committee of Journal Editors (ICJME) has developed a framework for data sharing to be used by journals (Warren, 2016). It is important that nursing engages in these discussions in order to capture opportunities and to make the significant contributions for which it has the potential.

Bakken makes a very compelling case for the importance of, advantages of, and the necessity of becoming familiar with these new data science approaches, either singly or, more aptly, as part of a team in order to capitalize on the opportunities emerging. She stresses the importance of getting the major nursing organizations involved and helping to underscore the importance of emerging opportunities.

Implementation Science

The importance of implementation of science is underscored by Titler and Shuman in Chapter 3. Despite additional resources developed over the past few decades to help in translating research to policy making and decision making, limited progress has been made. She also points out that despite the availability of evidence-based recommendations for health policy and practice, evidence-based care is delivered only about 70% of the time, according to a 2014 National Healthcare Quality and Disparities

Report (Agency for Healthcare Research and Quality [AHRQ], 2015). Implementation can be facilitated when tied to national programs such as the Centers for Medicare and Medicaid Services (CMS) value-based programs, which reward systems with incentive payments for quality of care; or credentialing bodies such as the Joint Commission for Accreditation of Healthcare Organizations (The Joint Commission), which sets standards of care for accreditation. Titler and Shuman also give examples of how local and state governments can facilitate progress in areas such as childhood obesity by implementing sound nutritional policies for school lunch programs. Barriers to implementation are identified and strategies to overcome them are elucidated as well. Titler underscores the facts that it is difficult to change attitudes and that change does not happen quickly, even in the face of new knowledge. Relationship building and trust are required to get individuals or groups to endorse change, and that trust must be maintained in order for change to be sustained.

FACTORS THAT INFLUENCE CLINICAL PATTERNS AND PROVIDE TIES THAT BIND RESEARCH

In progressing forward, changes are made over a range of parameters. Important factors that influence clinical patterns and provide ties to bind research to policy include: *identified gaps, timing, changes in technology, health disparities, new knowledge and emerging scientific areas,* and *adaptation of existing models and tools*. A number of innovative clinical patterns, as developed and described by senior researchers, are highlighted within the chapters of this text.

The first of these, *identifying gaps*, is an important factor in setting the stage for change. The absence of satisfactory health care options for our older populations is noted by both Rantz and Szanton in Chapters 12 and 13. Each has addressed the issues, while keeping the patient central to the equation. Szanton focused her work on enabling individuals to remain in their homes through adaptation of those environments. Unique to her approach was the idea of creating innovative, nurse-led teams that could help to modify the environment. She included a handyman as well as others who could help to bring a more external environment to modify the one in which her patients were living. Examples included occupational therapists and social workers. Rantz developed a creative approach to extended care at TigerPlace, a facilitated living environment for those who were not able to remain at home. This approach involved the use of wearable and environmentally placed sensors that could serve as activity monitors. Thus, those living at TigerPlace could safely and freely move around, with the sensors noting and reporting any changes in activity patterns that might indicate a need for assistance.

Several examples illustrate the importance of *timing*. Innovative clinical approaches are often required in order to make change, and those changes often lead to changes in policy. However, change can be greatly facilitated or impeded by timing. Readiness of the health care system, health team members, our communities, and legislative groups are all examples of how timing can play a role. Some innovations described were created to make more immediate changes, such as the examples of Rantz, and Szanton, in responding to changing demographic imperatives; or Grey, in her work, addressing the near-epidemic increase of diabetes in teenagers. Other examples set the stage for change, such as the work of Cashion, Williams, and Dorsey in the area of genomics and Finkelstein in the use of technology. It is worth noting that gaps and timing are often closely tied together.

Changes in technology also influence clinical patterns. The ability to use emerging technologies to better deliver care, monitor health or response to therapy, or provide improved access are all potential advantages. As the population ages, but still remains relatively active, new ways of maintaining health become important. Finkelstein and his colleagues have pioneered the use of technology in their telehealth studies as a way of meeting these new and emerging needs for more accessible ways to obtain care and maintain good health. This is a creative way to approach the changing health care landscape and has the added advantage of increasing access to health care for many populations, both rural and urban.

Health disparities continue to plague society. An added advantage of approaches using emerging technologies is that they may help to address the health disparities currently present in our society, by reaching hard-to-reach populations. Other creative clinical approaches highlighted that address health disparities include those of Moser and her team in addressing the needs of rural populations with cardiovascular issues, and the pioneering work of Martha Hill and her team in addressing health disparities in inner-city populations using community-based approaches.

New knowledge in emerging scientific areas is another important tie. One of the unique aspects of nursing research is that nurses engage in both basic and clinical research and thus have a collective expertise with a wide span of influence. This is a particular advantage for using nursing research to shape health policy. Emerging scientific areas addressed in this text include genetics, end-of-life and palliative care, and caregiving for the aging population. The latter two areas, although they have not just emerged, are emerging in new ways and with additional urgency due to the increased numbers and new care circumstances.

An interesting example of the confluence of basic science and clinical expertise is in the area of genomics. The NIH Symptom Science Model, described by Cashion and Austin in Chapter 2, demonstrates this dynamic and provides a unique approach to collect data in a comprehensive fashion, providing the ability to synergize both basic and clinical knowledge acquired.

In terms of clinical models, the approach of addressing symptoms rather than disease has long been a hallmark of nursing and nursing research. Heitkemper's program of research on the symptoms of gastrointestinal distress is a good example. This approach can be a powerful tool in the health policy arena, as it is symptoms that typically get the attention of patients and the general public. Addressing symptoms can be an important catalyst for change related to issues surrounding chronic illness and in circumstances in which self-management is an important driver.

Within the emerging area of end-of-life and palliative care, there are several good examples in this text. The research of Hinds with children experiencing life-limiting illnesses, and their families, is breaking new ground. Her programs are producing an evidence base for clinical care and informing the national conversation at a time when policies are being developed in this important area of health. Hinds's work is novel in the extent to which she is incorporating the family as integral members of the team for children with life-limiting illness. This is a good example of being at the beginning of policy formation or even slightly ahead of the curve, although it is not ahead of national need.

Creative clinical approaches are often developed out of necessity, just as policy is often developed for the same reason. This necessity is usually preceded by changing demographics or circumstances. Gitlin describes this well when she talks about the need for improved models to address caregiver needs. Because the changing demographics of age and medical advances led to shorter hospital stays, caregiving shifted from hospitals and medical centers to home or residences for older adults. Historically, health care systems have been based on acute care paradigms, and the changing structure of families, decreased number of caregivers available, and increased women in the workforce have created a need for patterns of caregiving that differ from the previous norm. Her studies address this need in new and creative ways, and form the basis for policy change.

The forces shaping Gitlin's work differ markedly from those prevailing at the time Riegel began to develop her self-care model in the 1990s, and serve as an interesting example of change over time. Early in her career, Riegel noticed that patients appeared to improve in the hospital, but experienced frequent readmissions following discharge. Her observations and determination to do something to change the situation were met with resistance and what she refers to as a "fill the beds mindset." However, her research showed positive outcomes and led to her development and the acceptance of the self-care model used today.

Clinical *innovation through adaptation of existing models* is demonstrated by several examples in this text. This approach may be met with less resistance, since the change is less extensive and the benefit more obvious. Another example provided in this text is the POLST strategy of Hickman and her team in end-of-life or acute life-limiting illness. Much of the important work in this area has been done by nurses, showing that advance directives (ADs) successfully determine that a patient's wishes are followed more often if an AD is in place, and periods of bereavement are often shortened for survivors. However, an AD is a minimal approach to supportive care, so Hickman and team have developed a more comprehensive approach to supportive care called POLST, which helps the patient and caregiver mutually determine what the patient wishes.

Another example of adaptation of a previously existing model that was successful in adults, but not teens, is the work of Grey. Knowing your audience is important when attempting to make change. One creative innovation exemplifying both of these concepts is shown in Chapter 7 by Grey and Rechenberg, which describes the work of Grey and her team in developing the Coping Skills

Training (CST) model for teens to better manage their diabetes. Teens, even when they know what they should do, do not always do it, and the protocol, as originally developed, placed serious limitations on a teen lifestyle. What the team did was to take the successful model from the Diabetes Complications and Control Trial (DCCT), which worked well in adults, and add a CST module for teens that helped them maintain good blood sugar control while still being allowed to act like teenagers. This is also a good example of adapting a successful model to fit specific circumstances. A further innovation the team added was to scale up the programs and test them using Internet approaches. Finding out which programs lend themselves to this approach, and which do not, helps to set the stage for new approaches in telehealth, or precision telehealth, using the most current terminology. This is an example of a scientist further adapting his or her own successful model to a different set of circumstances, and in doing so, becoming able to reach the target audience effectively.

LESSONS LEARNED

Throughout this text, a number of threads emerge, which when tied together create a tapestry of lessons learned to serve as a guide to shaping health policy. Among these include: *selection of a pressing need or public health issue; timing; barriers; constituency or stakeholders; sustainability; evaluation and refinement; and translation.* The examples in this text demonstrate most, several, or all of these approaches in successfully using nursing research to shape health policy.

Pressing Need or Issue

Major public health problems, disorders affecting large segments of our population, acceleration of a previously dormant issue, or an emerging public health issue all garner more attention and provide a greater potential for active change. Szanton advises to fit your interests in with what society needs. Making change in these areas is generally facilitated by the urgency of the problem and the higher number of invested stakeholders. Any of these factors can lead to a greater demand for action. As our population ages, the issues surrounding end of life are a good example of increasing attention and demand for change. With an emerging public health problem, there are often unexpected opportunities. As the technology in the area of genomics has become more available, genetic screening is increasing. Williams cites an example of a study of the problems experienced by parents while awaiting the results of newborn screening. Results showed that a major hardship was the anxiety created during the extensive waiting period between testing and results; a rapid change in policy was made to considerably shorten the time, thereby creating a rapid improvement for parents. This also led to a better understanding of the importance of genetic counseling.

Timing

Timing is an important factor in successful efforts to shape health policy. Identifying a pressing issue or need can facilitate change because the urgency provides momentum. Altered circumstances may cause an issue to emerge suddenly or over time. Examples are provided in this text in which timing is facilitated, such as with Gitlin's work, where the need for caregiving is increasing due to changes in population demographics of aging and earlier discharge changes in the health care system. Examples are provided in which the push is uphill at first, followed by increasing demand, such as in the research areas of self-management described by Riegel and the efforts in telehealth pioneered by Finkelstein. A recent review highlights the importance of timing for the use of telehealth (E. R. Dorsey & Topol, 2016). Telehealth use is being facilitated now because it is not only providing better access to care, but also convenience and economy; it is expanding from acute care applications to episodic and chronic conditions; and it is migrating from hospitals and satellite clinics to the home and mobile devices.

Other researchers are in the position of being ahead of the curve, and able to anticipate what might be needed. They potentially have the advantage of being able to plan ahead and even be proactive, such as in the areas of genomics as described by Cashion and Austin, Williams, Dorsey, and Miller, Hickman, and Hinds in end of life. In another example, Bakken and colleagues are literally helping to forge an emerging field of data science, not widely discussed even 10 years ago.

Societal issues may often push a policy agenda, so that there is increased receptivity for research to inform emerging policies. Hickman, Hinds, and Miller, working in the area of end of life, provide examples of this. As the societal push for more autonomy during this phase of life grows, there is a demand for information about the best way to deliver care, rules governing patient autonomy, and regulations governing access to facilities over the period of this trajectory.

Windows of opportunity do occur, and should be captured, but they do not always occur at convenient times. Lack of data, incomplete data, and other factors may challenge one's skills to provide timely advice based on best professional judgment informed by available data. Lessons learned from interdisciplinary teams and data science may help to mitigate these challenges.

Barriers

Inevitably, barriers will be present when making change. Barriers to the use of research evidence in health policy, well described by Titler and Shuman in Chapter 3, include beliefs and attitudes, knowledge and skills, relevance, and organizational context. It is important to develop successful strategies to address these barriers in order to promote the use of research for evidence-based policies. Such strategies include capacity building, provision of research findings for use by policy makers, relationship building, and models for knowledge translation to the public and policy makers. The section on how best to provide research information to policy makers clearly addresses this challenge.

In some cases, barriers may not be related to information as much as emotional overtones surrounding an issue. Research involving children, genomics, and end-of-life issues is a good example of this. Miller talks in Chapter 19 about addressing the emotional component and the intellectual component of issues before being able to move forward. These considerations can be seen in the work of both Hinds and Hickman. Framing a context becomes key in such instances to help facilitate understanding and provide a basis for change.

Constituency or Stakeholders

Constituents are those concerned about an issue, and their specific interests around an issue can vary widely. Before moving forward, assessment of who has a vested interest and the nature of that interest is key to success. Constituents can provide history, expertise, context, and even economic resources. They can also provide opposition. Some intriguing partnerships over a wide range of constituencies and participants are described in the chapters within this text.

Community members, health care team members, congressional representatives, professional associations, and legal representatives, as well as a variety of other groups, can constitute one's constituency. It is essential to engage the commitment and imagination of these groups to pave the way for success. An interesting example of creating engagement is that of Rantz and her team when naming their health care facility. Because the facility was developed under the auspices of the University of Missouri, whose mascot is the tiger, using the name TigerPlace immediately provided a sense of investment of the university campus and its associates. Another example of strategic engagement of constituency is that of Hickman. Knowing that end-of-life issues are very sensitive to religious communities, Hickman and her team engaged in discussions with the Indiana Catholic Bishops to help get a passable bill drafted in the Indiana legislature for the use of the POLST instrument in situations of life-limiting illness. Also sensitive to the myriad legal issues, the team started discussions early with the American Bar Association to help with any subsequent legislation.

Sustainability

Planning for sustainability to the extent possible is an important factor. Ideally, the information gained from successful research studies will provide compelling rationale for policy or regulation change, but that is not always the case. Finkelstein and Cady in Chapter 16 provide several examples of successful telehealth interventions that were not sustained due to lack of reimbursement. His chapter also provides a good example of how timing can work favorably. There is now a greater impetus for incorporating telehealth approaches into the health care system, and the persistence in this area appears to be paying off. Incorporating constituents also helps to build sustainability. Naylor involved third-party payers in piloting her transitional care work, thus paving the way for eventual reimbursement and sustainability. Building upon what is already in place or adapting something already in use may be a positive factor. Examples of this include Hickman refining the concept of ADs in developing the POLST and Grey in adding CST to an accepted DCCT protocol.

Evaluation and Refinement

Once changes in policy have been made, it is also important to evaluate whether the changes have been successful and to be sensitive to changes over time. This helps to maintain the relevance of changes made and to maintain currency and sustainability. This is described well by Titler and Shuman in Chapter 3.

Translation

Despite the availability of evidence-based practice recommendations for health policy and practice, evidence-based care is delivered only about 70% of the time, as discussed by Titler. She points out that this demonstrates a gap between availability of evidence-based recommendations and their application to improve population health. Translating research into practice and policy is a necessary step to realize the benefits of new knowledge, and many of the factors that can facilitate that translation are discussed in this text. Communication of new knowledge as widely as possible with specific attention to target audiences and tailoring the message so that it is best received by intended audiences are key ingredients to translation.

Being a member of a professional, civic, or advocacy organization can also help in the quest to implement and affect national policy. Grey, with her expertise as a pediatric nurse practitioner, networked with practitioners and practices across the country to implement her CST program for teens with diabetes.

Incorporating key constituents in the design and implementation of research and policy activities can be helpful in translation, as these individuals have a vested interest in seeing or experiencing the benefit from results. This strategy was described in several chapters in the text. A strategy used by Szanton was that of obtaining funding from the CMS Innovations Laboratory, which was designed to facilitate translation by streamlining reimbursement provision for research studies with successful outcomes.

Context is also an important factor in translation of research to policy. Finkelstein gave several examples of successful outcomes, but at the time was addressing future needs in a system geared to traditional methods. This poses a challenge for adoption of new and innovative ways.

As it may be difficult to translate research to policy change, it is important to note that persistence pays off. As mentioned by many contributors, sometimes with innovation, it is a waiting game. The system may not be ready and has to be primed or updated. In this spirit, it is worth noting that several authors spoke implicitly or explicitly about what fueled the determination that inspired them. It was noted specifically by Riegel, Rantz, and Szanton, in that early clinical experiences inspired them to attack a challenging issue and make change. So, when considering the next generation, it is noteworthy that early experiences often spark an interest that is sustained over time, resulting in the passion to make a difference. Regardless of the special circumstances, it is clear from the examples in this text that perseverance is a key ingredient required to shape health policy.

HEALTH POLICY DIRECTIVES: RECIPROCAL RELATIONSHIP WITH NURSING RESEARCH

A reciprocal relationship between nursing research and health policy is evident in many of the nursing research examples provided by the senior scientists writing for this text. Just as such a relationship is understood with professional practice, the same dynamic, cyclical relationship exists with health policy. Research, as one of the many factors that shapes health policy, is, in turn, influenced by such policy. Three national health policy statements have been examined in terms of their being shaped by nursing research and having also informed the research: the Affordable Care Act (ACA), the Institute of Medicine (IOM)/National Academy of Medicine (NAM) *Future of Nursing* report, and the genomic nursing science blueprint. For example, the reciprocal relationship is evident with Hickman's development of the POLST as a research team endeavor. The POLST facilitates an individual's end-of-life ADs being honored by having them signed by a qualified health provider, such as a physician or a nurse practitioner and clearly recorded. The POLST has shaped national and state policy of ADs. In turn, as the POLST has been adopted in a number of states, research has been conducted to refine and protect the ethics of the program.

As with the practice–research relationship, the policy–research relationship may be more or less direct. The POLST example provides understanding of a direct relationship, but often the research may be removed several steps from immediate shaping of health policy. The condition of the directness of the relationship varies by many factors, including the type of research such as laboratory or intervention level and the length of time in the research program. For example, Dorsey's study, using genomics in her nursing research quest for a new intervention for neuropathic pain in patients with spinal cord injury (SCI), has yet to progress through the development and testing of an intervention. She is laying the genetic foundation for the possible intervention, as is appropriate. Dorsey's work provides an excellent example of nursing research with strong potential for influencing clinical guidelines for SCI patients in the future.

This section examines the reciprocal relationship between nursing research and health policy within the context of the three national health policy directives cited earlier. The numerous strategies employed by the nurse scientists in their endeavors to shape health policy are addressed.

The Affordable Care Act

Nursing research has informed, as one of many factors, two of the major directives of the ACA: that is, the development of new models of care that provide high-quality care at lower or reasonable costs and the shift to community health care with an emphasis on health promotion and disease prevention, especially for chronic health conditions. In turn, the Innovative Care Center at the CMS has funded several of the nursing studies that are developing new models of care, particularly those situated in the community with chronic illnesses.

Rantz and her co-investigators (Rantz, Popejoy, Musterman, & Miller, 2014) have created and tested a new model of care for older adults under the concept of Aging in Place. Through 20 years of research, studying clinical and cost outcomes when individuals are able to age in place with the facilitation of nurse care coordination and home care (Sinclair Home Care) and ultimately in an independent living facility (TigerPlace), the evidence was clear. Stronger clinical outcomes, such as cognition, activities of daily living (ADLs), and less depression, were achieved in conjunction with lower costs for the care. Forming a public/private partnership with Americare, the TigerPlace facility was sustained. This research program is an excellent example of the nursing research/health policy relationship. In order to start the Sinclair Home Care and TigerPlace program for aging in place, legislation was required at the state level and in turn, a new model for long-term care of the older adult has been demonstrated with stronger clinical outcomes and lower costs. Medicare regulations have been changed to reimburse some nurse care coordination services. This team of investigators, including nurses, physicians, social workers, engineers, and management/informatics, wranglers, has provided a new model of care; the research was funded partly by the National Institute of Nursing Research (NINR) and partly by the CMS, to address the "explosion" of older adults needing long-term care, allowing them to remain in their homes as long as possible.

Riegel, Dickson, and Faulkner (2015) are known for their development and study of the concept of self-care and self-management with adults who experience heart failure. As one of the early pioneers in this area, Riegel has generated a middle range theory of self-care that incorporates the processes of maintenance and management of the chronic illness. As she and the team conducted a series of studies, the evidence showed stronger health outcomes, such as with clinical congestion concurrent with fewer rehospitalizations among patients with heart failure who practiced self-care maintenance and management. One of the ways Riegel has influenced health policy is through professional organizations, such as the International Self-Care organization, and marketing awareness programs, such as a Self-Care Day, acknowledged by the U.S. Senate. This program of research provides information for shaping the health management of individuals with heart failure, a prevalent chronic illness in our society.

While the three examples provided earlier illustrate how nursing research shapes health policy, several of the investigators and their teams also address the issue of community care for individuals and families. Hill and her team of researchers developed a community-based intervention to facilitate the health of African American men with hypertension.

Nursing research, because it focuses on problems of concern to the American people, often provides important insight for health policy makers. Not only does the research target critical health problems, but it is almost always conducted by multidisciplinary teams of scientists. This brings many diverse expert opinions to focus on the identified health problems, which are quite complex. These are the characteristics of research, in general, that garner the attention of policy makers (Hinshaw, 2011).

The Future of Nursing: Leading Change, Advancing Health

The IOM/NAM report on the future of nursing outlined a number of recommendations. The research programs addressed in this text strongly illustrate two of the major recommendations: the need for nursing to provide leadership in (a) redesigning the health care system, as called for in the ACA; and in (b) building interprofessional teams to generate and conduct those endeavors. The nurse investigators in this text, reporting their research programs and how they have shaped health policy, are exemplary in how they have met the criteria for providing leadership in redesigning the health care system with new models, as well as having built strong multidisciplinary or interprofessional teams. Several examples are considered.

Grey, Knafl, Schulman-Green, and Reynolds (2015) are studying how to assist teens with type 1 diabetes in coping with and engaging in self-management. Both the chronic condition and the self-management process are challenging for teens to relate to, comply with, and value. A CST program has been developed and tested to provide a community-based intervention. The research program has shown that clinical outcomes are improved in teens who participate in the CST; for example, increased glycemic control, self-efficacy, and quality of life. The CST program has also involved families of the teens and teens at risk for type 2 diabetes. Being innovative, the researchers chose to put the CST program into an online intervention (i.e., TEEN COPE). This delivery of the intervention greatly appealed to teens and was as effective as any other. Grey and her team's studies have informed the American Diabetes Association (ADA) recommendations for screening teens with type 1 diabetes for depressive symptoms yearly. The CST program is being used in more than 150 clinics with teens with chronic illnesses and stands as an example of practice shaping policy.

Szanton et al. (2011) investigated a new community-based intervention program for older adults living in their homes (CAPABLE, or Community Aging in Place, Advancing Better Living for Elders). Building on Gitlin and Rose's studies (2016) focusing on older adults, Szanton especially targeted the person–environment fit for elders. She cited an example of an older woman in a wheelchair who could not enter her kitchen because of the door size and had to crawl around the room to get food. With this tragic example in mind, Szanton formed a research team of nurses, occupational therapists, and handymen to build and test an intervention that focused on functional ability and making the environment fit the older adults (e.g., repairing doors and stabilizing banisters). Randomized clinical trials indicated that stronger outcomes were achieved with the CAPABLE program; for example, less difficulty with ADLs, lower pain levels, and improved handling of falls. These studies have been funded by NINR and the CMS Innovations Center. They have major potential for influencing Medicare reimbursement for services beyond the usual in health care. Data now exist to suggest that reimbursement for handyman repairs would be to the patients' long-term benefit. As Dr. Szanton suggests: How can you control or manage your diabetes if you cannot move about your kitchen with reasonable ease? The other "lesson" to be learned is how to be creative with research and practice teams; including a handyperson on these teams is unusual. This type of leadership is an excellent example of what *The Future of Nursing* report called for: creative leadership in redesigning the health care system with innovative practice and research multidisciplinary teams.

Two studies mentioned earlier are excellent examples focused on redesigning the health system through new models and the use of multidisciplinary, interprofessional teams to address complex issues and problems. Rantz's and others' research with the aging in place program of home care and independent living facility has the potential to change the face of long-term care for older adults. A strong multidisciplinary team contributed to the generation and testing of this community-based program. Hickman's studies with the POLST have had extensive state and national influence on the use of ADs for older adults and their families. Again, a multidisciplinary team representing several disciplines brought diverse, needed expertise to the research program.

Blueprint for Genomic Nursing Science

The genomic nursing science blueprint (Calzone et al., 2013) was generated by the Advisory Panel for Genomic Nursing Science. The goal was to identify the priority areas for research through a comprehensive review of the current science and expert evaluations of that scientific base. The priorities were aligned with the strategic plan of the NINR. Williams's chapter in this text, addressing the blueprint, acknowledges its contribution to the discipline in providing guidelines for needed areas of genomic nursing science. As a pioneer in genomic nursing research, Williams addresses the interrelationship of such research with health policy.

S. G. Dorsey et al. (2006) are laying the genetic foundation for understanding neuropathic pain with SCI patients. This is a type of pain that is unusual and often does not appear until months after the injury. Understanding the genetic difference in such pain and especially the genetic underpinnings for a viable intervention is critical. Dorsey's research program is an excellent example of the integration of genetics into nursing research. Its potential for shaping health policy is excellent because the studies underlie a major research field for nursing: symptom assessment and management. Symptom assessment and management is an integral area for research in the nursing discipline. Beginning to integrate genomics in this field will greatly add to our ability to understand and intervene with symptoms that are experienced by patients.

A number of examples have been provided of the reciprocal relationship between nursing research and health policy. The relationship is a dynamic, cyclical one with mutual ability to shape both health policy and the discipline's research.

Strategies Used by Nurse Researchers to Shape Health Policy

In 2011, Hinshaw outlined the multiple strategies that senior nurse researchers reported using to inform policy makers about the information gleaned from their studies. Those strategies included:

- Informing local practices in acute care organizations (e.g., hospitals) and communities
- Shaping state health policies
- Informing national health guidelines and standards
- Informing national health policies through federal testimony, NAM report recommendations
- Shaping health science policy (Hinshaw, 2011, p. 11)

The authors in this text utilized the strategies identified in the 2011 study and added several others. The strategies show sophistication and goal-driven productivity. It is evident that nurse researchers understand that their research should shape health policy, so they engage in actions to make their information available to policy makers at the local, state, national, and international levels.

A number of the nurse investigators reporting their research programs in this text informed organizational practice policies in their local acute care or community agencies. Grey and her colleagues implemented the CST program for teens with chronic illnesses in more than 150 clinics across the country. Rantz and her team have established a demonstration program for home care and independent living for older adults who wish to age in place.

State health policies have been influenced by Hickman and her colleagues' series of studies refining and implementing the POLST program for facilitating ADs for older adults and their families. This program is implemented in a number of states, and the NAM recommends that it be part of the policies for all states. Gitlin's research with the caregivers of older adults is being tested in an additional state (Connecticut).

Several national/international guidelines have been informed by these nursing research programs. Grey and her team have contributed to the guidelines and standards for the ADA regarding the annual screening of teens with chronic illnesses for depression. In the 2011 text *Shaping Health Policy Through Nursing Research* (Hinshaw, 2011), this was also one of the major strategies cited for nursing studies to influence health policy.

In this text, a number of additional strategies were cited in terms of informing health policies. Riegel, collaborating with an international organization on self-care of which she is the leader, has promoted a "Self-Care Day" to enhance client and professional awareness. A U.S. Senate resolution was sought to highlight this concept and type of care. Hickman and her team shaped a recommendation for the NAM that POLST be implemented in every state in the country. Finkelstein and his colleagues' research program is shaping new federal policies about the reimbursement of telehealth. The strategies being used by nurse investigators to shape health policy are expanding and becoming more sophisticated in nature.

Shaping science policy for health is another critical area in which nursing has been quite effective. The NINR is the lead institute for the NIH for research on palliative care and end-of-life issues. Miller's chapter outlines an infrastructure that has been implemented to compile the research funded across the institutes in this field of study. The Office of End-of-Life and Palliative Care Research provides such compiled information to multiple sources, at their request; for example, for congressional testimony and NAM study committees and reports. In addition, the information is used by the nursing scientific community and other disciplines to examine the state of the science and identify future areas for study.

Nurse investigators are actively seeking ways of shaping health policy. Awareness days, congressional testimony, and NAM recommendations are examples of effective ways of garnering the attention of policy makers. A number of strategies are evident for informing health policy at the local, state, national, and international levels.

CONCLUSION

There are burgeoning opportunities for using nursing research to shape health policy as we move forward into the future. The health care system is changing in ways that focus more on wellness, self-management of chronic illness, and using new and emerging technologies. Additional emphases on shared infrastructure, interdisciplinary and team science, as well as community involvement are increasing. All of these aspects are a part of the fabric of nursing science and tie us to health policy for the future. The impetus is for us to provide the data that will drive safe, progressive evidence-based polices. This volume provides some outstanding examples of what has been done, and provides a snapshot of what can and should be done in order to meet these challenges. It is imperative for nursing science to play an essential role in the policy changes that will help to determine the future health of individuals and of the nation. It is up to nurse researchers, from both current and future generations, to tie nursing science to that healthy future.

REFERENCES

Agency for Healthcare Research and Quality. (2015). *2014 national healthcare quality and disparities report* (AHRQ Publication No. 15-0007). Rockville, MD: U.S. Department of Health and Human Services.

Ahalt, S. C., Bizen, C., Evans, J., Erlich, Y., Ginsburg, G. S., Krishnamurthy, A., & Wilhelmsen, K. (2014). *Data to discovery: Genes to health* (White Paper from the National Consortium for Data Science). The National Consortium for Data Science, University of North Carolina, Chapel Hill, NC.

Calzone, K. A., Jenkins, J., Bakos, A. D., Cashion, A. K., Donaldson, D., Feero, W. G., . . . Webb, J. A. (2013). A blueprint for genomic nursing science. *Journal of Nursing Scholarship, 45,* 96–104.

Cashion, A. K., & Grady, P. A. (2015). The National Institutes of Health/National Institutes of Nursing Research intramural research program and the development of the National Institutes of Health Symptom Science Model. *Nursing Outlook, 63,* 484–487.

Dorsey, E. R., & Topol, A. J. (2016). State of telehealth. *New England Journal of Medicine, 35*(2), 154–161.

Dorsey, S. G., Renn, C. L., Carim-Todd, L., Barrick, C. A., Bambrick, L., Krueger, B. K, . . . Tessarollo, L. (2006). In vivo restoration of physiological levels of truncated TrkBT1 receptor rescues neuronal cell death in a trisomic mouse model. *Neuron, 51,* 21–28.

Gitlin, L. N., & Rose, K. (2016). Impact of caregiver readiness on outcomes of an intervention to address bio-behavioral symptoms in persons with dementia. *Journal of Geriatric Psychology, 31*(9), 1056–1063.

Grey, M., Knafl, K., Schulman-Green, D., & Reynolds, N. (2015). A revised self and family management framework. *Nursing Outlook, 63,* 162–170.

Hinshaw, A. S. (2011). Science shaping health policy: How is nursing research evident in such policy changes. In A. S. Hinshaw & P. A. Grady (Eds.), *Shaping health policy through nursing research* (pp. 1–16). New York, NY: Springer Publishing.

National Institutes of Health. (2016). *Health data initiative.* Retrieved from http://www.healthdata.gov

Rantz, M., Popejoy, L., Musterman, K., & Miller, S. J. (2014). Influencing public policy through care coordination research. In G. Lamb (Ed.), *Care coordination: The game changer; How nursing is revolutionizing quality care* (pp. 203–220). Silver Spring, MD: American Nurses Association.

Riegel, B., Dickson, V. V., & Faulkner, K. M. (2015). The situation specific theory of heart failure self-care: Revised and updated. *Journal of Cardiovascular Nursing, 23*(3), 190–196.

Starkweather, A. R., Ramesh, D., Lyon, D. E., Siangphorn, U., Deng, X., Sturgill, J., . . . Greenspan, J. (2016). Acute low back pain: Differential somatosensory function and gene expression compared to healthy no-pain controls. *Clinical Journal of Pain, 32*(11), 933–939.

Szanton, S. L., Thorpe, R. J., Boyd, C., Tanner, E. K., Leff, B., Agree, E., & Gitlin, L. N. (2011). Community aging in place, advancing better living for elders: A biobehavioral environmental intervention to improve function and health-related quality of life in disabled older adults. *Journal of the American Geriatric Society, 59*(12), 2314–2320.

Warren, E. (2016). Strengthening research through data sharing. *New England Journal of Medicine, 375*(5), 401–403.

Index